THE
LITTLE BLACK BOOK
OF NEUROLOGY

A Manual for Neurological House Officers

THE
LITTLE BLACK BOOK
OF NEUROLOGY

A Manual for Neurological House Officers

Editor

STEPHEN E. THURSTON, M.D.

Contributors

Orlando L. Avila, M.D.
Michael F. Bahntge, M.D.
Richard H. Civil, M.D.
Gerald E. Grossman, M.D.
Susan K. Klein, M.D.
Norman W. Lefkovitz, M.D.
Bernd F. Remler, M.D.
Barbara M. Weissman, M.D.
Crispin W. Wilhelm, M.D.

*From the Neurology House Staff of Case Western Reserve University,
University Hospitals of Cleveland, and the Cleveland V.A. Medical Center, Cleveland, Ohio*

Illustrations by **Sundee L. Morris, M.D.**

YEAR BOOK MEDICAL PUBLISHERS, INC.
Chicago • London • Boca Raton

Copyright © 1987 by Year Book Medical Publishers, Inc.
All rights reserved. No part of this publication may be
reproduced, stored in a retrieval system, or transmitted, in
any form or by any means—electronic, mechanical, pho-
tocopying, recording, or otherwise—without prior written
permission from the publisher. Printed in the United States
of America.

1 2 3 4 5 6 7 8 9 0 C M 91 90 89 88 87

Library of Congress Cataloging-in-Publication Data

The little black book of neurology.

Includes bibliographies and index.
1. Nervous system—Diseases—Handbooks, manuals,
etc. 2. Neurology—Handbooks, manuals, etc.
I. Thurston, Stephen E. II. Avila, Orlando L.
III. Case Western Reserve University. IV. University
Hospitals of Cleveland (Ohio) V. Cleveland V.A.
Medical Center (Ohio) [DNLM: 1. Neurology—
handbooks. WL 39 L778]
RC355.L58 1986   616.8   86-15827
ISBN 0-8151-6350-9

Sponsoring Editor: Richard H. Lampert
Manager, Copyediting Services: Frances M. Perveiler
Production Project Manager: R. Allen Reedtz
Proofroom Supervisor: Shirley E. Taylor

PREFACE

Many trainees keep pocket-size loose-leaf notebooks containing useful information. These are continuously revised and expanded to satisfy their changing needs through the residency years and, often, thereafter. *The Little Black Book of Neurology* is designed to provide, in an easy-access, pocket-reference form, basic information that neurology housestaff need at their fingertips as they begin their training. The contents represent what the current residents and fellows in neurology at Case Western Reserve University wish they had available to them during their first year on the neurology wards. Each contributor was guided by what, in retrospect, he or she would like to have had readily available in the middle of the night to institute appropriate initial management and write an intelligent admission note before presenting the patient. Written ''by residents, for residents'' as a source of ready reference, it is not an all-inclusive text. Rather, it is a book of lists, tables, definitions, and concise reviews of clinical topics to aid in localization, differential diagnosis, and management. It is in no way a substitute for sound clinical training or familiarity with the literature. Bibliographical references are limited to accessible definitive source material.

The book is organized alphabetically into subject headings. Cross-referencing should facilitate quick access. An index of eponyms is included at the end of the book. Although a manual for adult neurology, we included topics thought to be particularly useful during the child neurology rotation.

The Little Black Book of Neurology is the result of a collaborative endeavor. I join the contributing residents in appreciation of the efforts of Dr. Robert B. Daroff who organized this project and provided continuous guidance and support. Dr. Robert L. Ruff and other members of the neurology faculty critically reviewed much of the material.

Our neurosurgical housestaff and faculty also gave helpful suggestions. The staff of Year Book Medical Publishers was extremely cooperative in providing advice and instruction during the writing and preparation of the manuscript. In particular, we thank Richard H. Lampert, Editor-in-Chief, and James A. Ross, Director of Editing and Production. Susan Landgraf deserves special credit for her devotion of time and energy to preparing the photo-ready copy. Finally, I thank my wife, Nan, who has been most patient and supportive throughout.

STEPHEN E. THURSTON, M.D.

ABSCESS (see also Encephalitis, Meningitis)

Brain abscesses are located, in order of decreasing frequency in: frontal, temporal, parietal, cerebellar, and occipital areas. Diencephalic and brainstem locations are rare. The most common causes are head trauma; neurosurgery; infections of contiguous structures (otitis, mastoiditis, sinusitis, dental abscess); and hematogenous spread (often resulting in multiple and loculated abscesses) secondary to pulmonary infection, endocarditis, and congenital heart disease. All bacteria and fungi are potential culprits but streptococci, bacteroides, staphylococci, enterobacteria, and pseudomonas are the most common.

Since spread is often via diploic or emissary veins, epidural abscess or subdural empyema may result. Alteration in consciousness is the rule; headache is present in 70%, fever in 50%, focal neurological deficits in 50%, nausea and vomiting in 50%, and focal or generalized seizures in 30%. The classic triad of fever, headache, and focal neurological deficit is present in less than 50%.

CT scans show ring enhancement with contrast infusion but this is a nonspecific finding which can occur with tumors, infarction, or other processes. The EEG is often focally abnormal. LP is contraindicated in suspected or proven cases of abscess as herniation may result and the diagnostic yield is minimal. In the face of a CNS infection, an LP should only be performed if the CT is negative. If the CT shows a suspected abscess, blood, throat, nasopharyngeal, urine, and other pertinent cultures should be obtained and antibiotics begun. In addition, skull, sinus, mastoid, chest, and dental x-rays should be obtained. Arteriography is required if mycotic aneurysm is suspected and, usually, prior to neurosurgical treatment. If the CT scan is negative, a radionuclide brain scan may be more sensitive in detecting early cerebritis.

Treatment involves prolonged IV antibiotics (4-6 weeks) and surgical drainage or excision. In the absence of positive cultures, penicillin is the mainstay of therapy in doses of 20 million units IV daily. Chloramphenicol, 1-5 gm IV q6h, has been the traditional anaerobic coverage. Early neurosurgical consultation is mandatory. Cerebritis (implying the absence of a capsule formation) may be treated by prolonged antibiotics alone.

With present modes of therapy, mortality is between 15-20%. Poor prognosis is associated with multiple or multiloculated abscesses, ventricular rupture, coma, inappropriate antibiotic usage, and fungal infection.

Spinal epidural abscess usually presents with spine and radicular pain progressing to weakness over hours to days. Occasionally, a more protracted course occurs. The thoracic spine is the most common site in adults. The most common organism is *staph aureus*, followed by streptococci and Gram-negatives. If the diagnosis is suspected, an emergency myelogram is indicated. Treatment consists of surgical drainage and appropriate antibiotic coverage.

Ref: Mandell GL, et al. Principles and Practice of
        Infectious Diseases, 2nd ed. New York: Wiley, 1985.

ACALCULIA

The loss of previously acquired arithmetic ability secondary to a cerebral lesion. It is often a part of Gerstmann's syndrome.

ACIDOSIS (see Electrolyte Disorders)

AGNOSIA

Failure to recognize a stimulus (visual, auditory, tactile) that cannot be attributed to anomia, in an individual whose primary sensory modalities are demonstrably intact. The most common agnosia is tactile, manifested by the inability to recognize objects placed in a hand (astereognosia) or identify figures or numbers traced upon the skin (agraphesthesia). These usually occur in the limb contralateral to a cerebral hemispheric lesion.

Visual agnosias are rare and controversial. Almost all patients with this disorder have a demonstrable primary visual deficit (impaired acuity and/or visual field loss) and some degree of dementia. Prosopagnosia is a form of visual agnosia in which there is an inability to recognize familiar faces; this is invariably associated with an altitudinal hemianopsia and is indicative of bilateral occipital disease.

Finger agnosia is the inability to recognize fingers; it is usually secondary to a lesion of the dominant parietal lobe and is part of Gerstmann's syndrome.

In auditory agnosia, also called "pure word deafness", a nonaphasic individual cannot understand the spoken word but can understand the written word.

Anosagnosia is used to describe the denial of a deficit usually secondary to a nondominant parietal lesion.

AGRAPHIA

Loss of a previously learned ability to write in a limb that is not paretic. It is almost always associated with an aphasia.

AIDS (ACQUIRED IMMUNODEFICIENCY SYNDROME)

Decreased cellular and humoral immunity due to infection with a retrovirus (human immunodeficiency virus, HTLV III/LAV). In adults, defined as the occurrence of malignant tumors, most commonly Kaposi's sarcoma or non-Hodgkins lymphoma, and/or opportunistic infections, in previously healthy persons under 60 years of age who are not known to have any other immunosuppressive disorders. Neurological manifestations occur in up to 60 and are the presenting complaint in up to 30 The virus is neurotropic as well as lymphotropic. The virus may directly cause meningitis, encephalitis, myelopathy, peripheral neuropathy. Indirect effects are related to immunosuppression metabolic disorders, and opportunistic infection. Viral syndromes include subacute encephalitis (headache, progressive dementia, focal motor deficits, and, occasionally, hemianopsia, myoclonus or seizures), atypical aseptic meningitis, herpes simplex encephalitis, progressive multifocal leukoencephalopathy, viral myelitis, and varicella zoster encephalitis. Nonviral infections of the nervous system have been caused by *Toxoplasma gondii, Cryptococcus neoformans, Candida albicans, Mycobacteria, Treponema pallidum, Coccidioides, Mycobacterium tuberculosis, Aspergillus, and E. coli.* Neoplasms have included primary CNS lymphoma, systemic lymphoma with CNS involvement, and metastatic Kaposi's sarcoma. Cerebrovascular complications have included hemorrhage and infarction. Patients may have more than one intracranial pathological process. Cranial neuropathies may be due to chronic inflammatory polyneuropathy, lymphoma, or aseptic meningitis. Peripheral neurological complications include chronic inflammatory polyneuropathy, distal symmetric polyneuropathy, herpes zoster radiculitis, myalgias, myopathy and polymyositis.

Treatment of secondary infections depends upon the particular organism(s). Azidothymidine has been used to treat primary infection with the human immunodeficiency virus.

Ref: Levy RM. J Neurosurg 62:475, 1985.

3

ALCOHOL (see also Nutritional Deficiency Syndrome)

Neurological complications of alcohol include intoxication, withdrawal syndromes, deficiency states, and miscellaneous other conditions.

Intoxication with alcohol produces cognitive dysfunction as well as cerebellar and vestibular symptoms. There is also a positional vertigo related to diffusion of alcohol into the cupula. This results in acute vertigo when a recumbent position is assumed.

Withdrawal syndromes may be early or late. The early symptoms occur 12-24 hours after cessation of drinking and most commonly present as tremulousness. Treatment consists of sedation with benzodiazepines. A less common early withdrawal symptom is hallucinosis which may be visual, tactile, or auditory. Auditory hallucinations may become chronic and require treatment with neuroleptics. Withdrawal seizures usually occur within the first 24 hours but may occur after several days and are usually generalized. Focal seizures imply a structural lesion and should not be attributed to alcohol withdrawal. Treatment of withdrawal seizures is controversial. Those who recommend treatment suggest loading acutely with phenytoin and then discontinuing anticonvulsants several days later. Thiamine is routinely given as is magnesium if the serum magnesium is low. The late symptoms of alcohol withdrawal include delirium tremens which has a peak incidence between 72 and 96 hours after cessation of drinking and consists of vivid hallucinations, tremors, agitation, and increased autonomic activity (tachycardia, fever, hyperhidrosis). Treatment consists of sedation with benzodiazepines, hydration with IV fluids, and administration of thiamine, multivitamins, and magnesium as above.

Wernicke-Korsakoff's syndrome is the most common deficiency syndrome secondary to chronic alcoholism. Wernicke's syndrome represents the acute phase of the triad of ocular motor disturbance (nystagmus, ophthalmoplegia, gaze palsy), cerebellar ataxia, and mental confusion. Korsakoff's syndrome is a more chronic condition and includes an anterograde amnesia (inability to incorporate ongoing experience into memory). Wernicke and Korsakoff syndromes are attributed to thiamine deficiency. Treatment consists of thiamine, 100 mg/day for three days parenterally, followed by oral thiamine indefinitely. IV glucose should never be given without thiamine in a chronic alcoholic due to the risk of precipitating Wernicke's encephalopathy. Again, as with most alcohol-related syndromes, supplemental vitamins and magnesium may be beneficial.

Other deficiency syndromes include alcoholic cerebellar degeneration, peripheral neuropathy, and optic neuropathy. <u>Cerebellar degeneration</u> invariably involves the anterior vermis and paravermian regions with truncal and gait ataxia. Chronic thiamine and multi-vitamin treatment are indicated. A "dying back" sensory-motor <u>neuropathy</u> usually is heralded by complaints of numb, burning feet. Minor motor signs may evolve. Thiamine and multi-vitamins are appropriate treatment. <u>Nutritional amblyopia</u> (previously called tobacco-alcohol amblyopia) consists of a gradual visual loss which improves with improved nutrition and vitamin supplementation. It is not secondary to the toxic effects of alcohol.

Conditions of somewhat uncertain etiology seen in chronic alcoholics are central pontine myelinolysis, Marchiafava-Bignami syndrome, alcoholic myopathy, and cortical atrophy. <u>Central pontine myelinolysis</u> presents with progressive quadriparesis, horizontal gaze palsy, and obtundation leading to coma. It is presently regarded as secondary to excessively rapid correction of hyponatremia. <u>Marchiafava-Bignami syndrome</u> is a rare demyelinating disease of the corpus callosum associated with excessive consumption of crude red wine. It presents clinically as a frontal lobe dementia. <u>Alcohol myopathy</u> is of both an acute and chronic form. The acute form occurs during a binge and is associated with muscle pains and rhabdomyolysis. The chronic form, consisting of a slowly progressive proximal atrophy, is somewhat controversial. The existence of a dementia secondary to cortical atrophy in chronic alcoholics, not explained by a Korsakoff's syndrome, is not accepted by most authorities. The CT appearance of "atrophy" may be related to fluid shifts in the brain and may reverse with abstinence.

Alcoholics have an increased incidence of stroke related to a variety of factors including rebound thrombocytosis, altered cerebral blood flow, and hyperlipidemia.

Ref: Nokada T, Knight RT. Med Clin North Am 68:121, 1984.

ALEXIA

A disturbance of the previously acquired ability to read secondary to a cerebral lesion. The three common alexias are anterior (frequently associated with Broca's aphasia), central (associated with agraphia), and posterior ("alexia without agraphia"). The latter is usually secondary to a lesion of the left occipital lobe and splenium of the corpus callosum; in addition to the alexia there is a right homonymous hemianopsia and difficulty naming colors.

ALKALOSIS (see Electrolyte Disorders)

AMAUROSIS FUGAX

The symptom of monocular visual loss (partial or complete) consequent to retinal ischemia, also called transient monocular blindness. The latter term is more descriptive, as "amaurosis fugax" is used by some in referring to episodes of transient cortical blindness. It is of sudden onset and short duration (seconds to rarely longer than 5-30 minutes), and consists of a negative visual phenomenon (black or gray). The most common cause is embolization from the internal carotid artery (57-67%) or the heart. It may also result from hemodynamic changes due to carotid or ophthalmic artery stenosis. Other etiologies include giant cell arteritis, hyperviscosity syndromes, hypertensive crisis, migraine, and glaucoma. Transient monocular visual loss may also occur in disorders of the optic nerve such as papilledema, demyelination and drusen. The evaluation and treatment of amaurosis as a manifestation of embolic disease, similar to other TIA's in the anterior circulation, is controversial.

Ref: Savino PJ, et al. Retinal stroke. Arch Ophthalmol 95:1185, 1977.

Ellenberger C, Epstein AD. Ocular complications of atherosclerosis: What do they mean? Seminars in Neurology 6:185, 1986.

AMNESIA (see Memory)

AMYOTROPHIC LATERAL SCLEROSIS (see Motor Neuron Disease)

ANEURYSMS (see also Hemorrhage)

Intracranial aneurysms are classified as saccular ("berry"), mycotic, arteriosclerotic, traumatic, dissecting, and neoplastic. Atherosclerotic aneurysms tend to thrombose rather than rupture. The most common cause of subarachnoid hemorrhage after age 20 is ruptured saccular aneurysms. The most common sites are depicted on page 7.

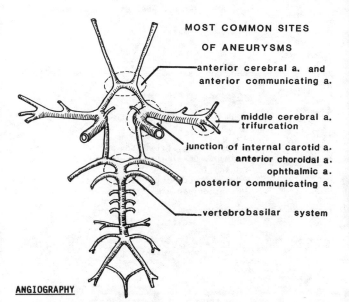

MOST COMMON SITES

OF ANEURYSMS

anterior cerebral a. and
anterior communicating a.

middle cerebral a.
trifurcation

junction of internal carotid a.
anterior choroidal a.
ophthalmic a.
posterior communicating a.

vertebrobasilar system

ANGIOGRAPHY

Complications of arteriography (angiography) can be classified as local, systemic, or neurological. Local complications include puncture site hematomas, intimal tears, pseudoaneurysms, and arteriovenous fistulas. Systemic complications include urticaria, laryngospasm, shock, and cardiac dysrhythmia. Many forms of CNS (and ocular) dysfunction have been reported ranging from diffuse encephalopathy to focal ischemia resulting, for example, in monocular or binocular blindness, hemiparesis, or aphasia. Most neurological complications are transient. Complication rate is greater with increasing age and preexisting cerebrovascular disease. The incidence of complications is approximately 8.5% with neurological complications accounting for 2.6%. Most of the latter are transient; permanent neurological deficit occurs in only 0.3%. Patients who are having angiography for evaluation of symptomatic cerebrovascular disease, however, have a 0.6% incidence of permanent neurological deficit.

Angiographic anatomy is depicted on pages 8-10.

Ref: Earnest F, et al. AJR 142:247, 1984.

ANGIOGRAPHIC ANATOMY

INTERNAL CAROTID CIRCULATION

A_1–A_5:	Segments of anterior cerebral artery
ACH:	Anterior choroidal artery
ANG:	Angular artery
ASFP:	Ascending frontoparietal artery
ATV:	Anterior terminal vein
BVR:	Basal vein of Rosenthal
C_1–C_5:	Segments of internal carotid artery
FPR:	Frontopolar artery
ICV:	Internal cerebral vein
ISS:	Inferior sagittal sinus
M_1–M_5	Segments of middle cerebral artery
PC:	Pericallosal artery
PCR:	Posterior cerebral artery
PP:	Posterior parietal artery
PTV:	Posterior terminal vein
SRS:	Straight sinus
SSS:	Superior sagittal sinus
SV:	Septal vein
TS:	Transverse sinus
VG:	Great cerebral vein of Galen

VERTEBROBASILAR CIRCULATION

AICA:	Anterior inferior cerebral artery
AT:	Anterior temporal artery (branch of PC)
BA:	Basilar artery
CALC:	Calcarine artery (branch of PC)
LPCh:	Lateral posterior choroidal artery
MPCh:	Medial posterior choroidal artery
PC:	Posterior cerebral artery
PICA:	Posterior inferior cerebellar artery
PO:	Parieto-occipital artery (branch of PC)
PT:	Posterior temporal artery (branch of PC)
SCA:	Superior cerebellar artery
TP:	Thalamoperforate artery
VA:	Vertebral artery

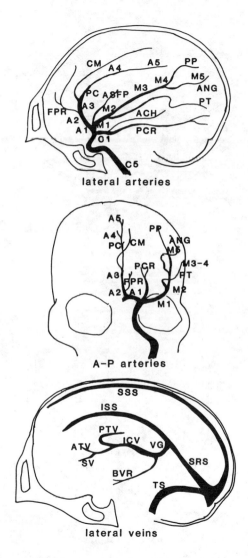

lateral arteries

A-P arteries

lateral veins

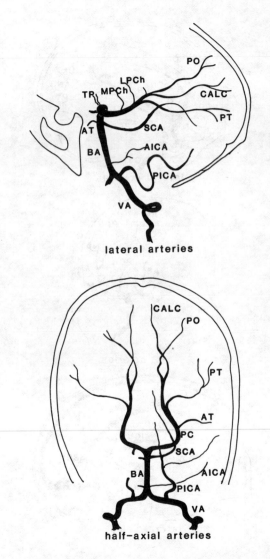

lateral arteries

half-axial arteries

ANGIOMAS

Vascular malformations due to abnormal embryogenesis. The following is McCormick's classification of five types of angiomas.

Arteriovenous malformation (AVM): Although AVM's comprise 12% of angiomas, they are the most symptomatic. Symptoms are caused by local ischemia, distant ischemia due to the "stealing" of blood flow, direct pressure, and hemorrhage. Pathology consists of vascular clusters forming direct arteriovenous shunts without intervening capillaries, with abnormal gliotic parenchyma between the vessels. Ninety percent occur in the cerebral hemispheres with the remainder in the brainstem, cerebellum, and spinal cord. AVM's may be seen on contrast CT, but are best defined with angiography. Patients presenting with seizures have a 1-2%/year rate of hemorrhage. Patients presenting with hemorrhage rebleed at a rate of 6% in the first year and 2-3%/year thereafter. Mortality is 10% for the first hemorrhage and 20% for subsequent hemorrhages. Various embolization and surgical procedures, and radiation therapy are used in management.

Telangiectasia: Small (0.3-1.0 cm) angiomas containing capillary-like vessels, commonly occurring in the brainstem but also in the cortex and spinal cord. Hemorrhage is uncommon but fluctuating neurological symptoms, simulating multiple sclerosis, are frequent. They are not visualized on angiography.

Varix: A single, often large, dilated vein with mural thrombosis. They may cause symptoms as a mass lesion and may be seen during contrast CT or the venous phase of angiography.

Cavernous angioma: A circumscribed mass of sinusoidal vessels packed together, with mural fibrosis, without intervening CNS parenchyma. They may hemorrhage. They do not visualize well at angiography.

Venous angioma: These comprise 62% of all angiomas and are usually asymptomatic. They consist of groups of anomalous veins separated by neural parenchyma.

Ref: McCormick WF, Schochet SS. Atlas of Cerebral Vascular Disease. Philadelphia: Saunders, 1976.

Luessenhop AJ, Rosa L. Cerebral arteriovenous malformations. J Neurosurg 60:14, 1984.

ANISOCORIA (see Pupils)

ANTICOAGULATION (see Ischemia)

ANTICONVULSANTS (see Antiepileptic Drugs)

ANTIDEPRESSANTS

The table on page 13 summarizes the relative side effects of antidepressant drugs of significance in making initial selections. Anticholinergic side effects include blurred vision, dry mouth, constipation, urinary retention, memory dysfunction and exacerbation of narrow angle glaucoma. Depressed patients with dementia or tardive dyskinesia may worsen due to anticholinergic effects. Parkinsonian patients may improve. Patients with migraine or chronic pain may benefit from antidepressants with a relatively higher affinity for serotonin receptors.

Ref: Richardson JW, Richelson E. Mayo Clin Proc 59:330, 1984.

ANTIEPILEPTIC DRUGS (see also Epilepsy, Pregnancy)

Use of antiepileptic drugs begins with the appropriate selection of a single drug based on clinical and electro-graphic identification of the seizure type(s). The dose is increased until seizures are controlled or toxicity develops. The lowest dose that will control seizures is used. Consider adding a second drug if control is not attained or adverse effects occur.

Drug levels provide useful guidelines in the management of seizure patients, although the endpoints of therapy remain clinical - side effects or seizure control. Total (free plus unbound) plasma levels are most widely used (see table). There is now increasing emphasis on monitoring free (unbound) levels of more highly protein-bound drugs such as phenytoin, carbamazepine, and valproic acid. Use of free levels should be considered when protein binding is altered (usually decreased) due to hypoalbuminemia (renal or hepatic disease, pregnancy, cardiac failure, cancer, sepsis, burns) or to the abnormal presence of substances in the plasma such as free fatty acids, bilirubin, urea, uric acid, certain hormones and various drugs. Side effects may correlate more closely with free than total phenytoin levels. For valproic acid and carbamazepine there is not yet clear evidence that side effects or therapeutic effects correlate better with free than total levels.

Ref: Levy RH, Schmidt D. Utility of free level monitoring of antiepileptic drugs. Epilepsia 26:199, 1985.

RELATIVE SIDE EFFECTS OF ANTIDEPRESSANT DRUGS

Antidepressant Generic (Trade)	Sedation	Anticholinergic	Postural Hypotension	Serotonin Affinity	Decreased Seizure Threshold
Tertiary amine tricyclics					
Amitriptyline (Elavil)	+	+	+		
Imipramine (Tofranil)	+	+	-	+	+
Trimipramine (Surmontil)	+	+		+	
Doxepin (Sinequan)	+	+		+	
Secondary amine tricyclics					
Nortriptyline (Aventyl)	(+)	+		+	
Desipramine (Norpramin)					
Protriptyline (Vivactyl)		+			
Dibenzoxazepine					
Amoxapine (Asendin)					+
Tetracyclic					
Maprotiline (Ludiomil)	(+)			+	+
Triazolopyridine					
Trazodone (Desyrel)					+

13

COMMON ANTIEPILEPTIC DRUGS:

Drug	Preparations	Therapeutic Plasma Concentration
Phenytoin	30 mg, 100 mg caps 50 mg tabs 30 mg/5 ml elixir 125 mg/5 ml elixir	10-20 µg/ml (6-14 µg/ml in neonates to 12 weeks)
Phenobarbital (Luminal)	15,30,60,130 mg tabs 20 mg/5 ml elixir 10 mg/ml for injection	15-40 µg/ml
Primidone (Mysoline)	50 mg, 250 mg tabs 250 mg/5 ml elixir	5-12 µg/ml Primidone is also metabolized to phenobarbital
Carbamazepine (Tegretol)	100 mg, 200 mg tabs	6-12 µg/ml
Ethosuximide (Zarontin)	250 mg caps 250 mg/5 ml elixir	40-100 µg/ml
Valproic acid (Depakene)	250 mg caps 125 mg, 250 mg, 500 mg enteric-coated tabs 250 mg/5 ml elixir	50-100 µg/ml

Dose (Initial and Maintenance)	Approximate Half-life
Neonates: 15-20mg/kg, then 3-5 mg/kg/day in divided doses IV	Variable
Infants: 15 mg/kg, then 3-5 mg/kg/day in 3-4 doses	4-11 hrs
Children: 15 mg/kg, then 5-15 mg/kg/day in 2 doses	4-11 hrs
Adults: 15 mg/kg, then 5 mg/kg/day in single dose	20-40 hrs
Infants, children: 6-16 mg/kg, then 3-8 mg/kg/day in 2 doses	40-70 hrs
Adults: 4-8 mg/kg, then 2-4 mg/kg/day in single dose	50-120 hrs
Children: 50 mg/d, incr 50 mg q3 days to 10-25 mg/kg in 2-4 doses	10-12 hrs
Adults: 250 mg/d in 2 doses, incr 125 mg q3 days to 10-20 mg/kg/day in 2-4 doses	
Children: 100 mg bid, incr 100 mg qod to 15-20 mg/kg/day in 3-4 doses	5-27 hrs
Adults: 200 mg bid, incr 100 mg qod to 7-15 mg/kg/day in 3-4 doses	5-27 hrs
Children: 250 mg/d, incr 250 mg q4-7 days to 15-40 mg/kg/day in 3-4 doses	30 hrs
Adults: 250 mg bid, incr 250 mg q4-7 days to 15-30 mg/kg/day in 3-4 doses	50-60 hrs
Children: 10-15 mg/kg/day, incr 5-10 mg/kg/day q1 week to 15-100 mg/kg/day in 3-4 doses	4-14 hrs
Adults: 10-15 mg/kg/day, incr 5-10 mg/kg/day q1 week to 15-45 mg/kg/day in 3-4 doses	6-17 hrs

FACTORS AFFECTING SERUM CONCENTRATIONS OF ANTIEPILEPTIC DRUGS

Antiepileptic	Change in Level	Other Antiepileptics	Other Drugs	Clinical State
Phenytoin	Increased by	Phenobarbital Valproic acid Ethosuximide	Chloramphenicol Disulfiram Isoniazid Dicumarol Amphetamines Tolbutamide Chlordane Phenylbutazone Alcohol (acute) Aminosalicylic acid Chlorpromazine Estrogens Methylphenidate Prochlorperazine Sulfaphenazole	Hepatic disease
	Decreased by	Phenobarbital Carbamazepine Clonazepam	Alcohol (chronic) Reserpine	Pregnancy Renal disease Mononucleosis Acute hepatitis

16

Drug		Increased by / Decreased by		
Phenobarbital	Increased by	Valproic acid, Phenytoin	Furosemide, Amphetamines	Renal disease, Hepatic disease, Acidic urine
	Decreased by	Clonazepam		Alkaline urine
Primidone	Increased by	Valproic acid, Clonazepam		
	Decreased by	Phenytoin		
Carbamazepine	Increased by		Propoxyphene, Erythromycin	Hepatic disease
	Decreased by	Phenobarbital, Phenytoin, Primidone		Pregnancy
Valproic acid	Increased by			Hepatic disease
	Decreased by	Carbamazepine, Phenytoin, Phenobarbital, Primidone		
Clonazepam	Increased by	Phenytoin		
	Decreased by	Phenobarbital		

PHARMACOLOGICAL ADVERSE SIDE EFFECTS
OF ANTIEPILEPTIC DRUGS
(From Dreifuss, 1983)

Phenytoin

Acute: Drowsiness, ataxia, diplopia, nystagmus, gastrointestinal complaints, choreoathetosis, nausea, hypotension (after injection)

Chronic: Gingival hyperplasia, hypertrichosis, coarse facies, Dupuytren's contractures, folate deficiency, megaloblastic anemia, osteomalacia with Vitamin D deficiency, peripheral neuropathy, encephalopathy, cerebellar dysfunction, endocrine dysfunction (adrenal, thyroid, diabetogenesis), pseudolymphoma, immunosuppression, agranulocytosis, hemorrhage in the newborn

Phenobarbital

Acute: Sedation, behavior disturbances, ataxia

Chronic: Difficulty with concentration, cognitive deficit, loss of initiative, hemorrhage in newborn

Primidone

Acute: Sedation, vertigo, nausea, unsteadiness

Chronic: Behavior disturbances in the young, loss of libido, difficulty with concentration, hemorrhagic disease in newborn

Carbamazepine

Acute: Diplopia, drowsiness, vertigo, blurred vision, dry mouth, stomatitis, SIADH, dehydration, headache, diarrhea, constipation, paresthesiae

Chronic: Enzyme induction, aplastic anemia, leukopenia, hepatic enzyme elevation, nervousness

Ethosuximide

Acute: Nausea, vertigo, loss of appetite, vomiting, hiccups, headache

Chronic: Loss of sleep, nervousness, occasional psychotic behavior, hiccups, headache, reported exacerbation of major seizures

Valproic Acid	**Acute**: Drowsiness, gastrointestinal disturbances (nausea and vomiting) **Chronic**: Alopecia, weight gain, weight loss, tremor, ankle swelling, amenorrhea, hyperammonemia, unexplained stupor, granulopenia, hepatic enzyme elevation, thrombocytopenia, occasional psychosis
Benzodia- zepines (clonazepam, clorazepate)	**Acute**: Sedation, ataxia, irritability, increased salivation, tonic seizures **Chronic**: Behavior disturbances, loss of initiative, tolerance to the drug with breakthrough seizures

IDIOSYNCRATIC ADVERSE EFFECTS OF ANTIEPILEPTIC DRUGS
(From Dreifuss, 1983)

Skin rash: All antiepileptic drugs

Erythema multiforme: All, more likey with ethosuximide

Stevens-Johnson syndrome: All, except valproic acid

Exfoliative dermatitis: All

Systemic lupus erythematosus: phenytoin, ethosuximide

Bone marrow depression: Most all, including phenytoin, primidone, carbamazepine, ethosuximide, valproic acid

Thrombocytopenia: All, though rare with phenytoin, phenobarbital, clonazepam

Lymphadenopathy: phenytoin, ethosuximide

Hepatic toxicity: valproic acid (usually in first 6 months of therapy), phenytoin, carbamazepine

Pancreatic toxicity: valproic acid

Ref: Dreifuss FE. Adverse effects of antiepileptic drugs. In, Ward AA, Penry JK, Purpura D (eds). Epilepsy. New York: Raven Press, 1983.

LABORATORY MONITORING OF ANTIEPILEPTIC DRUGS

Phenytoin, mephenytoin	CBC every 6 months Calcium every 6 months Folate, B_{12}, if anemic
Phenobarbital, mephobarbital	CBC every 6 months Calcium every 6 months Folate, B_{12}, if anemic
Primidone	CBC every 6 months Folate, B_{12}, if anemic
Carbamazepine	CBC weekly for 4 weeks, then monthly for 1 year, then every 3 months LFT every 3 months
Ethosuximide, methosuximide, phensuximide	CBC monthly for 6 months, then every 3 months LFT every 6 months
Valproic acid	CBC and platelets monthly for 6 months, then every 3 months LFT monthly for 6 months, then every 3 months
Acetazolamide	Electrolytes every 3 months Calcium every 6 months
Paramethadione, trimethadione	CBC every 3 months LFT every 6 months Urinalysis every 6 months

CBC = complete blood count, LFT = liver function tests

ANTIEPILEPTIC AGENTS

Class	Generic Name	Trade Name
Hydantoins	phenytoin	Dilantin
	mephenytoin	Mesantoin
	ethotoin	Peganone
Barbiturates, Desoxybarbiturates	phenobarbital	Luminal
	mephobarbital	Mebaral
	metharbital	Gemonil
	primidone	Mysoline
Oxazolidinediones	trimethadione	Tridione
	paramethadione	Paradione
Succinimides	phensuximide	Milontin
	methsuximide	Celontin
	ethosuximide	Zarontin
Acetylurea	phenacemide	Phenurone
Iminostilbene	carbamazepine	Tegretol
Benzodiazepines	diazepam	Valium
	lorazepam	Ativan
	clonazepam	Clonopin
	clorazepate	Tranxene
	nitrazepam	Mogadon
Branched-chain carboxylic acid	valproic acid	Depakene
Sulfonamide	acetazolamide	Diamox
Adrenocorticotropic hormone	ACTH corticotropin	
Paraldehyde	paraldehyde	Paral
Bromides		

ANTIPLATELET DRUGS (see Ischemia)

ANTIPSYCHOTIC DRUGS (see Neuroleptics)

APHASIA

A disturbance of communication caused by damage to certain areas of the cerebrum. Common to all aphasias is a disturbance in speech as well as other aspects of symbolic communication (writing, typing, and various coding systems such as sign language). In the vast majority of right-handed individuals, aphasia is secondary to a lesion in the left cerebral hemisphere. A hemisphere in which a lesion produces aphasia is considered "dominant" for language. In left-handed and ambidextrous individuals, either hemisphere may be dominant or there may be mixed dominance with each hemisphere sharing a portion of language function.

Necessary for the diagnosis of aphasia is paraphasic speech output and/or anomia. Paraphasias consist of using incorrect words or neologistic sounds; for example, "the grass is greel" or "give me the plieber". Anomia is the inability to correctly name common objects.

There are numerous aphasia classifications, none of which are entirely satisfactory. The most commonly used classification is that of Geschwind and Benson which is based upon speech fluency, repetition ability, and comprehension and permits the definition of eight aphasic syndromes.

There is generally, but not always, a parallelism between language output (writing, speaking) and comprehension (written word, spoken word).

Ref: Strub RL, Black FW. The Mental Status Examination
        in Neurology, 2nd ed. Philadelphia: FA Davis,
        1985.

APRAXIA (see also Ocular Motor Apraxia)

The inability to perform previously learned motor activities in the presence of intact motor and sensory systems, attentiveness, cooperation, and comprehension.

"Ideomotor" apraxia is the inability to voluntarily complete an act, which can be performed spontaneously, in response to a motor command. It may be due to lesions of the dominant parietal or frontal lobes as well as the corpus callosum ("callosal" apraxia).

"Ideational" apraxia is the inability to use common objects in a proper manner. This form of apraxia is rare, controversial, and not of specific localizing significance.

Other apraxias involve the inability to construct geometric figures (constructional apraxia), dress (dressing apraxia), or walk normally (gait apraxia). The latter is probably secondary to bifrontal dysfunction and is often seen in "normal pressure hydrocephalus".

Apraxia testing includes: making simple facial expressions to command such as "blow out a match", "lick your lips"; performing tasks with the left and right upper limbs such as combing hair, saluting, brushing teeth; drawing a house or various two and three dimensional figures; taking off and putting on a robe or coat; and following various whole body commands such as standing up, walking, assuming the boxer's pose.

ARTERIOGRAPHY (see Angiography)

ARTERITIS (see Vasculitis)

ASTERIXIS

An abrupt, dysrhythmic loss of voluntary tone in antigravity muscles. It is usually elicited by having the seated patient extend his arms and forcibly dorsiflex his wrists. Originally described in hepatic encephalopathy, it occurs in a variety of encephalopathies including drug intoxication (sedatives, anticonvulsants), sepsis, electrolyte abnormalities, hypercarbia, hypoxia, and encephalopathy following metrizamide myelography.

Unilateral asterixis is less common and is secondary to a structural CNS lesion, usually an infarction, contralateral to the movement disorder.

Ref: Reinfeld H, et al. NY State J Med 83:206, 1983.

ATAXIA (see also Spinocerebellar Degeneration)

A lack of muscular coordination and precision of movement. It is often used to refer to abnormal midline (truncal) or limb movements or abnormal ("scanning") speech seen in patients with cerebellar disease. The following are loosely considered to be manifestations of ataxia:

1. Decomposition of movement
2. Dysmetria, the inability to gauge the velocity, force, or distance of a movement is manifested by over-shooting, undershooting, or inability to check a movement
3. Dysdiadokokinesia, the impairment of rapid alternating movements

4. Intention (action) tremor
5. Abnormalities of posture and gait including leaning or falling to one side, and/or walking with a broad base

Ataxia may result from cerebellar dysfunction, impaired sensation (especially proprioception), vestibular dysfunction, and loss of motor power. Sensory ataxia is usually secondary to a peripheral neuropathy or lesions of the posterior roots. It is characterized by a wide-based gait worsened by eye closure. Romberg's sign is present. Vestibular ataxia is associated with vertigo and nystagmus.

ATHETOSIS (see also Choreoathetosis)

A movement disorder characterized by slow, sinuous, writhing movements which are irregular and patterned. All groups of muscles may be involved but the movements tend to be most pronounced in the distal extremities. Athetosis is often associated with varying degrees of weakness and/or rigidity. It may be unilateral or bilateral and, as with most other movement disorders, is aggravated by stress and disappears during sleep. Athetosis should be distinguished from the pseudo-athetoid movements of the outstretched hands that occur in patients with impaired proprioception. When athetoid movements become increasingly sustained, differentiation from dystonia may be difficult (see Dystonia). Athetosis is slower than chorea. Both frequently occur together. For differential diagnosis, see Choreoathetosis.

AUDIOMETRY (see Hearing)

AUTONOMIC DYSFUNCTION

Manifestations include: impotence in males; urinary frequency and urgency; constipation or diarrhea; orthostatic hypotension and syncope; loss of thermo-regulatory sweating; and pupillary abnormalities including mydriasis, Horner's syndrome, and anisocoria.

The table on page 26 divides progressive autonomic failure into those with and without associated signs of CNS dysfunction. Peripheral neuropathy is the most common etiology in cases without CNS signs. Familial dysautonomia (Riley-Day) is a genetically determined disorder beginning in infancy. Idiopathic orthostatic hypotension occurs without peripheral neuropathy or CNS dysfunction; it generally begins in the fifth and sixth decades.

Progressive autonomic failure with CNS signs is seen in a variety of disorders. Multiple system atrophy

(Shy-Drager) is associated with either a progressive cerebellar disturbance (see Spinocerebellar Degeneration) or striato-nigral degeneration (see Parkinson's Disease), or both. A variety of physiological and biochemical tests are available to clarify the etiology of the autonomic dysfunction. Numerous pharmacological agents have been used therapeutically.

DRUGS USED IN TREATING ORTHOSTATIC HYPOTENSION
(Modified from Polinsky)

Drugs*	Possible Mechanisms of Action
Fludrocortisone (A,b,j)	a. Increase sodium and fluid retention
Indomethacin (a,b,f,G)	b. Sensitization of vascular α-adrenergic receptors
Propranolol (e,H)	c. Indirectly acting sympathomimetic drug
Ephedrine (C,d)	d. α-agonist drug
Phenylephrine (D)	e. Blockade of neuronal uptake
Amphetamine (C,d,K)	f. Block presynaptic inhibitory adrenergic receptor
Methylphenidate (d,K)	g. Decrease circulating vasodilator prostaglandins
MAO inhibitors (L)	h. Inhibit β-adrenergic activity
Dihydroergotamine (I)	i. Nonadrenergic vasoconstrictor
Vasopressin (I)	j. Inhibits extraneuronal catecholamine uptake
Metoclopramide (M)	k. CNS "stimulant" drug
Clonidine (D)	l. Diminish norepinephrine catabolism
Prednisone (A,b,J)	m. Blocks dopamine receptors

*Mechanism of action is in parentheses; primary mechanism is capitalized

---

Ref: Polinsky RJ. Multiple system atrophy: clinical aspects, pathophysiology, and treatment. Neurologic Clinics 2:487-498, 1984.

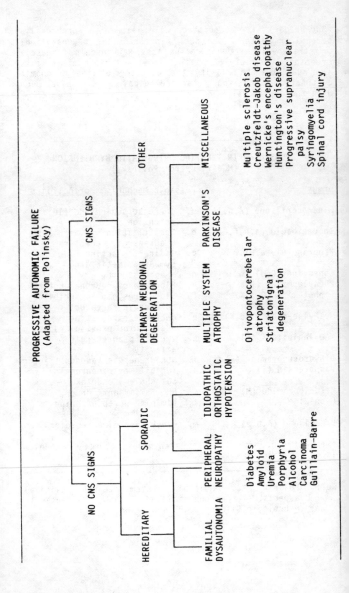

PROGRESSIVE AUTONOMIC FAILURE
(Adapted from Polinsky)

NO CNS SIGNS

HEREDITARY

FAMILIAL
DYSAUTONOMIA

SPORADIC

PERIPHERAL
NEUROPATHY

Diabetes
Amyloid
Uremia
Porphyria
Alcohol
Carcinoma
Guillain-Barre

IDIOPATHIC
ORTHOSTATIC
HYPOTENSION

CNS SIGNS

PRIMARY NEURONAL
DEGENERATION

MULTIPLE SYSTEM
ATROPHY

Olivopontocerebellar
atrophy
Striatonigral
degeneration

PARKINSON'S
DISEASE

OTHER

MISCELLANEOUS

Multiple sclerosis
Creutzfeldt-Jakob disease
Wernicke's encephalopathy
Huntington's disease
Progressive supranuclear
palsy
Syringomyelia
Spinal cord injury

BLADDER

NEUROANATOMY OF BLADDER CONTROL

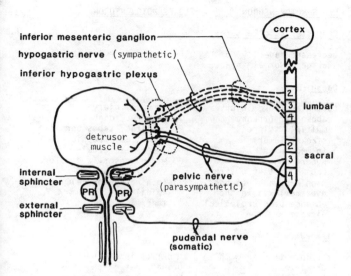

The micturition reflex:

1. Bladder filling to critical intravesical pressure.
2. Activation of stretch receptors (sympathetic, α-adrenergic)
3. Reflex detrusor contraction, with coordinated reflex internal sphincter relaxation (sympathetic, α-adrenergic antagonism; parasympathetic, cholinergic agonism)
4. Activation of sensory receptors for urethral urine flow (parasympathetic, cholinergic)
5. Contraction of bladder wall (sympathetic, β-adrenergic antagonism; parasympathetic, cholinergic agonism)
6. Voluntary relaxation of external sphincter (cortex→ anterior horn cell→pudendal nerve→striated muscle→contraction of external sphincter)

BLADDER DYSFUNCTION

UPPER MOTOR NEURON	LOWER MOTOR NEURON

Characteristic Feature:

Decreased capacity for storage. Normal infant.	Decreased emptying ability

Cause:

Cortex and cord injury above T12 (trauma, multiple sclerosis, stroke, tumor) In men, prostatic hypertrophy causing outlet obstruction may cause bladder hyperreflexia in the absence of neurological disease	Lower cord injury 1. Sensory: diabetes mellitus, tabes dorsalis 2. Motor: amyotrophic lateral sclerosis 3. Mixed sensory and motor: spinal dysraphism (meningomyelocele), spinal cord, trauma, tumor

History:

Urge incontinence with dry intervals Wet at night	Overflow incontinence Urinary retention Straining to void Wet or dry at night

Bulbo-cavernous Reflex:

Present	Absent

Cystometrogram:

"Hyperreflexic bladder" Small bladder capacity Small residual volumes Vesicoureteral reflux (and upper tract damage) may occur at peak pressures.	"Flaccid bladder" Large bladder capacity Large residual volumes Vesicoureteral reflux and upper tract damage can occur with persisting urinary retention.

UPPER MOTOR NEURON	LOWER MOTOR NEURON

Treatment Goal:

Increase storage capacity	Increase bladder tone; avoid storage of large urinary volumes; promote bladder emptying

Treatment:

Oxybutynin (Ditropan)
  cholinergic antagonist
Dose:
  child: 2.5 mg PO bid-tid
  adult: 15 mg PO tid-qid
Side effects:
  dry mouth, blurred
  vision

Propantheline bromide
  (Pro-Banthine)
  cholinergic antagonist
Dose:
  child: not currently
  approved for use
  adult: 15-30 mg PO
  tid-qid
Side effects:
  dry mouth, blurred vision

Imiprimine (Tofranil)
  α and β-adrenergic
  agonist
Dose:
  child: 1.5-2 mg/kg/
  dose qid
  adult - 25 mg PO qid
Side effects:
  dry mouth, blurred
  vision, constipation,
  tachycardia, sweating
  fatigue, tremor

Intermittent self-
  catheterization

Bethanechol (Urecholine)
  cholinergic agonist
Dose:
  child - 5 mg qd,
  increase as below
  adult: 5-10 mg SQ tid
  initially, then 50 mg PO
  qid chronically
Side effects:
  contraindicated in asthma,
  hyperthyroidism, coronary
  artery disease, ulcer
  disease

Phenoxybenzamine (Dibenzyline)
  α-adrenergic antagonist
Dose:
  child: 0.3-0.5 mg/kg/d
  adult: 10-30 mg/d
Side effects:
  retrograde ejaculation,
  drowsiness, orthostatic
  hypotension

Intermittent self-
  catheterization, or
  crede maneuver

Ref: Wein AJ, et al. Management of neurogenic bladder
       dysfunction in the adult. Urology 8:432, 1976.

McGuire EJ. Clinical evaluation and treatment of neurogenic vesical dysfunction. In, Libertino JA (ed). International Perspectives in Urology, Vol II. Baltimore: Williams and Wilkins, 1984.

BRACHIAL PLEXUS (see also Neuropathy, Peripheral Nerve)

Brachial plexus neuropathy (idiopathic brachial neuritis, neuralgic amyotrophy) is characterized by acute onset of shoulder (occasionally arm) pain which is not affected by neck movement or Valsalva maneuver. Pain may persist for up to 2-3 weeks and is followed rapidly by variable weakness and atrophy. Weakness may be in the distribution of a root, trunk, or cord of the brachial plexus or of a peripheral nerve, either singly or in combination. There may be dissociated involvement of muscles innervated by the same nerve. Approximately 1/3 of cases are bilateral. Prognosis for recovery is good. Treatment is supportive with range of motion exercises to prevent a shoulder arthropathy. EMG may be helpful in localization and in excluding a cervical radiculopathy.

Traumatic or compressive brachial plexopathy may be due to penetrating or blunt trauma, stretch injury, or sustained compression. Causes include dislocation of the humeral head, sequelae of clavicular fracture, malpositioning during surgery, birth trauma, nerve blocks, wearing heavy backpacks, firearm recoil, and contact sports. Upper brachial plexus (C5-C6, Erb-Duchenne palsy) injuries are more common than those of the lower plexus (C8-T1, Klumpke-Dejerine palsy).

Neoplastic brachial plexopathy is typically associated with pain and a Horner's syndrome.

Radiation brachial plexopathy occurs 5 months to 20 years after radiation. Pain is less common and Horner's syndrome is rare.

Ref: Tsaris P, et al. Natural history of brachial plexus neuropathy. Arch Neurol 27:109, 1972.

Lederman RJ, Wilbourn AJ. Brachial plexopathy: recurrent cancer or radiation? Neurology 34:1331, 1984.

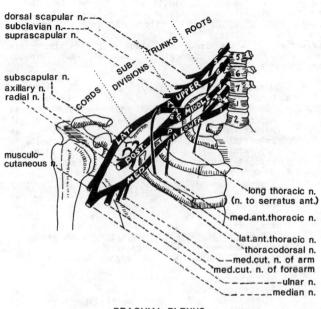

BRACHIAL PLEXUS

BRAIN DEATH (see also Coma)

Definitions vary from center to center. Legal criteria of death vary from state to state. The following are guidelines to the determination of irreversible brain function in adults. Particular caution is advised in the application of brain death criteria to young children; a pediatric neurologist should be consulted. The clinical criteria for brain death are mandatory; once these are met, supplementary laboratory studies may provide additional support.

I. Clinical criteria (mandatory)
   A. Coma of known cause due to an irreversible cerebral process. Must not be due to CNS depressant or neuromuscular blocking drugs, hypothermia (<32°C/90°F), or metabolic or endocrine disturbances. Blood pressure should be maintained, if possible. Pooling of blood in retinal vessels indicates arterial stasis.
   B. No cerebral function. No behavioral or reflex responses involving structures above the cervical spinal cord can be elicited by stimuli to any part of the body. No spontaneous movement or posturing to deep pain. Spinal reflex withdrawal is permissible. Deep tendon (spinal) reflexes may be present if all other criteria are met.
   C. No brainstem function (reflexes)
      1. Pupils unreactive to light (midposition or dilated)
      2. Corneal reflexes absent
      3. Vestibular-ocular reflexes absent. No response to oculocephalic maneuvers ("dolls-head") and 50cc ice water caloric stimuli in each ear
      4. Gag reflex (pull on endotracheal tube) absent
      5. No other brainstem reflexes (e.g., blink, ciliospinal, jaw jerk, snout)
      6. No spontaneous respiration during apneic oxygenation for 10 minutes or with a pCO_2 >60. Patients are ventilated for 10-30 minutes with 100% O_2 and then disconnected from the ventilator while 100% O_2 is supplied by tracheal catheter at 6 L/min. Blood gases are drawn before and 5 minutes after disconnecting the respirator.
   D. Criteria should be present over 6-24 hours

II. Laboratory criteria (confirmatory)
   A. Toxic screen or specific drug levels
   B. Isoelectric EEG according to standards established by the American EEG Society
      1. Minimum of 8 scalp electrodes and ear reference electrodes
      2. Interelectrode distances of at least 10 cm
      3. Interelectrode resistances <10,000 ohms but >100 ohms
      4. Test recording system by deliberate creation of electrode artifact by manipulation
      5. Gains increased during most of the recording from 7.0–2.0 μV/mm
      6. Use of 0.3–0.4 time constants during part of the recording
      7. Recording with EKG and other monitoring devices (e.g., pair of electrodes on dorsum of hand) to detect extracerebral responses
      8. Tests for reactivity to pain, loud noise, and light
      9. At least 30 minutes total recording time
      10. Recording by qualified technician
      11. Repeat record if doubt about electrocerebral silence
      12. Do not transmit EEG's by telephone
   C. Brainstem auditory and somatosensory evoked potentials can provide additional evidence of absent brainstem functions
   D. Absence of cerebral circulation may be demonstrated by cerebral arteriography, bolus radioisotope angiography, or intracranial pressure (ICP) monitoring showing ICP above mean systolic pressure for 1 hour

Ref: Black PM. NEJM 299:338, 299:393, 1978.

Neurology 32:395, 1982.

BRAINSTEM

MIDBRAIN CROSS SECTION

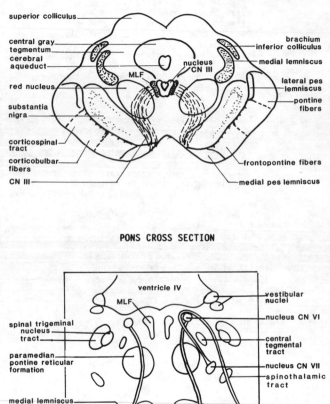

superior colliculus

central gray
tegmentum
cerebral
aqueduct

MLF

red nucleus

substantia
nigra

corticospinal
tract

corticobulbar
fibers

CN III

nucleus
CN III

brachium
inferior colliculus

medial lemniscus

lateral pes
lemniscus

pontine
fibers

frontopontine fibers

medial pes lemniscus

PONS CROSS SECTION

ventricle IV

MLF

spinal trigeminal
nucleus
tract

paramedian
pontine reticular
formation

medial lemniscus
lateral lemniscus

corticospinal tract

vestibular
nuclei

nucleus CN VI

central
tegmental
tract

nucleus CN VII

spinothalamic
tract

CN VII

CN VI

34

MEDULLA CROSS SECTION

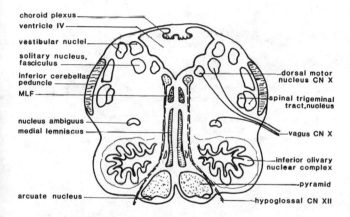

Brainstem syndromes are best described in the terms of precise neuroanatomical localization. Eponymic descriptions in the literature vary. I=ipsilateral. C=contralateral. Roman numerals indicate cranial nerves. br.=branch. a.=artery. MLF=medial longitudinal fasciculus. INO=internuclear ophthalmoplegia. CTT=central tegmental tract. CBT=corticobulbar tract. CST=corticospinal tract. ML=medial lemniscus. sup.=superior. mid. cerebell. ped.=middle cerebellar peduncle.

BRAINSTEM SYNDROMES

Syndrome	Localization	Clinical Features
Chiray-Foix-Nicolesco's	Midbrain tegmentum, upper red nucleus	C: Hemiataxia, intention tremor, hemiparesis, sensory disturbances
Benedikt's	Midbrain tegmentum, red nucleus, III, peduncle	I: III palsy, C: Hemiataxia, intention tremor, hyperkinesia, hemiparesis
Claude's	Midbrain tegmentum, red nucleus, III, ± peduncle	I: III palsy, C: Hemiataxia, rubral tremor, hemiparesis
Weber's	Ventral midbrain, III, peduncle	I: III palsy, C: Hemiparesis
Parinaud's	Dorsal rostral midbrain	Paralysis of upgaze and accommodation, light-near dissociation of pupil, lid retraction, convergence-retraction nystagmus
Nothnagel's	Dorsal midbrain, brachium conjunctivum, III nucleus, MLF	Ataxia, III palsy, INO, vertical gaze
Koerber-Salus-Elschnig	Dorsal midbrain, superior periaqueductal grey	III palsy, nystagmus, INO, altered mental status, spasticity, abnormal respiration
	Medial superior pons (paramedian br. of upper basilar a.), sup. and mid. cerebellar ped., MLF, CTT, CBT, CST, variable ML	I: Ataxia, INO, palatal myoclonus (late), C: Hemiparesis (face, arm, leg), variable sensory

Syndrome	Localization	Clinical Features
Raymond-Cestan	Medial mid-pons (paramedian br. mid basilar a.), mid. cerebell. ped. CBT, CST, variable ML	I: Ataxia, C: Hemiparesis (face, arm, leg), variable sensory, variable ocular motor
	Lateral mid-pons (short circumferential a.), mid. cerebell. ped., V	I: ataxia, paralysis of muscles of mastication, facial hemihypesthesia
One and a half	Paramedian pontine reticular formation MLF	I: Horizontal gaze palsy, C: INO
Foville's	Paramedian pontine reticular formation, VI, VII, CST	I: Horizontal gaze palsy, facial palsy, C: Hemiparesis (sparing face)
Millard-Gubler	Ventral paramedian pons, VI and VII fascicles, CST	I: VI palsy, facial palsy, C: Hemiparesis
Raymond's	Ventral pons, VI fascicles, CST	I: VI palsy, C: Hemiparesis
Brissaud's	Ventral pons, VII, CST	I: Facial spasm C: Hemiparesis
Babinski-Nageotte	Dorsolateral ponto-medullary junction	I: Ataxia, hemihypesthesia in face, Horner's, C: Hemiparesis, hemihypesthesia in body

Syndrome	Localization	Clinical Features
Wallenberg's	Dorsolateral medulla, vestibular nucleus, restiform body, V (spinal tract and nucleus), IX, X, descending sympathetics, spinal lemniscus	Vertigo, vomiting, nystagmus, I: lateropulsion, ataxia, loss of pain and temperature in face, paralysis of soft palate, posterior pharynx and vocal cord, Horner's, C: loss of pain and temperature in body
Cestan–Chenais	Lateral medulla	I: Ataxia, paralysis of soft palate, posterior pharynx and vocal cord, Horner's, C: Hemiparesis, hemihypesthesia in body
Avellis'	Lateral medulla, IX, X	I: Paralysis of soft palate, posterior pharynx, and vocal cord, C: Hemiparesis, hemihypesthesia
Vernet's	Lateral medulla, IX, X, XI	I: Paralysis of soft palate, posterior pharynx, and sterno-cleidomastoid, decreased taste over posterior 1/3 of tongue, hemi-hypesthesia of pharynx, C: Hemiparesis
Jackson's	Lateral medulla, IX, X, XI, XII	I: Paralysis of soft palate, posterior pharynx, vocal cords, sternocleido-mastoid, upper trapezius, and tongue, C: Hemiparesis, hemihypesthesia

Syndrome	Localization	Clinical Features
Tapia's	Lateral medulla, IX, X, XII (more commonly there is extracranial involvement)	As in Schmidt's except sternocleido-mastoid and trapezius not involved
Preolivary	Anterior medulla, XII, pyramid	I: Tongue atrophy or weakness C: Hemiparesis

Ref: Wolf JK. The Classical Brain Stem Syndromes. Springfield: Charles C Thomas, 1971.

BULBAR PALSY

A syndrome of weakness or paralysis of muscles supplied by cranial nerves IX, X, XI and XII secondary to lesions of the nuclei or nerves (see Pseudobublar Palsy for lesions of the supranuclear pathways). Involved muscles include those of the pharynx and larynx, sternocleido-mastoid, upper trapezius, and tongue. Patients may present clinically with dysarthria, dysphagia, hoarseness, nasal voice, palatal deviation, diminished gag reflex, or weakness of the sternocleidomastoid, upper trapezius or tongue (may have atrophy and fasciculations). Etiologies include motor neuron disease ("progressive bulbar palsy" is one form), cerebrovascular lesions of the brainstem, intra- and extramedullary tumors, syringobulbia (may be associated with syringomyelia), meningitis, encephalitis, herpes zoster, poliomyelitis, diphtheria, aneurysms (uncommon), granulomatous disease, bone lesions (platybasia, Paget's, foramenal syndromes). Guillain-Barre syndrome, myasthenia gravis, and other neuromuscular disorders affecting bulbar innervated muscles must also be considered.

CALCIFICATION

Benign Intracranial Calcifications:

Pineal: If displaced more than 3 mm laterally on a good, nonrotated frontal skull film, a unilateral mass lesion should be sought. Large pineal calcification suggests a pineal tumor.

Choroid plexus: Seen in the lateral ventricles in about 10% of patients on routine skull films, more commonly on CT.

Habenular commissure: Delicate C-shaped calcification approximately 3-5 mm anterior to the pineal.

Dura: Flat, oval homogeneous densities appear in the falx (usually anteriorly), tentorium, or over the convexities in about 10% of skull films. The petroclinoid ligament is frequently calcified.

Carotid arteries: Carotid calcification should be differentiated from that seen with carotid aneurysms.

Pathologic Intracranial Calcifications:

Endocrine: Hypo- and hyper-parathyroidism.

Vascular: Arteriovenous malformation (30% on plain skull films), aneurysm, chronic subdural (rarely), chronic epidural (rarely), chronic intracerebral hematoma (rarely).

Infectious: Brain abscess, granuloma, cysticercosis, echinococcosis, toxoplasmosis (widespread calcifications in the neonate), cytomegalovirus (periventricular calcification in the neonate).

Neoplastic: Chordoma, craniopharyngioma (calcification in 60-70%, curvilinear or speckled calcification above enlarged sella, differentiate from carotid aneurysm or pituitary adenoma), glioma (calcification occurs in approximately 54% of oligodendrogliomas, 27% of ependymomas, 13% of astrocytomas, and 5% of glioblastomas), meningioma (18%, adjacent bony sclerosis), brain metastasis, osteochondroma, pinealoma (20%), lipoma.

Phakomatoses: Tuberous sclerosis, Sturge-Weber.

Multiple calcifications suggest metastases, parathyroid disorders, infections, tuberous sclerosis.

Basal ganglia calcifications may be seen on skull films with the following disorders:

Infectious:	Cytomegalovirus, toxoplasmosis, viral encephalitis (measles, chickenpox), cysticercosis
Toxic-anoxic:	Birth anoxia, carbon monoxide, lead encephalopathy, radiation therapy
Endocrine:	Hypoparathyroidism, pseudohypoparathyroidism, and pseudopseudohypoparathyroidism
Developmental:	Familial cerebral ferrocalcinosis (Fahr's disease), tuberous sclerosis, oculocraniosomatic disease, Cockayne syndrome

On CT, basal ganglia calcification is seen more frequently (about 1% of scans), than on plain skull films. Further investigation is indicated when they are seen in patients under 40 years of age or when they are not restricted to the globus pallidus.

Ref: Taveras JM, Wood EH. Diagnostic Neuroradiology, 2nd ed. Baltimore: Williams and Wilkins, 1976.

Baker HL. JAMA 247:883, 1982.

CALCIUM

Hypocalcemia may result in increased neuromuscular irritability, tetany, positive Chvostek's and Trousseau's signs, and seizures. If hypocalcemia develops slowly, encephalopathy may develop, with irritability and lethargy, possibly mimicking psychiatric disease. Progression of the mental status changes to coma is rare. Increased intracranial pressure and papilledema occur occasionally.

The EKG shows QT lengthening which should be distinguished from pseudo QT lengthening in hypokalemia resulting from flattening of the T wave and misinterpretation of the later U wave as the T.

When evaluating hypocalcemia, bear in mind: 1) the association between hypomagnesemia and hypocalcemia in hypoparathyroidism (see hypomagnesemia); 2) when corrected for hypoalbuminemia, the patient may be normocalcemic (0.8 mg/ml decline in calcium is accounted for by a 1.0 gm/l drop in albumin).

Hypercalcemia may present with encephalopathy, which, like hypocalcemia, can mimic psychiatric disease, or it may present with systemic symptoms such as anorexia, nausea and vomiting, and nephrogenic diabetes insipidus. In contrast to hypocalcemia, coma is seen in severe hypercalcemia, but seizures are uncommon. Clinical status can be roughly correlated with calcium level as follows:

12-16 mg/ml	Personality changes, affective disorders
16-19 mg/ml	Impaired cognition and level of consciousness, psychosis
>19 mg/ml	Stupor and coma

In hyperparathyroidism, proximal muscle weakness and muscle atrophy have been described. EMG may be normal. Note that lithium may produce a reversible hyperparathyroid state; the mental status changes may be mistakenly attributed to the psychiatric disease for which the lithium was given.

The EKG shows QT interval shortening, characteristically with abrupt T wave up slope.

CALORICS (see also Vestibulo-ocular Reflex)

Water colder or warmer than body temperature, applied to the tympanic membrane, changes the firing rate of the ipsilateral vestibular nerve and causes ocular deviation and nystagmus. In normals, cold water induces a slow ipsilateral deviation with contralateral "corrective" fast phases. Warm water induces a slow contralateral deviation and ipsilateral fast phases. The direction of nystagmus is conventionally described as that of the fast phase. The mnemonic COWS ("cold opposite, warm same"), indicates the direction of caloric nystagmus for cold and warm stimuli respectively. Bilateral irrigation induces vertical nystagmus. Here the mnemonic is CUWD ("cold up, warm down").

Caloric testing may be done quantitatively in a laboratory or at the bedside. Quantitative calorics are used to test vestibular function. Bedside calorics are used to 1) establish the integrity of the ocular motor system in patients with an apparent gaze paresis and 2) to evaluate altered states of consciousness. Caloric stimulation may be used to elicit vestibular eye movements if oculocephalic maneuvers (see Vestibulo-ocular Reflex) are negative or when a cervical injury is suspected.

Bedside calorics are performed after the external auditory canal is examined, impacted cerumen removed, and possible continuity with the inner ear or intracranial spaces excluded. The head is elevated 30° from horizontal. Water is gently injected with a syringe through a soft catheter inserted in the external auditory canal. One cc of ice-water is usually sufficient and should be used in alert patients to minimize discomfort. In unresponsive patients, up to 100 cc of ice-water should be used and several minutes allowed for a response. Irrigation is repeated in the opposite ear after waiting at least 5 minutes for vestibular equilibration. Warm water (44°C) may also be used. Hot water should never be used due to the risk of thermal injury.

Eye movements elicited by vestibular stimuli, whether passive head rotation (see Vestibulo-ocular Reflex) or caloric, allow localization within the ocular motor system. Impaired movement of both eyes to one side occurs with lesions of the ipsilateral abducens nucleus. Impaired abduction alone suggests a VI nerve palsy. Impaired adduction is seen in third nerve palsies and in the eye ipsilateral to the medial longitudinal fasciculus lesion of an internuclear ophthalmoplegia; the former may be differentiated by the presence of pupillary dilation.

Bilateral internuclear ophthalmoplegias cause, in addition to bilateral adduction weakness, impaired vertical vestibular eye movements. These vertical eye movements are also impaired by midbrain lesions, especially in the region of the posterior commissure. Horizontal vestibular eye movements may remain intact in spite of absent vertical vestibular eye movements if the lesion is rostral to the sixth nerve nucleus. Eye deviation may occur in directions unrelated to the semicircular canals being stimulated in certain patients with drug intoxication or structural disease of central vestibular connections.

As consciousness declines, fast phases are progressively lost, resulting in only a tonic deviation of the eyes. In acute coma due to brainstem lesions, horizontal fast phases are absent because of involvement of the burst cells in the paramedian pontine reticular formation. Vertical fast phases are lost due to involvement of burst cells in the rostral interstitial nucleus of the medial longitudinal fasciculus. The occurrence of nystagmus in an acutely unresponsive patient suggests a psychogenic cause.

Absent vestibular eye movement may result from lesions of vestibulo-ocular reflex pathways in the eighth nerve, medulla, pons or midbrain. Absent responses may also be due to disease of the labyrinth or drug effects. Drug effects may occur with ototoxic agents (aminoglycosides), vestibular suppressants (barbiturates, phenytoin, tricyclic antidepressants, major tranquilizers), and neuromuscular blockers (succinylcholine, pancuronium).

Ref: Plum F, Posner JB. The Diagnosis of Stupor and
        Coma, 3rd ed. Philadelphia: FA Davis, 1982; 54-64.

CARDIOPULMONARY ARREST (see also Coma)

Duration of coma and degree of functional recovery after in-hospital cardiac arrest are directly related to duration of anoxia. Coma is uncommon following prompt resuscitation in an intensive care unit. Prearrest morbidity affects survival. Pneumonia, hypotension, renal failure, cancer or home-bound lifestyle are predictive of a poor prognosis. Following in-hospital cardiac arrest, roughly 14% of patients survive to be discharged. Arrest for longer than 15 minutes has a very poor prognosis.

Survival after out-of-hospital arrest is related to prompt resuscitation and efficient paramedical support. Up to 50% of patients not awake on arrival at the hospital after arrest survive to be discharged, approximately 1/3 of these with persistent brain damage. Neurological responses at the time of admission have been correlated with outcome in various studies.

In nontraumatic coma, if 2 of 3 of the following are absent on admission to the hospital, only 1% will achieve moderate disability or a good recovery: corneal reflex, pupillary reaction, or vestibulo-ocular reflex.

Seventy-eight percent of patients who recover have awakened by 10 hours, and 90% have awakened by 24 hours. Persistent coma for 48 hours is usually associated with death or a chronic vegetative state.

Ref: Bates D, et al. Ann Neurol 2:211, 1977;
       Snyder et al. Neurology 27:807, 1977;
       Levy et al. Ann Int Med 94:293, 1981;
       Bedel et al. NEJM 309:569, 1983;
       Bass E, Ann Int Med 103:920, 1985.

CARPAL TUNNEL SYNDROME (see also Neuropathy, Peripheral Nerve)

Compression of the median nerve as it courses under the transverse carpal ligament, usually due to thickening or fibrosis of the ligament or of the synovia of the flexor tendons. It is bilateral in as many as 50%. It is often associated with obesity, diabetes, trauma, pregnancy, rheumatoid arthritis, thyroid disease, lupus erythematosus, sarcoidosis, mucopolysaccharidosis, or amyloidosis and may be familial.

Clinically, there is intermittent numbness and paresthesias, especially at night. Sensory symptoms are restricted to the distribution of the median nerve. Pain may radiate up the forearm. Symptoms may be reproduced by extreme flexion of the wrist (Phalen's signs) or by tapping over the course of the nerve in the wrist (Tinnel's sign). Weakness of opponens pollicis, abductor pollicis brevis, and first two lumbricals and thenar atrophy may occur after weeks or months.

Differential diagnosis includes C6 or C7 radiculopathy, brachial plexopathy, peripheral neuropathy, and median neuropathy other than at the wrist.

Nerve conduction studies reveal prolonged (>4.5 ms) distal motor latencies of the median nerve and the median nerve distal motor latency minus the ulnar nerve distal motor latency is >1.8 ms. EMG may demonstrate denervation.

Treatment consists of avoiding activities that precipitate symptoms and wearing a wrist extension splint at night. Local steroid injections are not clearly beneficial. Indications for surgery are weakness, atrophy and EMG evidence of denervation. Surgery is not indicated in pregnancy as the symptoms usually resolve after delivery.

Ref: Nakano KK. Muscle Nerve 1:264, 1978.

CAUDA EQUINA/CONUS MEDULLARIS (see page 46)

CEREBELLUM (see Ataxia, Spinocerebellar Degeneration)

CEREBRAL CORTEX

   Brodmann's cytoarchitectural map of cerebral cortex, indicating major functional areas, is depicted on page 47.

CEREBRAL PALSY

   A nonprogressive disorder, usually of movement and posture, due to brain injury occurring in the period of early brain growth, generally under three years of age (i.e., static encephalopathy). No active CNS disease should be present at the time of the diagnosis. The two basic categories are "spastic" and "extrapyramidal" (choreoathetosis, rigidity, or ataxia). Mixtures of the two types are frequent. The common patterns of the spastic variety are: hemiplegic, double hemiplegic (four limbs with uppers more affected), quadriplegic (four limbs with lowers more affected), and diplegic (four limbs with lowers markedly more affected than uppers). Factors associated with increased risk of CP include: low birth weight, multiple pregnancies, and neonatal difficulties such as anoxia, seizures, and cyanotic episodes. See also Encephalopathy, Perinatal Hypoxic-Ischemic.

Ref: Vinning EPG, et al. Child 130:643, 1975.

CLINICAL DIFFERENTIATION OF CAUDA EQUINA AND CONUS MEDULLARIS SYNDROMES

CONUS MEDULLARIS (lower sacral cord)	CAUDA EQUINA (lumbosacral roots)

Sensory Deficit:

Saddle distribution	Saddle distribution
Bilateral, symmetric	Asymmetric
Sensory dissociation present	Sensory dissociation absent
Presents early	Presents relatively later

Pain:

Uncommon	Prominent, early
Relatively mild	Severe
Bilateral, symmetric	Asymmetric
Perineum and thighs	Radicular

Motor Deficit:

Symmetric	Asymmetric
Mild	Moderate to severe
Fasciculations may be present	Fasciculations absent
Atrophy absent	Atrophy more prominent

Reflexes:

Achilles reflex absent	Reflexes variably
Patellar reflex normal	involved

Sphincter Dysfunction:

Early, severe	Late, less severe
Absent anal and bulbo cavernosus reflex	Reflex abnormalities less common

Sexual Dysfunction:

Erection and ejaculation impaired	Less common

Adapted from DeJong RN. The Neurologic Examination, 4th ed. New York: Harper and Row, 1979, p 587.

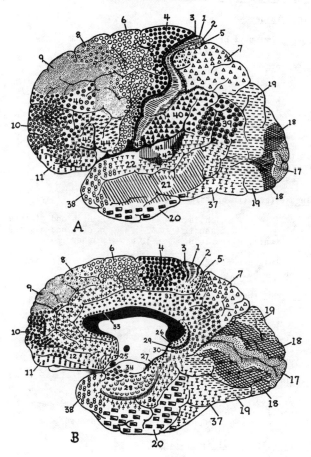

A

B

Functional areas: 4-primary motor strip, 3,1,2-sensory strip, 17-primary visual cortex, 18, 19-visual association cortex, 8-frontal eye fields, 6-premotor cortex, 41 and 42-auditory cortex, 5,7 somaesthetic association cortex.

From: Carpenter MB. Human Neuroanatomy 7th ed. 1976:554.

CEREBROSPINAL FLUID (see also Meningitis)

Normal Values

Protein (mg/ml):				
preterm	mean 115	prealbumin	4%
term	mean 90	albumin	65%
child	5-40	α-1-globulin	4%
adult	20-40	α-2-globulin	8%
ventricular fluid	6-15	β-globulin	12%
cisternal fluid	15-25	γ-globulin	7%
		Ig>>IgA>IgM	

Decremental gradient of CSF protein between 1st and 25th cc removed: 15%

IgG index upper limit: 0.66
IgG/alb ratio upper limit: 0.27
Myelin basic protein: <4 ng/ml

Glucose (mg/ml):		
preterm	mean 50	
term	mean 52	
child	40-80	50% of blood glucose
adult	50-70	60% of blood glucose
ventricular fluid	6-18 mg/ml higher	

CSF glucose follows blood glucose changes with latency of 1-2 hours.

Cell count (WBC/cu mm):		
preterm	9	57% PMN
term	8	61% PMN
adult	0-5	0% PMN

Degradation of WBC at room temperature after 2 hours: 40%
Degradation of WBC at 4°C after 2 hours: 15%

Pressure: (mmH$_2$O) Newborn 80-100
                child/adult 60-200

Pregnancy: No change in CSF profile
Obesity: No significant increase in CSF pressure

CSF profiles in disease states

Abbreviations:
    PMN = polymorphonuclear cells
    L+M = lymphocytes and mononuclear cells
    ↑/↓ = slight to moderate increase/decrease
    av   = average
    NL   = normal

CSF PROFILES IN VARIOUS DISEASE STATES

	Pressure	Cell count	Protein	Glucose
Purulent meningitis	↑ in 90% 200-1500	100-10000 90-95% PMN	NL-2200, av 418	40-10

Rapid ↓ cell count and ↑ glucose with therapy. Persistent pleocytosis (>30 WBC) may occur in adequately treated children. Counterimmunoelectrophoresis (CIE) may aid in early diagnosis, especially in partially treated cases.

	Pressure	Cell count	Protein	Glucose
Aseptic meningitis	↑ acutely	few to 1000 L + M	NL-400, av 77	NL

PMN may predominate in acute stage. Lymphocytic choriomeningitis presents with up to 3000 WBC. Chemical meningitis may be associated with marked hypoglycorrhachia. See page 172.

Tuberculous meningitis	↑ in 80%	50-500 L + M	NL-1140, av 200	<30, NL acutely

Fungal meningitis:

Cryptococcus	NL	↑ PMN+L+M	NL-500	40-10

Positive India ink, cryptococcal antigen

Candida	NL	↑ PMN+L+M	50-200	NL acutely, then ↓
Coccidio-idomycosis	NL	50-200 M, >1000 in late stage	90-300	20-4
Neuro-syphilis	NL or ↑	↑ L+M	NL->1000	NL or ↓

CSF profile varies greatly among the different syndromes and stages

	Pressure	Cell count	Protein	Glucose
Herpes simplex encephalitis	NL	50-500L	50-90	NL or ↓

CSF profile is not pathognomonic. RBC and xanthochromia may exist

CNS infection in immunocompromised host

	NL or ↑	mostly <5	NL-↑	NL or ↓

Fever and mental status changes may be the only symptoms in bacterial meningitis; meningeal signs are uncommon. CSF in CMV infection is characteristically normal. Beware of thrombocytopenia in neutropenic patients (LP complications).

	Pressure	Cell count	Protein	Glucose
Infectious mononucleosis meningitis	↑	10-150L, some atypical	↑	NL
Mollaret's meningitis (attack)	NL or ↑	200-1000M	70-1000	NL
SSPE	NL	NL	NL or ↑	NL

Striking elevation of gamma globulin to 20-50% of total protein. Oligoclonal bands are present.

	Pressure	Cell count	Protein	Glucose
Brain abscess	NL or ↑	10->500 PMN or L	NL or ↑	NL

Rupture may cause rapid changes in CSF profile.

	Pressure	Cell count	Protein	Glucose
Toxoplasmosis	↑	10-50 M some eos	↑	NL

	Pressure	Cell count	Protein	Glucose
Polio-myelitis	↑ up to 600	100-200 PMN	NL-366, av 70	NL

↓ cell count with progression.
L's predominate during paralytic phase.

	Pressure	Cell count	Protein	Glucose
Arach-noiditis	↓ in presence of block	↑ L, few eos and PMN	↑	NL or ↓
Brain tumor	NL or ↑	NL or ↑	↑	NL

Pleocytosis and positive cytology generally requires extension to the ventricular system. Primary CNS lymphomas present with pleocytosis and, frequently, evidence of immunoglobulin production.

	Pressure	Cell count	Protein	Glucose
Carcino-matous meningitis	NL, ↑ in late stages	0-500 PMN,L	↑ or ↑↑	NL or↓
Spinal block	↓ or ↓↓	NL or ↑	↑ or ↑↑	NL or ↓

Clotting (Froin's syndrome) occurs when protein >1000 with sufficient content of fibrinogen. Lower level blocks produce higher protein levels.

	Pressure	Cell count	Protein	Glucose
Intramedullary tumor	NL	<10	NL or ↑	NL
Subacute combined degeneration	NL	few M	NL or ↑	NL
Syringo-myelia	NL	<10	NL	NL
ALS	NL	<10	NL	NL
Vasculitis	NL	<500 PMN,L,M	NL or ↑	NL

	Pressure	Cell count	Protein	Glucose
Cerebral hemorrhage	↑	NL->1000	NL-2000, av 270	NL or ↓
Subarachnoid hemorrhage	↑	↑	<150	NL

Lysis of RBC begins after 2-4 hours. Xanthochromia visible after 8-10 hours, may persist for weeks.

	Pressure	Cell count	Protein	Glucose
Vogt-Koyanagi-Harada syndrome	NL	4-700 L	NL or ↑	NL
Behcet's disease	NL	10-200 L	NL or ↑	NL

Acute disseminated encephalomyelitis

	Pressure	Cell count	Protein	Glucose
	NL or ↑ at onset	50-150 PMN	<100	NL
Optic neuritis	NL	5-30 M in 60%	NL or ↑	NL
PML	NL	0 or few WBC	NL	NL
Guillain -Barre	NL	rarely >25L	NL->1000	NL

Protein is maximal between days 4-18. Gamma globulin increased. Oligoclonal bands frequently present.

	Pressure	Cell count	Protein	Glucose
Seizure	NL	rarely >5 PMN	NL or ↑	NL

Pleocytosis tends to be related to prolonged or repeated seizures.

	Pressure	Cell count	Protein	Glucose
Migraine	NL or ↑	5-15L	NL or ↑	NL

A migrainous syndrome with cell counts >200 has been described.

	Pressure	Cell count	Protein	Glucose
Uremia	NL or ↑	NL	NL→>100	NL
Pseudotumor cerebri	>250	NL	often ↓	NL
Myxedema	NL	NL	NL–240	NL
Parkinson's disease	NL	NL	NL	NL

Oligoclonal bands may occur in patients with postencephalitic parkinsonism.

| Multiple sclerosis | NL | <16 L+M | NL–130 in 95% (see below) | NL |

Multiple sclerosis special studies

	IgG/alb ratio	IgG index	Oligoclonal bands
Definite MS	61%	91%	83%
Probable MS	52%	70%	81%
Possible MS	21%	44%	39%

Cell count probably does not increase with exacerbation. Percentage of T-lymphocytes in CSF is higher than in blood. Gamma globulins are increased in 95%. Myelin basic protein may increase with exacerbation.

Special considerations

Oligoclonal bands: If present, usually 2–5, rarely >10. Occur in multiple neurological diseases indicating inflammatory process in the CNS. Gamma globulin levels may be normal.
Decreased lumbar CSF protein (<20 mg/ml): Normal in children, age 6 months–2 years. Also seen with removal of large CSF volume, post-LP CSF leak, hyperthyroidism, leukemia, 1/3 of patients with pseudotumor cerebri.
Xanthochromia: SAH, hypercarotinemia, hyperbilirubinemia, rifampin therapy, following traumatic tap.
Corrections for bloody tap (normal peripheral count): Reduce white count by one cell for every 700 RBC. Subtract 1 mg protein/ml for every 1000 RBC.

Tumor markers in CSF

Meningeal carcinomatosis: Increased β-glucuronidase, carcinoembryonic antigen. Choriocarcinomas, germinal cell carcinomas, teratomas: increase β-HCG (serum HCG/CSF <60 is highly suggestive of brain metastasis), increased α-fetoprotein.
Glioblastomas: Increased glial fibrillary acidic protein.
Medulloblastomas, gliomas: Increased putrescine and spermidine.

LDH, GOT, CPK, aldolase, phosphohexose isomerase, isocitrate dehydrogenase, adenylate kinase and lysozyme are nonspecifically elevated in CNS malignancy.

Complications of lumbar puncture

Headache: Incidence 10%. Onset 5 min to 4 days after LP. Duration 4-8 days. Characteristic relief from lying flat.
Brain herniation: Acute or delayed (within 12 hours) in 1-2% of patients with intracranial mass lesions. Occurrence favored by preexisting mass shifts.
Spinal subdural, epidural or subarachnoid hemorrhage: May occur in patients with bleeding diathesis, thrombocytopenia and anticoagulation.
Diplopia: Rare unilateral or bilateral 6th nerve palsy.
Others: Radicular irritation, meningitis, implantation of epidermoid tumor.

Contraindications to lumbar puncture include infection over site of entry, bleeding disorder, and intracranial mass lesion with increased ICP.

Ref: Fishman RA. Cerebrospinal Fluid in Diseases of the Nervous System. Philadelphia: Saunders, 1980.

CEREBROVASCULAR DISEASE (see Aneurysms, Hemorrhage, Ischemia)

NEUROTOXICITY OF VARIOUS CHEMOTHERAPEUTIC AGENTS

Agent	Toxicity
Intrathecal methotrexate	Acute: arachnoiditis, paraplegia Chronic: leukoencephalopathy, somnolence (associated with combined radiation therapy)
Cisplatin	Tinnitus, hearing loss, peripheral neuropathy, optic neuritis
Vincristine (and other alkaloids)	Peripheral (including autonomic) neuropathy, SIADH
Hexamethylmelamine	Peripheral neuropathy, mental status changes
5-fluorouracil	Acute cerebellar dysfunction, ocular motor disturbances
L-asparaginase	Encephalopathy, intracranial hemorrhage due to coagulopathy
Procarbazine	Encephalopathy, peripheral neuropathy
BCNU	Dizziness, transient confusion when given intra-arterially for brain tumor

Ref: Kaplan RS, Wiernik PH. Neurotoxicity of antineo-
plastic drugs. Seminars in Oncology. 9:103, 1982.

CHIASM (see Pituitary, Visual Fields)

CHILD NEUROLOGY (see also Cerebral Palsy, Chromosomal
Syndromes, Craniosynostosis, Degenerative Diseases of
Childhood, Developmental Malformations,
Encephalopathy, Fontanel, Hyperactive Child, Hypotonic
Infant, Immunization, Learning Disorders,
Macrocephaly, Metabolic Disorders of Childhood,
Microcephaly, Neurocutaneous Syndromes, and other
individual subject headings).

The <u>pediatric neurological exam</u> includes measurement of height, weight and head circumference (see pages 58-64) and general physical exam, with particular attention to skin, morphology of the extremities and cardiovascular exam.

A. <u>Premature neonates</u> (24-26 weeks gestation to 28 days corrected age)

1. <u>History</u>: Assessment of pregnancy, labor and delivery (drugs, illnesses, complications, etc.). If Apgar scores are not available, ask the parent if the baby cried or required help to breathe. Premature babies usually have pulmonary immaturity and are at risk for anemia, hyperbilirubinemia and sepsis.

2. <u>General exam</u>: Assess head size and shape. Transilluminate head. Look for external trauma such as a cephalohematoma, caput succedaneum, or subgaleal hematoma. Measure the size of the anterior and posterior fontanels and note whether they are bulging. Auscult head for bruits.

3. <u>Neurological exam</u>:

   a. <u>Mental status</u>: Assessment of pitch and volume of cry.

   b. <u>Cranial nerves</u>: Premies do not usually open their eyes until 26 weeks gestation. They have an inconsistent blink response to a bright light. Retinal hemorrhages may be seen soon after birth.

   c. <u>Motor/coordination</u>: Tone is difficult to assess. Compare patient with other "healthy premies" of the same gestational age in the nursery. Until 35 weeks gestation, premies do not hold arms and legs flexed at their sides. Premies of all ages should have spontaneous movements. None will be able to turn the head from side to side when placed face down. All will have head lag even with support of the examiner's fingers placed behind the shoulders as the baby is pulled from the supine to the sitting position. Note the placement of the extremities (internal or external rotation of the hips) in relationship to the trunk. Contractures are always abnormal.

   d. <u>Reflexes</u>: See table on pages 66-67.

   e. <u>Sensory</u>: Premies inconsistently withdraw and grimace to noxious stimuli.

B. <u>Full Term neonates</u> (1-28 days) should have very little head lag when pulled from a supine to a sitting position. Arching of the neck and back may be an early sign of increased tone. A full-term baby should be able to lift his head for short periods and turn it from a central face down position to one side. The normal full-term baby should flex his arms and legs and hold his head erect when held under the arms, facing the examiner. Hypotonic babies will allow their legs to flop apart in a frog leg position. Spastic babies may move the arms parallel to, but not in front of, the trunk.

C. <u>Infants and Children (1 month to 5 years)</u>
   1. <u>History</u>: Include feeding history and assessment of developmental milestones (see page 65). In general, girls may achieve developmental mile-stones earlier than boys.
   2. <u>Exam</u>:
      a. <u>Children less than 7 months</u>: Will generally cooperate for the whole exam, though you may want to auscult the heart or do funduscopy when the child is asleep (gently lifting the eyelids without exerting too much pressure on the forehead). Save the more active parts of the exam (motor and reflex testing) for the end.
      b. <u>Children 7 months to 2 years</u>: Again, certain parts of the exam, such as funduscopy, may be most easily done while the child is asleep. If the child is awake, save funduscopy until the end of the seated exam. Have the child sit on a parent's lap while obtaining the history and move slowly closer to the parent and child so you will not have to move suddenly to begin the exam. Begin the exam most distant from the face, e.g., examine the hands and feet for tone and reflexes. If the parent is adding to the child's frustration, excuse the parent from the room and get an impartial observer to help. After the seated exam is finished, allow the child to get down on the floor to play for the motor exam.

D. <u>Children greater than 2 years</u>: Most children ages 4 or older will cooperate for an exam. If they do not, this may signify developmental or psychosocial delay.

E. <u>School aged children 6-12 years</u>: Include assessment of school performance. In spite of their age, don't forget a drug and alcohol history if there has been a change in behavior.

F. <u>Adolescents</u>: Begin the history with the parent and patient in the examining room. Ask the parent to leave when the exam begins. Drug history, contra-ceptive history, etc., is best elicited during casual history-taking when the parent is out of the room.

FETAL AND INFANT NORMS
WEIGHT, LENGTH AND HEAD CIRCUMFERENCE

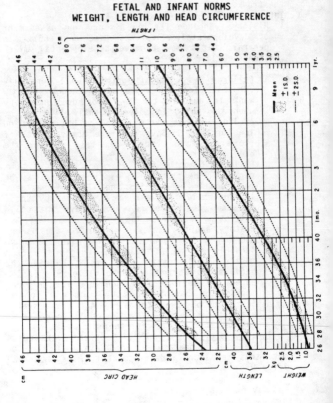

GIRLS
BIRTH TO 36 MONTHS
LENGTH AND WEIGHT

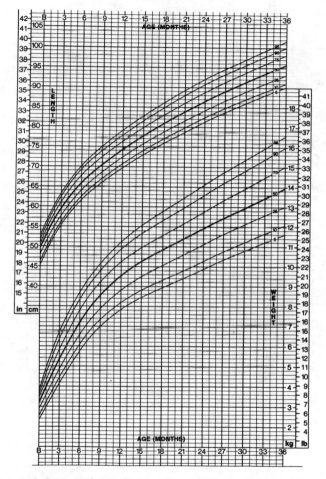

Adapted from National Center for Health Statistics data.
Copyright Ross Laboratories, 1976.

GIRLS
2 TO 18 YEARS
STATURE AND WEIGHT

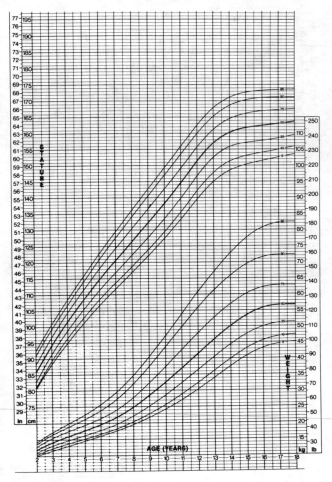

Adapted from National Center for Health Statistics data.
Copyright Ross Laboratories, 1976.

BOYS
BIRTH TO 36 MONTHS
LENGTH AND WEIGHT

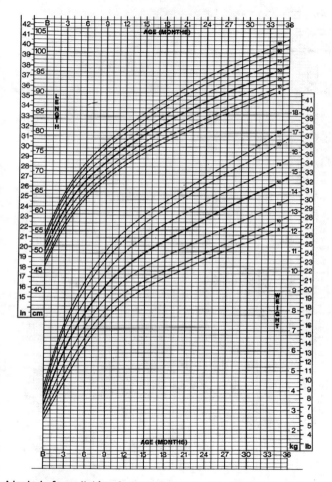

Adapted from National Center for Health Statistics data.
Copyright Ross Laboratories, 1976.

BOYS
2 TO 18 YEARS
STATURE AND WEIGHT

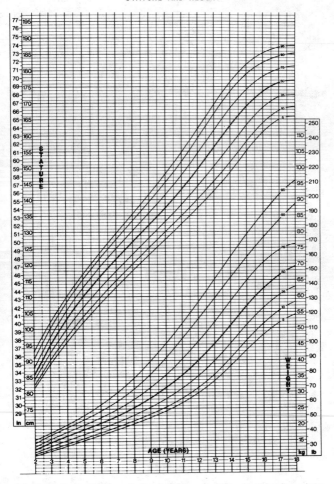

Adapted from National Center for Health Statistics data.
Copyright Ross Laboratories, 1976.

Reflex	Appears (gest. age)	Disappears
<u>Stepping/Placing</u>: Baby is held upright and the dorsal edge of the foot is brushed to the lower surface of a bed or table. The baby should flex the knee and lift the foot.	35 weeks	6 weeks
<u>Crossed adductor response</u>: Contraction of opposite adductor group with percussion of ipsilateral adductor group.	35 weeks	7 months
<u>Parachute</u>: Extension of arms at a 90° angle from the trunk and legs outward when the suspended, prone infant is lowered quickly on the examiner's supporting hand.	9 months	Persists
<u>Extensor Plantar Response (Babinski)</u>: Lateral aspect of foot is stroked. Great toe dorsiflexes.	Birth (Unilateral response may indicate corticospinal tract dysfunction)	10 months (Plantar flexor response established)
<u>Neck Righting</u>: When baby's head is turned, baby will roll trunk in the same direction.	4-6 months	2 years

CHOREA (see also Choreoathetosis)

A movement disorder characterized by involuntary, rapid, jerky, arrhythmic movements. Choreiform movements are often incorporated into deliberate movements by the patient to camouflage their disorder. Grimacing and respiratory grunts may be manifestations of chorea. The movements may be unilateral (hemichorea) or bilateral. As with most other movement disorders, chorea is aggravated by stress and disappears with sleep. Because of the frequent association of choreiform and athetoid movements, the differential diagnosis for both is listed below under Choreoathetosis.

CHOREOATHETOSIS

Drug induced:

1. Neuroleptics (see Neuroleptics)
2. L-dopa, apomorphine, bromocriptine
3. Oral contraceptives
4. Phenytoin
5. Chronic amphetamine abuse

Associated with neurological and other diseases:

1. Huntington's Disease: Choreoathetosis, progressive dementia and a mental disorder ranging from slight emotional disturbance to psychosis. Inheritance is autosomal dominant. Onset is usually in the fourth to fifth decades. Onset in 5-10% occurs before age 20. In the early onset form, rigidity and seizures may be more common, emotional disturbance may precede the movement disorder and dementia, and disease may be more severe. CT reveals convexity of the lateral ventricles due to the diminished size of the caudate nucleus and may show cortical atrophy, especially over the frontal lobes.
2. Tay-Sachs
3. Hallervorden-Spatz
4. Pelizaeus-Merzbacher
5. Lesch-Nyhan
6. Familial paroxysmal choreoathetosis
7. Chronic psychotic choreoathetosis
8. Chorea associated with dementia and acanthocytosis
9. Dystonia musculorum deformans
10. Congenital or postnatal encephalopathies due to hypoxia, developmental defects, birth trauma, kernicterus (cerebral palsy)

11. Sydenham's chorea (St. Vitus dance): Most common cause is rheumatic fever. Onset usually before age 20. Chorea follows rheumatic arthritis and carditis by several months, lasts 4-6 weeks, and usually recovers completely. Chorea is also reported in diphtheria, rubella, pertussis and other encephalitides.
12. Chorea gravidarum (see Pregnancy)
13. Hepatic encephalopathy
14. Systemic lupus erythematosus
15. Polycythemia vera
16. Vascular infarct or hemorrhage
17. Hypoparathyroidism, pseudohypoparathyroidism
18. Hyperthyroidism
19. Wilson's disease
20. Encephalitis
21. Postinfectious leukoencephalopathy
22. Carbon monoxide poisoning
23. Mercury poisoning
24. Henoch-Schonlein purpura
25. Fahr's disease
26. Meningovascular syphilis
27. Metastatic neoplasm to basal ganglia

Treatment consists of diagnosing and treating the underlying disorder, if possible. In some of these disorders the movements have been suppressed with haloperidol, tetrabenazine, reserpine, phenothiazines (chlorpromazine, perphenazine, trifluoperazine), or clonazepam.

Ref: Marsden CD, Fahn S (eds). Movement Disorders. London: Butterworth, 1982.

CHROMOSOMAL SYNDROMES (see page 70)

Ref: Smith DW. Recognizable Patterns of Human Malformation, 3rd ed. Philadelphia: Saunders, 1982.

CLINICAL FEATURES OF MOST COMMON CHROMOSOMAL SYNDROMES

	Trisomy 21 (Down's Syndrome)	Trisomy 18	Trisomy 13
Characteristic Features	Hypotonia Tend to keep mouth open Short neck	Failure to thrive Low birth weight (30% premature; 30% postmature)	Failure to thrive Capillary hemangioma
CNS	Mental retardation	Mental retardation Hypertonic after neonatal period	Mental retardation Holoprosencephaly Microcephaly Deafness Seizures EEG hypsarrhythmia
Craniofacial	Brachycephaly Upslanting palpebral fissures Medial epicanthal folds	Prominent occiput Narrow bifrontal diameter Small palpebral fissures Micrognathia, small oral opening	Sloping forehead Wide sagittal sutures and fontanelles
Eyes	Brushfield spots		Micro-ophthalmia Coloboma of iris Retinal dysplasia

COMA (see also Brain Death, Cardiopulmonary Arrest)

A state of unresponsiveness to external stimuli or inner need. Management of acute coma begins with evaluation of airway, circulation, temperature, glucose, and electrolytes.

I. History (from others): Onset, recent complaints, injuries, medical and psychiatric history, access to drugs

II. General physical exam: Vital signs, airway, trauma (exclude C-spine injury in cases of head trauma), infection, systemic illness, needle marks, odor on breath, nuchal rigidity, tympanic membranes, fundi (papilledema, vitreous hemorrhage, emboli)

III. Neurological exam:
   A. Level of consciousness: Clouding, delirium, stupor, coma, vegetative, locked-in, psychogenic unresponsiveness
   B. Brainstem function
      1. Pupils: Miosis, mydriasis, anisocoria, afferent defect (see Pupil)
      2. Eye movements: Spontaneous, conjugate horizontal deviations, vertical deviations, disconjugate deviation, oculocephalic reflex after C-spine injury excluded, calorics (see Calorics)
      3. Corneal reflex, lids
      4. Respiration: Cheyne-Stokes, central neurogenic hyperventilation (rare), tachypnea (common), apneustic, ataxic, sleep apnea (see Respiration)
   C. Motor
      1. Tone: Paratonia, extrapyramidal rigidity, spasticity, clonus, flaccidity
      2. Response to noxious stimuli: Localizes, flexion withdrawal, abnormal flexion (slow, stereotyped flexion of arm, wrist, and fingers with adduction of shoulder), abnormal extension (extension and pronation of the arm with adduction and internal rotation of shoulder; extension and internal rotation of leg with plantar flexion of foot), or no response (note any laterality)
      3. Spontaneous motor activity: Tremor, asterixis, multifocal myoclonus, seizures
   D. Reflexes: Hyperreflexia, areflexia

E. Glasgow coma scale is an attempt to quantitate level of consciousness. It is easy and reliable, with relatively low interobserver variation, but does not represent a complete exam (e.g., brainstem reflexes are not included).

GLASGOW COMA SCALE

EYE OPENING	Open	Spontaneously	4
		To verbal command	3
		To pain	2
	No response		1
BEST MOTOR RESPONSE	To verbal command	Obeys	6
	To painful stimulus	Localizes pain	5
		Flexion withdrawal	4
		Flexion-abnormal (decorticate)	3
		Extension-abnormal (decerebrate)	2
		No response	1
BEST VERBAL RESPONSE		Oriented and converses	5
		Disoriented and converses	4
		Verbalizes	3
		Vocalizes	2
		No response	1

Total (range: 3 to 15)

IV. Laboratory evaluation:
The following studies should be obtained immediately: blood glucose, Na, K, Cl, CO_2, BUN, creatinine, Ca, PO4, liver enzymes, PT, PTT, osmolality, and CBC; arterial blood gases (including notation of color and CO); CSF color, cell count, glucose, protein, and gram stain in the absence of a mass lesion; EKG. Although obtained at the same time as the above studies, the following may require a longer time to process: toxicology screen on blood, urine and gastric contents; T_4; cortisol; blood, urine, and other pertinent cultures; viral and fungal titers; spinal fluid cultures and cryptococcal antigen.

CT of the head should be obtained immediately (prior to skull films) in cases of suspected mass lesions; if acute meningitis is also suspected, treat with antibiotics (see Meningitis). EEG may be useful in differentiating certain types of coma, psychogenic unresponsiveness, and status epilepticus, and in prognostication.

V. Emergency Management:
  A. Oxygenation is assured by clearing airway, suctioning, ventilating with bag, and intubating as needed. Always be prepared for early intubation. Exclude cervical injury before extending neck. Atropine 1 mg IV may prevent cardiac arrest during intubation.
  B. Circulation is maintained with fluids and pressors to keep mean arterial pressure to 100 mm Hg. Continuously monitor EKG.
  C. Glucose 25 gm (50 cc D50%) is given with thiamine 100 mg IV immediately after blood is drawn.
  D. Intracranial hypertension is treated (see Intracranial Pressure)
  E. Exclude subdural or epidural hematomas by CT
  F. Stop seizures (see Epilepsy)
  G. Treat infection (see Meningitis)
  H. Restore acid base balance
  I. Normalize body temperature
  J. Treat drug overdose. For suspected narcotic overdose, give naloxone (Narcan) 0.4 mg IV, may repeat in 5 minutes. For suspected anticholinergic (e.g, tricyclic) overdose, give physostigmine 1 mg IV.
  K. Agitation should be controlled by reassurance if possible. Sedative drugs should be avoided. If sedation is necessary, as for CT, a rapid acting, short duration, reversible agent should be used, e.g, fentanyl 0.05-0.1 mg IV or morphine 2-10 mg IV. Respiratory status must be carefully monitored. More sustained sedation may be obtained with diazepam 5-10 mg IV or haloperidol 2-5 mg IM.
  L. Specific therapy for other causes is instituted as soon as a diagnosis can be established.

VI. Causes of Coma:
  A. Supratentorial
    1. Subcortical destructive lesion: thalamic infarct

    2. Hemorrhage: epidural, subdural, subarachnoid, intracerebral; hypertensive, vascular malformation, pituitary apoplexy

    3. Infarction: thrombotic or embolic arterial occlusion, venous thrombosis

    4. Tumor: primary, metastatic

    5. Abscess: intracerebral, subdural

    6. Closed head injury

B. Infratentorial

    1. Compressive: cerebellar hemorrhage, infarct, tumor, or abscess; posterior fossa subdural or extradural hemorrhages, basilar aneurysm

    2. Destructive: brainstem, infarction or demyelination, basilar migraine

C. Diffuse brain dysfunction

    1. Intrinsic: encephalitis, encephalomyelitis, subarachnoid hemorrhage, concussion, ictal or postictal state, meningitis, herniation

    2. Hypoxic, metabolic: anoxia/ischemia, nutritional (e.g., Wernicke's), hepatic encephalopathy, uremia, dialysis, pulmonary disease

    3. Endocrine: nonketotic hyperglycemic hyperosmolar coma, ketoacidosis, lactic acidosis, CNS acidosis, cerebral edema $2°$ to treatment, DIC, hypophosphatemia, hypoglycemia, Addison's disease, myxedema, thyrotoxicosis, panhypopituitarism

    4. Drug induced, toxic: (e.g., amphetamines, cocaine, psychodelics, tricylics, phenothiazines, lithium, benzodiazepines, methaqualone, glutethimide, barbiturates, alcohol, opiates).

    5. Ionic and acid base disorders: hypo/hyperosmolarity, hypo/hypernatremia, hypo/hypercalcemia.

    6. Hypo/hyperthermia.

    7. Remote effects of cancer: limbic encephalitis, thalamic degeneration, progressive multifocal leukoencephalopathy.

D. Psychogenic coma: conversion reaction, catatonic stupor, malingering

VII. Related disorders

A. Vegetative state (or coma vigil): Subacute or chronic condition after severe brain injury characterized by wakefulness, sleep-wake cycles, and eye opening to verbal stimuli, without cognitive function or localizing motor responses. Blood pressure and respirations are

maintained. Can follow coma and persist for years. May occur with forebrain occipital, hippocampal, or diffuse cerebral/cerebellar destruction.
B. Akinetic mutism: Subacute or chronic condition characterized by intact wake/sleep cycle, seeming alertness, or excessive somnolence, with little evidence of motor system damage, yet minimal vocalization or movement even with noxious stimuli. May occur with cingulate, limbic, corpus striatum, globus pallidus, thalamic, or reticular formation damage.
C. Locked-in syndrome: Intact consciousness plus quadriplegia and lower cranial nerve dysfunction. Usually occurs with ventral pontine infarcts, tumors, hemorrhages, and myelinolysis; ventral midbrain infarction; head injury; or severe neuromuscular disease.

VIII. Clinical findings in the differential diagnosis of coma.
A. Supratentorial mass with diencephalic or brain-stem compression
  1. Early focal cerebral dysfunction
  2. Rostral to caudal progression with signs referrable to one area at a given time
  3. Asymmetric motor signs
  4. Third nerve palsy precedes coma (early herniation)
B. Infratentorial mass or destruction
  1. Early brainstem dysfunction or sudden onset of coma with accompanying brainstem signs
  2. Vestibulo-ocular abnormalities present
  3. Cranial nerve palsies usually present
  4. Abnormal respirations common, appear early
C. Metabolic causes
  1. Confusion and stupor precede motor signs
  2. Motor signs symmetrical
  3. Pupillary reactions usually preserved (except with certain drugs and toxins, see Pupil)
  4. Asterixis, myoclonus, tremor, seizures common
  5. Acid base disturbance with hyper/hypo-ventilation common
D. Psychogenic unresponsiveness (pseudo-coma)
  1. Lids tightly closed
  2. Pupils reactive or dilated (factitious mydriatics)
  3. Oculocephalic responses highly variable, nystagmus present with caloric (and arousal may occur)
  4. Motor tone normal or inconsistent

5. Breathing normal or rapid
6. Reflexes nonpathologic
7. Normal EEG

IX. Prognosis (see Brain Death, Cardiopulmonary Arrest)

Ref: Plum F, Posner JB. The Diagnosis of Stupor and
        Coma, 3rd ed. Philadelphia: F.A. Davis, 1982.

COMPUTED TOMOGRAPHY

CT or Hounsfield numbers are relative attenuation or
absorption coefficients of tissues as calculated by the CT
scanner (see page 77). They range from -1000 for air to
+1000 for dense bone, with water set at 0. Normal brain
tissue covers a range of approximately 50 CT numbers.

Window width (WW) determines the range of CT numbers
which are displayed as shades of gray (there are
altogether 2000). Large window settings (>400), used
for the evaluation of bony structures, diminish contrast
between tissues. Smaller WW settings increase contrast.
Brain tissue is usually evaluated at WW 200 (high
resolution scanners).

Window level (WL) determines the center of the WW. If
the WW is 200 and the WL 50, the gray shades displayed on
the image range from -50 to +150 CT numbers. When the WW
is adjusted to its narrowest setting (= Measure) the image
can only consist of black and white dots. By adjusting
the WL until a structure in question begins to fill in
with white dots an actual measurement of its absorption
coefficient can be made.

Contrast enhancement is seen in normal vascular
structures such as large intracranial arteries, venous
sinuses, choroid plexus, tentorium, and falx. The
following also tend to enhance with contrast: meningiomas,
pituitary adenomas, chordomas, medulloblastomas,
lymphomas, sarcomas, metastases, optic nerve gliomas,
acoustic neurinomas, infarcts (from day 1 to several
months, typically after 3-4 days), and abscess capsules
(ring shaped enhancement also occurs in glioblastomas,
metastases, dermoid cysts, and other lesions). Little or
no enhancement is usually seen in normal brain tissue,
oligodendrogliomas, astrocytomas, ependymomas, fresh
infarcts, or edema. Variable degrees of enhancement may
be seen in glioblastomas, craniopharyngiomas, basilar
meningitis, encephalitis, and metastases.

Vascular anatomy of the brain in coronal CT sections
is depicted on page 78.

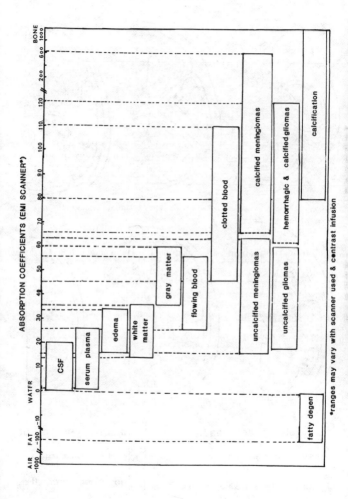

ABSORPTION COEFFICIENTS (EMI SCANNER*)

*ranges may vary with scanner used & contrast infusion

CSF · serum plasma · edema · white matter · gray matter · flowing blood · clotted blood · uncalcified meningiomas · calcified meningiomas · uncalcified gliomas · hemorrhagic & calcified gliomas · calcification · fatty degen

AIR FAT WATER BONE

VASCULAR DISTRIBUTIONS OF THE BRAIN
IN HORIZONTAL SECTIONS

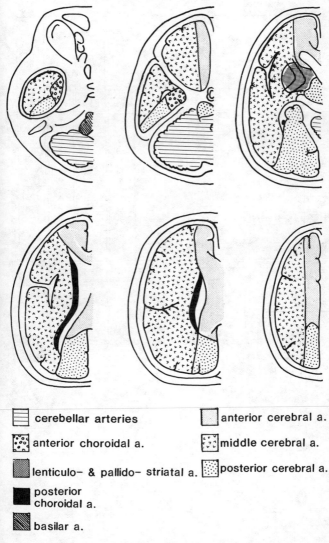

☰ cerebellar arteries	anterior cerebral a.
anterior choroidal a.	middle cerebral a.
lenticulo- & pallido- striatal a.	posterior cerebral a.
posterior choroidal a.	
basilar a.	

CONUS MEDULLARIS (see Cauda Equina/Conus Medullaris)

CORD (see Spinal Cord)

CORTEX (see Cerebral Cortex)

CRAMPS

I. Myopathic disorders
   A. Contractures are associated with glycogenoses
   (phosphorylase and phosphofructokinase deficiency) and carnitine palmityltransferase (CPT)
   deficiency. There is severe, intermittent, sharp
   muscle pain with palpable shortening and
   hardening of the affected muscles which may be
   precipitated by exercise (glycogenoses and CPT
   deficiency) or fasting (CPT deficiency). Cramps
   are associated with increased weakness and
   unaffected by curare or nerve block. They are
   due to a defect in uptake of calcium by sarcoplasmic reticulum. On EMG there is electrical
   silence during contractures. Treatment includes
   a high carbohydrate diet in phosphorylase
   deficiency; a high carbohydrate, low fat diet in
   CPT deficiency.
   B. Myotonia (see Myotonia)

II. Neurogenic disorders
   A. Tetany may result from hypocalcemia and
   alkalosis. Hypomagnesemia and hyperkalemia may
   cause carpopedal spasm. Severe tonic spasms are
   usually not painful but may be during a prolonged
   attack. They may be provoked by hyperventilation
   or nerve compression. There is a lowered
   depolarization threshold of motor nerve fibers.
   EMG reveals asynchronous grouped motor unit
   potentials discharging at a rate of 5-15/second
   separated by periods of electrical silence. Treat
   the primary cause.
   B. Myokymia with delayed relaxation (continuous
   muscle fiber activity)
   C. Motor neuron disease and denervation of muscle
   may be associated with cramp-like pain.

III. Central disorders
   A. Stiffman syndrome is a slowly progressive
   disorder characterized by axial greater than
   limb, continuous tonic contractures with normal
   strength. Associated painful spasms may be

initiated by voluntary movements, noise or other sensory stimuli. It is blocked with curare, general anesthesia, nerve block, and during sleep. The pathogenesis is unknown. EMG shows continuous activity in agonist and antagonist muscle groups wth normal motor unit morphology. Diazepam or baclofen may be helpful.

B. <u>Tetanus</u> is characterized by acute, usually rapidly progressive, generalized continuous tonic contractures wth superimposed painful spasms. Tonic spasms of the masticatory muscles (trismus and lockjaw) are common. They are due to loss of inhibitory postsynaptic potentials in spinal cord and are stopped with curare and during sleep. The EMG is as in the stiffman syndrome. Treatment includes tetanus antitoxin, diazepam, chlorpromazine, phenobarbital, and curare with mechanical ventilation.

IV. <u>Physiologic cramps in absence of pathology</u>: Painful muscle contractions may occur in normal subjects, usually at rest or after extreme exercise. They more commonly affect the lower extremities and are best treated with passive stretching of the muscle.

Ref: Layzer RB, Rowland LP. NEJM 285:31, 1971.

CRANIOCERVICAL JUNCTION

<u>Platybasia</u> refers to flattening of the base of the skull. The angle between the plane of the clivus and the plane of the anterior fossa is greater than 135°, or the basilar angle (nasion to tuberculum sellae to anterior lip of foramen magnum) is greater than 140°. It may be developmental or acquired (rickets, osteomalacia, Paget's). Spinal cord or medullary compression may cause progressive spastic quadriparesis and lower cranial nerve and cerebellar signs.

<u>Basilar impression (invagination)</u> refers to an upward protrusion of the odontoid peg into the foramen magnum. It may be associated with tonsillar herniation, syringomyelia, high arched palate, polysyndactyly, pes cavus, iris heterochromia, Sprengel's deformity, scoliosis, torticollis, or skull deformities. Clinical presentation may be asymptomatic or include hydrocephalus, headache, neckache, extremity weakness, paraesthesia, diplopia, facial pain, dysphagia, hearing loss, drop attacks, amaurosis fugax, short neck, facial asymmetry, nystagmus, palsy of cranial nerves X through XII, spastic paraparesis or cerebellar dysfunction.

On skull films, the odontoid tip extends >5mm above Chamberlains line, >7mm above McGregors line, and the A-P diameter of the foramen magnum is <19mm. Magnetic resonance imaging may be helpful.

Platybasia is seen in Down's syndrome, achondroplasia, mucopolysaccharidoses, Arnold-Chiari malformation, cleido-cranial dysplasia, osteogenesis imperfecta, or secondary to osteomalacia, Pagets (most common), fibrous dysplasia, rickets, low T_4, hypoparathyroidism, neoplasia, infection, or trauma.

The differential diagnosis of platybasia and basilar invagination includes foramen magnum, brainstem or cerebellar tumors, MS, cervical dislocation, degenerative joint disease of the spine, spinocerebellar degeneration, myelitis, ALS, and bulbar and pseudobulbar palsy.

Treatment for progressive disease consists of decompressive suboccipital craniectomy and cervical laminectomy. Basilar invagination may also be treated by removal of the odontoid with cervical fusion.

<u>Atlanto-axial subluxation</u> results in acute or chronic cord compression. It may be congenital, traumatic or secondary to rheumatoid arthritis.

<u>Arnold-Chiari malformation</u> is a congenital anomaly of the hindbrain with caudal displacement of the pons, medulla and cerebellar vermis.

Type I: Cerebellum is displaced into spinal canal, medulla is elongated, and myelomeningocele is rare. Hydrocephalus and syringomyelia may develop. Symptoms usually develop in the teens or young adulthood with headaches, neck pain, ataxia, dysphagia, dysarthria, diplopia, spasticity, papilledema, absent gag, downbeat and periodic alternating nystagmus, and/or dorsal column signs. Metrizamide myelography demonstrates cerebellar tonsillar herniation, cord compression, and associated syrinx. Cord atrophy is end stage. Angiography may demonstrate descent of the posterior inferior cerebellar artery. Magnetic resonance imaging may become the diagnostic procedure of choice.

Type II: Medulla and cerebellum are displaced inferiorly and deformed. An elongated medulla overlies the cervical cord, which may be small with upward directed cervical roots. Myelomeningocele is invariably present.

Hydrocephalus is most common presentation, usually in early childhood and is probably secondary to aqueductal stenosis or medullary obstruction. Polymicrogyria, heterotopias, syringomyelia, and hydromyelia are frequently associated. Recurrent apnea, stridor, or vocal cord paralysis may occur with activity and may become suddenly permanent. Medullary hemorrhage or infarction can cause abnormal respiratory drive. Degeneration of lower cranial nerve nuclei, and hypotonia or spasticity may occur. Skull films show cranial enlargement. A small posterior fossa is evident by low tentorial insertion and dural sinuses. Enlargement of foramen magnum, elongation of cervical arches, platybasia, basilar impression, assimilation of the atlas, and Klippel-Feil anomaly may be seen. Metrizamide myelography shows cerebellar displacement or hydromyelia. CT scan shows hydrocephalus, mesencephalic beaking, upward trans-incisural extension, and cerebellum wrapped around the brainstem.

Type III: Includes cervical spina bifida, cerebellar herniation through the defect and an open, dystrophic posterior fossa. Rarely compatible with postnatal life.

Type IV: Cerebellar hypoplasia. May be related to or equivalent to Dandy-Walker formation.

Chronic tonsillar herniation: Includes children and adults with chronic (sclerotic) herniation, in the absence of other hindbrain abnormalities. Bony deformities and syringomyelia may be present. Presentation includes dizziness, ataxia, diplopia, dysphagia, nystagmus, hearing loss, weakness, quadriparesis, dysesthesias, neck and arm pain, or sudden death.

Treatment of Arnold-Chiari malformations include shunting hydrocephalus, if present, posterior fossa decompression, and high cervical laminectomy. Deterioration may occur after intubation.

Ref: Gardner E, et al. The Dandy-Walker and Arnold-Chiari malformations. Arch Neurol 32:393, 1975.

Friede RL, Roessmann U. Chronic tonsillar herniation. Acta Neuropath 34:219, 1976.

CRANIOSYNOSTOSIS

Premature closure of one or more cranial sutures. Normal skull growth occurs perpendicular to suture lines. Primary, premature closure results in growth parallel to sutures producing characteristic cranial and/or facial deformities:

Suture Closed	Skull Deformity
Sagittal	Scaphocehaly (boathead)
Coronal	Brachycephaly (short head)
Single coronal or lambdoidal	Plagiocephaly (oblique head)
Metopic	Trigonocephaly (triangle head)
Coronal and Sagittal and/or Lambdoidal	Oxycephaly (pointed head)

Primary failure of brain development may result in secondary craniosynostosis (microcephaly, after shunting for hydrocephalus). Craniosynostosis is usually isolated, but may occur with associated anomalies as part of sporadic or genetic syndromes (Crouzon's, Apert's, Carpenter's, Chostzen's). It may result from disorders with bone marrow hyperplasia, abnormal calcium or phosphorus metabolism, and hyperthyroidism.

Surgical correction as early as possible is indicated in appropriate cases to prevent mental retardation (prevent increased intracranial pressure and allow normal brain growth), to improve appearance, and prevent visual or hearing deficits due to orbital or facial malformations.

Ref: Graham JM. Ped Ann 10:27, 1982.

CT (see Computed Tomography)

DEGENERATIVE DISEASES OF CHILDHOOD

A partial listing of degenerative syndromes presenting in childhood follows on pages 84-86.

DELIRIUM

A state of clouded consciousness with inattention, sensory misperception, disordered stream of thought, and disturbances of psychomotor activity. The onset is generally rapid and the total duration brief. Synonymous terms include "acute brain syndrome" and "acute confusional state". Most delirious patients are also agitated. Causes of delirium are many and include CNS infections, toxic and metabolic disorders, electrolyte imbalances, hepatic and renal disease, thiamine deficiency, and anoxic encephalopathy.

WHITE MATTER SYNDROMES

Disease	Age	Clinical Presentation	Pathology
Sudanophilic cerebral sclerosis	5-8 yrs	X-linked, gradual gait disturbance, intellectual decline, seizures, dysphagia, visual changes, adrenal insufficiency	Symmetrical demyelination of periventricular white matter, spares subcortical areas
Pelizaeus Merzbacher disease	Infant	__Type 1__ X-linked recessive, trembling, abnormal roving eye, movements cerebellar ataxia	Demyelination with spared myelinated "islands", oligodendrocytes have spherical lamellated inclusions
	Child	__Type 2__ Dominant inheritance, cerebellar ataxia, intention tremor, scanning speech	Same as above
Spongy white matter degeneration (Canavan's)	2-4 months	Hypotonia, optic atrophy, developmental delay, seizures, chorea, macrocephaly	Demyelination of white matter around convolutional areas, with spongy-appearing cyst formation

Disease	Age	Clinical Presentation	Pathology
Alexander's (hyaline degeneration)	Less than 1 year	Seizures, spasticity, macrocephaly, developmental delay	Leukodystrophy with eosino-philic material deposited on pial and perivascular surfaces
Metachromatic leuko-dystrophy (late infantile)	Less than 2 years	Strabismus, increased spasticity, hyporeflexia, intellectual deterioration, optic atrophy	Decreased urinary aryl-sulfatase A, diffuse demyeli-nation with metachromatically staining granules in brain, gall-bladder, kidneys, peripheral nerves, islet cells of pancreas, reticular zone of adrenal cortex, and liver
Metachromatic leukodys-trophy (juvenile)	5-7 years	Ataxia, spasticity, hyporeflexia	
Krabbe's disease (globoid cell)	4-6 months	Restlessness, progressive spasticity, infantile spasms, optic atrophy, hyporeflexia, peripheral neuropathy	Demyelination with mononuclear epithelioid cells and multinucleated globoid cells around blood vessels in the brain, cerebrosidase deficiency
Alper's disease	6 years	Intellectual decline, spasticity, opisthotonus	Decreased cerebral gray matter

Disease	Age	Clinical Presentation	Pathology
Cockayne's Syndrome	2 years	Autosomal recessive, growth failure, intellectual degeneration, hypersensitivity of skin to sunlight	Perivascular calcification in basal ganglia and cerebellum, patchy degeneration
Chediak-Higashi		Albinism, cranial neuropathies, progressive spinocerebellar degeneration, mental retardation, hepatomegaly	Intracytoplasmic inclusions in neurons and polymorphonuclear leukocytes
Infantile neuroaxonal dystrophy	2 years	Weakness, hypotonia, corticospinal tract dysfunction, urinary retention, seizures	Axonal swelling

Ref: Menkes   JH.   Textbook   of   Child   Neurology.
       Philadelphia: Lea and Febiger, 1980; 132-147.

DEMENTIA (see also Mental Status Testing)

A clinical state characterized by impairment of learning and memory, loss of cognitive and intellectual abilities, and disorientation. The diagnosis is made by mental status testing. The most common cause is Alzheimer's disease. Treatable causes must be excluded by appropriate studies. Such causes include infections (bacterial, fungal, luetic, tuberculous), deficiency disorders (B_{12}, thiamine), metabolic disorders (hypoglycemia), hepatic failure, uremia, Wilson's disease, endocrine disorders (myxedema, parathyroid abnormalities,

Cushing's syndrome), brain tumors, subdural hematomas, toxins and drugs, and hydrocephalus. Depression often presents as a so-called "pseudodementia".

Presently untreatable causes of dementia include Alzheimer's disease, Pick's disease, Huntington's chorea (see Choreoathetosis), progressive supranuclear palsy, spinocerebellar degeneration, Creutzfeldt-Jacob disease, multiple infarctions, Binswanger's disease, postanoxic and post-traumatic encephalopathy, demyelinating disorders, and dialysis dementia.

The laboratory evaluation of dementia should include CBC, SMA-20, FTA, vitamin B_{12} and folate, thyroid function studies, EEG, CT scan of the head, and, often, lumbar puncture.

DEMYELINATING DISEASE (see also Neuropathy)

These central disorders involve destruction of normally formed myelin and oligodendroglia in contrast to the dysmyelinating diseases (i.e., leukodystrophies) in which myelin is abnormally formed. Multiple sclerosis is the most common(see Multiple Sclerosis).

Classification of Demyelinating Diseases

I. Primary diseases of myelin
   A. Multiple sclerosis (MS)
   B. Devic's disease is a variant of MS consisting of optic neuritis and transverse myelitis.
   C. Schilder's disease is a rapidly progressive sporadic disease resulting in bilateral massive hemispheric demyelination seen mainly in children and adolescents.
   D. Balo's sclerosis is also a possible variant of MS resulting in acute demyelination in a concentric pattern.

II. Postinfectious encephalomyelitis refers to a rapid demyelination occurring shortly after measles, vaccinia, varicella, rubella, or other viral illnesses or after immunizations. Two forms are described: 1) acute disseminated encephalomyelitis; 2) acute necrotizing hemorrhagic leukoencephalitis. Improved vaccines have helped reduce the incidence of these disorders. Although controversial, steroids may be of benefit.

III. Nutritional (see Alcohol)
   1. Central pontine myelinolysis
   2. Marchiafava-Bignami syndrome

IV. Infectious
 1. Progressive multifocal leukoencephalopathy (PML)
 2. Subacute sclerosing panencephalitis (SSPE)

 V. Inherited CNS degenerative disorders
 1. Familial spastic paraplegia
 2. Hereditary ataxias
 3. Leber's disease

VI. Toxic/Metabolic
 1. Carbon monoxide
 2. Anoxia
 3. Radiation
 4. Methotrexate, especially with radiation

Ref: Pasternak JF, et al. Neurology 30:481, 1980.

DERMATOMES

Cutaneous sensory distribution of spinal roots are depicted on pages 89 (anterior view) and 90 (posterior view).
Cutaneous sensory distribution of peripheral nerves are depicted on pages 91 (anterior view) and 92 (posterior view).

CUTANEOUS SENSORY DISTRIBUTION
OF SPINAL ROOTS (ANTERIOR)

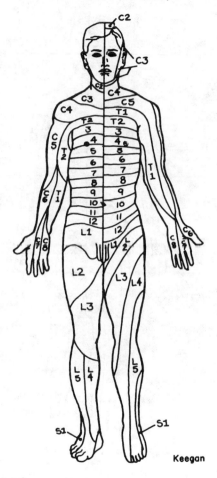

Keegan

Projections of Foerster and Keegan are contrasted.

From: Kopell HP, Thompson WAL. Peripheral Entrapment
Neuropathies. Huntington, NY: Robert E Krieger, 1976, p 8.

CUTANEOUS SENSORY DISTRIBUTION
OF SPINAL ROOTS (POSTERIOR)

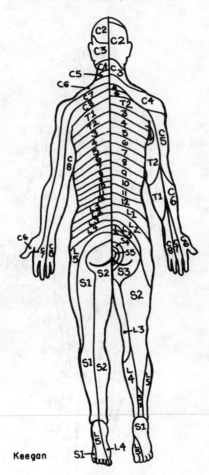

Keegan

Projections of Foerster and Keegan are contrasted.

From: Kopell HP, Thompson WAL. Peripheral Entrapment
Neuropathies. Huntington, NY: Robert E Krieger, 1976, p 8.

CUTANEOUS SENSORY DISTRIBUTION OF PERIPHERAL NERVES (ANTERIOR)

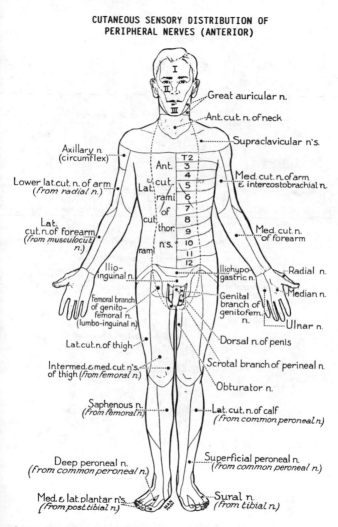

From: Haymaker W, Woodhall B. Peripheral Nerve Injuries: Principles of Diagnosis. Philadelphia: WB Saunders, 1953, p 43.

CUTANEOUS SENSORY DISTRIBUTION
OF PERIPHERAL NERVES (POSTERIOR)

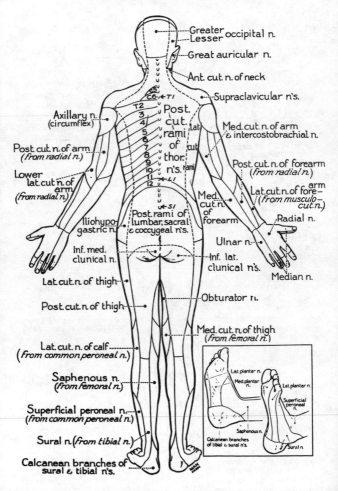

From: Haymaker W, Woodhall B. Peripheral Nerve Injuries: Principles of Diagnosis. Philadelphia: WB Saunders, 1953, p 40.

<u>DEVELOPMENTAL MALFORMATIONS</u> (see also Craniocervical
Junction)

I. Defective closure of neural groove (dysraphism)
   A. Spinal cord:
      1. Spina bifida aperta (myeloaraphia) - exposed
         neural tube without overlying leptomeninges,
         vertebral arch, or dermis.
      2. Spinal meningocele - meninges protrudes
         through defect in vertebral arch.
      3. Myelomeningocele - meninges and spinal cord
         protrude through defect in neural arch. May
         be associated with overlying dermal defects or
         Arnold-Chiari malformation. In addition to
         neurological deficit, may have hydrocephalus,
         meningitis, and recurrent urinary tract
         infections.
      4. Congenital dural sinus - communication between
         meninges and dermis via incompletely closed
         vertebral arch.
      5. Spina bifida occulta - closure defect of
         vertebral arch only, usually L5,S1. Commonly
         diagnosed radiographically. No clinical
         symptoms. May have overlying tuft of hair,
         discoloration, dimple, or dermal sinus.
      6. Diastematomyelia - septum protrudes through
         cord in anterior-posterior direction.
   B. Brain:
      1. Anencephaly - absence of cranial vault and its
         contents. Incompatible with life.
      2. Cranial meningocele - meninges protrudes
         through defect in skull.
      3. Meningoencephalocele - meninges and brain
         parenchyma protrudes through defect in skull.

II. Defective segmentation, cleavage, proliferation, and
    migration
   A. Brain (most common):
      1. Holoprosencephaly - failure of segmentation
         and cleavage of embryonic forebrain into
         paired cerebral hemispheres resulting in
         absence of interhemispheric fissure, large
         single ventricle, and marked absence of
         cerebral parenchyma.
      2. Arhinencephaly - absence of olfactory bulb and
         tracts.
      3. Porencephaly - cavitation due to focal
         agenesis of cerebrum resulting in communi-
         cation between lateral ventricle and convexity
         lined with ependyma or malformed grey matter.

4. Schizencephaly - bilateral porencephaly.
5. Hydranencephaly - cavitation due to a focal destructive process which may communicate with the lateral ventricle and is not lined with ependyma.
6. Hydrocephalus - enlarged ventricles lined with ependyma.
7. Lissencephaly (agyria) - absence of gyri.
8. Pachygyria - abnormally wide and thick gyri with abnormal lamination.
9. Heterotopias - ectopic collections of grey matter.
10. Microgyria, polymicrogyria - areas of small gyri, usually markedly increased in number, with abnormal lamination.
11. Agenesis of various structures such as septum pellucidum, corpus callosum, or cerebral hemispheres.
12. Persistence of fetal structures such as cavum septum pellucidum.

DEVELOPMENTAL MILESTONES (see Child Neurology)

DIABETES INSIPIDUS (see Sodium)

DIABETES MELLITUS (see Glucose, Neuropathy)

DIALYSIS (see also Uremia)

Subdural hematoma occasionally occurs following dialysis and is thought to result from osmotic shifts and complications of heparinization.

Dysequilibrium syndrome results from fluid and electrolyte shifts in the extracellular fluid, resulting in seizures or transient encephalopathy.

Dialysis dementia is a progressive, fatal disorder characterized by myoclonus, dysarthria, aphasia, and memory disturbance. It occurs in geographic clusters and is attributed to the concentration of aluminum and, possibly, tin in the dialysate and oral phosphate binders. There have been a few reports of remission of the condition with dialysis against a low aluminum dialysate. The development of seizures is a bad prognostic sign. Sometimes, dialysis dementia is accompanied by vitamin-D resistant osteomalacia, proximal muscle weakness, and normochromic normocytic anemia. EEG may show slowing with bursts of high frequency waves in the frontal regions. Renal patients are also prone to infections, electrolyte abnormalities, and drug intoxication; these should be excluded before the diagnosis of dialysis dementia is made.

DIC (DISSEMINATED INTRAVASCULAR COAGULATION)

A disorder of blood coagulation resulting in excessive bleeding or clotting. Causes include amniotic fluid embolism, snake bites, tumors, burns, infections, heat stroke, organ grafts, extra-corporeal circulation, transfusion reactions, and microangiopathic hemolytic anemia. Clinical findings include petechiae and ecchymoses. Lab evaluation reveals thrombocytopenia, schistocytes on smear, prolonged PT and PTT, decreased fibrinogen, and the presence of fibrin split products.

Neurological complications include arterial occlusion causing infarction, intraparenchymal and subarachnoid hemorrhage, and obtundation and coma (may be secondary to metabolic derangement).

About 10% of nonbacterial thrombotic endocarditis (NBTE) is associated with DIC. One third will have emboli and infarction (50% hemorrhagic). NBTE is associated with malignancy, most commonly adenocarcinoma, leukemia, and lymphoma. NBTE is also associated with rheumatic, atherosclerotic and congenital heart disease, cardiomyopathy, hepatitis, cirrhosis, colitis, COPD, pulmonary fibrosis, glomerulonephritis, organ transplantation, polyarteritis, rheumatoid arthritis, barbiturate overdose, diabetes, burns, and thrombotic thrombocytopenic purpura.

DIPLOPIA (see Eye Muscles, Ophthalmoplegia)

DISC DISEASE (see Radiculopathy, Spinal Cord)

DIZZINESS (see also Syncope, Vertigo)

Nonspecific term commonly used to describe a variety of subjective experiences. Elicit an accurate description of what the patient means and place the complaint into one of the following four categories:

1. The sensation of impending faint or loss of consciousness (syncope or presyncope). Etiologies include cardiac dysrhythmia, postural hypotension (diabetic autonomic neuropathy; side effect of antihypertensive, diuretic, dopaminergic, and other drugs), anemia, Addison's disease (see Syncope).
2. Dysequilibrium or loss of balance without various subjective movement sensations of head. May occur with cerebellar or proprioceptive disturbances or muscle weakness.
3. Dizziness due to causes other than 1 and 2 above and other than true vertigo may be described as lightheadedness, floating, wooziness, faintness, or some other sense of altered consciousness. Etiologies include:

A. Hyperventilation syndrome. One of the most common causes of dizziness or lightheadedness. Circumoral and digital paresthesias are frequently associated. Symptoms may be reproduced during hyperventilation. Occasionally, a patient will experience positional vertigo with hyperventilation (see Vertigo).

B. Multiple sensory deficits. Two or more of the following are usually present: visual impairment (often due to cataracts), neuropathy, vestibular dysfunction (see also Vertigo), cervical spondylosis, or orthopedic disorders interfering with ambulation. Patients may complain of lightheadedness when walking and turning. Holding the examiner's finger lightly may provide enough additional sensory input to relieve the symptoms. Patients are often elderly and/or diabetic.

C. Psychogenic dizziness (not associated with hyperventilation). Patients complain of vague lightheadedness, mental fuzziness, or difficulty thinking. They may be depressed or anxious. Dizziness is usually continuous rather than episodic. Patients may state that all or none of the maneuvers done during physical examination produce dizziness.

D. Severe anemia or polycythemia may cause symptoms of lightheadedness or dizziness.

E. Drugs may produce symptoms of dizziness that are not necessarily related to orthostatic changes in blood pressure or presyncope. These include: antiarrhythmics, anticonvulsants, antidepressants, antihistamines, antihypertensives, anti-Parkinsonian agents, hypnotics, hypoglycemics, phenothiazines, alcohol, and tobacco.

F. Endocrinologic disorders (hypoglycemia, Addison's disease, hypopituitarism, insulinoma).

G. Carotid sinus hypersensitivity.

4. Vertigo (see Vertigo)

Treatment of dizziness due to disorders in categories 1, 2, and 3 will depend on the underlying cause. For evaluation and management of dizziness and vertigo, see Vertigo.

DOLL'S HEAD MANEUVER (see Vestibulo-ocular Reflex)

DYSARTHRIA (see also Bulbar Palsy, Pseudobulbar Palsy)

A disorder of speech produced by disturbances of the muscles of articulation. Six patterns of dysfunction have been distinguished: flaccid, spastic, ataxic, hypokinetic, hyperkinetic, and mixed. Although each has differing sound characteristics to the trained ear, most clinicians rely on associated neurological signs such as extremity ataxia; involvement of cranial nerves VII, IX, X, or XII; or brisk jaw jerk or gag reflex to distinguish the speech patterns (ataxic, flaccid, and spastic, respectively).

Ref: Teppermann PS, Thacker RC.   Postgrad Med 68:86, 1980.

DYSKINESIA

A general term for abnormal involuntary movements. For descriptions of specific movement disorders, see: Asterixis, Athetosis, Chorea, Choreoathetosis, Dystonia, Myoclonus, Neuroleptics, Parkinson's Disease, Progressive Supranuclear Palsy, Rigidity, Tremor. Dyskinesias should be classified into these descriptive categories, although many patients display more than one type of movement (as in tardive dyskinesias, see Neuroleptics). Drugs are a common cause of many of the above movement disorders.

DYSPHAGIA

Difficulty swallowing, often associated with discomfort or pain. Difficulty swallowing liquids greater than solids generally reflects neurological disease, whereas dysphagia for solids greater than liquids suggests physical obstruction. There may be specific history of gagging, choking, or nasal regurgitation of liquids. Voice changes are common. Neurological examination of lower cranial nerves should focus on soft palatal movement and reflexes, phonation (see Dysarthria) and ability to cough and swallow. Careful ENT exam is important to exclude mass lesions and previous oropharyngeal surgery. Barium studies may help identify specific swallowing abnormalities.

Neurological causes of dysphagia include any process affecting the lower brainstem, lower cranial nerves or the muscles they innervate (see also Bulbar Palsy, Pseudobulbar Palsy). These include polymyositis, myotonic dystrophy, oculopharyngeal dystrophy, myasthenia gravis, botulism, local compressive neoplasms, some neuropathies, motor neuron diseases, multiple sclerosis, syringobulbia, brainstem tumors, and certain choreic disorders. Rabies and tetanus may cause pharyngeal muscle spasm resulting in dysphagia.

Therapy is aimed at the underlying cause. Other therapeutic modalities include elevation of the head of the bed, nasogastric feeding (may predispose to gastro-esophogeal reflux and aspiration), feeding gastrostomy (may also predispose to reflux), feeding jejunostomy, physical therapy, dilation procedures, and cricopharyngeal myotomy.

DYSTONIA

Involuntary movements characterized by sustained twisting which may affect different muscle groups in the limbs, trunk, neck, or face. The movements are usually slow, but can be more rapid, so-called dystonic spasms; these spasms may be repetitive. Dystonic movements may build up to an intense, sustained muscular contraction such that the involved body part remains in a fixed posture. Dystonia may be generalized (affecting the entire body), segmental (affecting just one or two limbs or the neck and one limb) or focal (affecting localized muscle groups, as in writer's cramp or oromandibular dystonia). It may be present continuously or may be brought out only by voluntary movements (action dystonia) or specific motor acts such as playing the piano, writing, chewing, or speaking. Dystonia is usually made worse by fatigue and stress, improves with relaxation and sleep, and may occur together with chorea, athetosis, or tremor.

Classification of Dystonias

A. __Hereditary__
   1. __Dystonia musculorum deformans__ (hereditary torsion dystonia, idiopathic torsion dystonia). The recessive form tends to occur in Jews in early childhood and tends to progress over a few years. The dominant form is not limited to ethnic group, begins in late childhood and adolescence, and progresses more slowly. Dystonia may begin with a single limb, but with time, other limbs, the spine, shoulders, and pelvic girdle become involved. The spasms become more frequent until they are continuous and the body is contorted. Other manifestations may include torticollis, gait disturbance, tremor, myoclonic jerks during movement and mild choreoathetosis. Excitement makes the dystonia worse, but sleep improves it.

2. <u>Familial paroxysmal choreoathetosis</u> (periodic dystonia). Paroxysmal attacks of dystonic spasms and choreoathetosis of the limbs and trunk that last minutes to hours. The dystonic form is autosomal recessive, while the choreoathetotic form is autosomal dominant. It occurs in children and young adults. It may be precipitated by startle or sudden movements. Paroxysmal dystonia and choreoathetosis also are seen with perinatal anoxia, basal ganglia disease, multiple sclerosis, hypoparathyroidism, and thyrotoxicosis.

3. <u>Hereditary form associated with Parkinson's disease</u>

B. <u>Idiopathic nonhereditary dystonias</u> are mainly adult onset. The disease tends to remain limited as focal or segmental dystonia and does not usually become generalized.

1. <u>Torticollis</u> consists of involuntary contractions of the sternocleidomastoid, trapezius, and scalenus muscles resulting in a slow turning, twisting head movement. Head flexion (antero-collis), or extension (retrocollis) may also occur. Duration of the contraction is variable. Involved muscles may hypertrophy. Additional muscles may be involved. It may remit after a few months or progress to total disability. It can affect patients of all ages, but is most common during the third to sixth decades. Most cases are idiopathic. It may occur as a result of antipsychotic medication or as part of dystonia musculorum deformans or an extrapyramidal syndrome following encephalitis lethargica. Similar appearing head postures may be seen with eye muscle imbalance, cervical spine disease or posterior fossa mass lesions.

2. <u>Blepharospasm</u> is an involuntary, spasmodic closure of the eyelids, often preceded by increasing frequency and force of blinking. It is usually bilateral. It occurs in the middle or older age range, somewhat more frequently in women. It may increase with sunlight, wind, noise, movement of the head, or stress. The orbicularis oculi spasms may increase in frequency and severity to the point of rendering the patient functionally blind.

3. <u>Blepharospasm plus oromandibular dystonia (Meige syndrome)</u> includes blepharospasm plus a variety of involuntary movements of the lower face, jaw, and neck that may consist of chewing, lip pursing, opening of the mouth, spasmodic deviation of the jaw, and retractions and protrusions of the tongue. It is exacerbated by stress and fatigue.

It may be temporarily relieved by pinching the
neck, talking, or singing. The cause is unknown.
Other forms of dystonia such as torticollis and
arm dystonia may occur. Oromandibular movements
may occur without blepharospasm.

4. <u>Other disorders associated with blepharospasm</u>
include tardive dyskinesia (see Neuroleptics),
Parkinson's disease (especially the postencephalitic form), Huntington's disease, Wilson's
disease, PSP, myotonia, Schwartz-Jampel syndrome,
tetany, tetanus, ocular disorders (conjunctival
and corneal disease, iritis), midbrain infarction
or demyelination, drugs (antihistamines, sympatho-
mimetics, L-dopa), reflex blepharospasm (in
response to bright light, noise, or eating), and
functional disorders.

5. <u>Writer's cramp</u> occurs upon attempting to write;
the muscles of the thumb and fingers go into
spasms or develop a feeling of stiffness or pain.
This may spread into the forearm and shoulder. On
stopping writing, the disturbance disappears. At
all other times, the hand is normal. Similar
disturbances have been reported during other
activities, such as when playing musical
instruments. The problem persists with varying
degrees of severity.

6. <u>Spasmodic dysphonia</u> (spastic dysphonia) consists
of contraction of all the speech muscles when
attempting to speak. The voice is strained and
speaking is a great effort. Shouting is much
easier than quiet speech, and whispering is not a
problem. Swallowing and singing are not affected.
It usually occurs in middle-aged or older
individuals and is usually nonprogressive.

C. <u>Associated with other hereditary syndromes</u>:
Wilson's disease, Huntington's disease, Hallervorden-
Spatz disease, juvenile neuronal ceroid-lipofuscinoses

D. <u>Secondary to acquired neurological disorders or toxins</u>:
Perinatal cerebral injury, infection (especially
encephalitis), postinfectious syndromes, head trauma,
focal cerebrovascular disease, tumor, toxins (carbon
monoxide, carbon disulfide, manganese), drugs (see
Neuroleptics).

<u>Treatment of Dystonia</u>

At least 50% of patients do not gain any benefit
from drug therapy. Benefit is often the result only of
empirical drug trials. Many patients, especially those
with the focal forms, may do better living with a mild

disability than going through multiple drug trials. If therapy is indicated:

Medical: Start with an anticholinergic such as trihexyphenidyl in low doses and gradually build up to the maximum dose that the patient can tolerate (children often tolerate higher doses than adults). Other drugs that have been used include diazepam, clonazepam, carbamazepine, L-dopa preparations, haloperidol, phenothiazines, baclofen (especially for focal dystonias), lithium, and choline. It is worthwhile trying these drugs in sequence, though many patients gain no useful benefit from any of them.

Surgical: For blepharospasm, orbicularis oculi extirpation and section, alcohol injection, or thermolysis of the facial nerve are variably effective, not always permanent and have complications and side effects. Injection of botulinum toxin is also used. Thalamotomy in unilateral dystonia has produced variable results. Spinal cord stimulation has also been used with variable results.

Ref: Fahn S, Eldridge R. Definition of dystonia and classification of the dystonic states. Adv Neurol 14:1, 1976.

Jankovic J, et al. Blinking and blepharospasm: mechanism, diagnosis, and management. JAMA 248:3160, 1982.

Marsden CD, Fahn S (ed). Movement Disorders. London: Butterworth, 1982.

EDEMA (see Computed Tomography, Intracranial Pressure)

EEG (ELECTROENCEPHALOGRAPHY)

I. Normal activity
  A. Alpha: Frequency 8-13 Hz. Location maximal occipitally. Voltage 15-50 μV in adults, 50-60 μV in children age 3-15. Amplitude may be up to 50% higher on right side, up to 30% on the left. Present during wakefulness. Attenuates with eye opening and mental stimulation. Reaches 8 Hz around age 3.
  B. Beta: Frequency 14-35 Hz. Location fronto-central. Voltage up to 35 μV. Accentuated by barbiturates, benzodiazepines, and other drugs. Increased over skull defects. Depressed over focal brain lesions. May be attenuated with contralateral movement or tactile stimulation.

C. <u>Theta</u>: Frequency 4-7 Hz. Location variable. Voltage variable but normally lower than alpha in adults. Normal in waking records of young children and the elderly (depending on frequency and abundancy) and during drowsiness and sleep.

D. <u>Delta</u>: Frequency <4 Hz. Location variable. Voltage variable. Normal during sleep. Abnormal in adult waking record or focally during sleep.

E. <u>Mu</u>: Frequency 7-11 Hz. Location central or centro-parietal. Voltage similar to or lower than alpha rhythm. Does not attenuate with eye opening and may be asymmetrical. Attenuates with contralateral movement or intended movement.

F. <u>Lambda waves</u>: Single sharp transient (wave) with duration of 160-250 ms. Location occipital. Voltage up to 65 µV, often surface positive. Occurs during scanning (saccadic) eye movements. Can be eliminated by staring at blank wall without pattern.

G. <u>Posterior slow waves of youth</u>: Seen most frequently in children 8-14, but may be seen from ages 2-20. Consists of single, random, irregular theta and delta waves of moderate voltage, behaving like alpha.

II. Normal sleep activity

A. <u>POSTS</u>: "<u>P</u>ositive <u>O</u>ccipital <u>S</u>harp <u>T</u>ransients of <u>S</u>leep." May be seen in all ages during light sleep, singly or repetitively.

B. <u>Spindles</u>: Short bursts of 12-14 Hz activity of increasing, then decreasing, amplitude, maximal over the central regions, during Stage II and III of sleep. Spindles may be present at birth and are usually present by 2-3 months of age. May be asynchronous up to age 2 years.

C. <u>Vertex sharp transients</u>: Symmetrical, bilaterally synchronous sharp waves seen over the vertex during Stage I and the onset of Stage II sleep.

D. <u>K-complexes</u>: Seen during sleep spontaneously or with sensory stimuli, consisting of high voltage biphasic vertex slow wave followed by sleep spindles.

E. <u>Hypnogogic hypersynchrony</u>: Seen in children up to age 13-16, consisting of high voltage, bilaterally synchronous and symmetric. Sinusoidal waves and occasional spikes, maximal over the central and frontal regions.

F. <u>Benign epileptiform transients of sleep</u>: Spikes seen in the anterior and midtemporal regions during Stage I and II sleep.

G. **Rhythmic temporal theta:** Sharp notched theta rhythm of approximately 6 Hz seen over the temporal regions during drowsiness. Also called psychomotor variant.

III. Abnormal patterns
   A. **Generalized theta and delta:** Nonspecific change seen with metabolic, toxic, and degenerative encephalopathies.
   B. **Triphasic waves:** Medium to high amplitude bilaterally synchronous waves with a frequency of 1.5-2.5 Hz, often frontally predominant. Most commonly seen with hepatic encephalopathy or renal failure but also seen with other metabolic encephalopathies.
   C. **Frontal intermittent rhythmic delta activity (FIRDA):** Intermittent sinusoidal waves with a frequency of 1.5-3 Hz. Found frontally in adults and occipitally in children (OIRDA). Present when the eyes are closed and during drowsiness and REM sleep. May be seen with lesions of the mesencephalon, diencephalon, cerebellum, third and fourth ventricle, deep frontal regions, or with diffuse cortical and subcortical gray matter encephalopathies, metabolic encephalopathies, encephalitis and cerebral trauma. Unilateral FIRDA suggests a lateralized lesion.
   D. **Dysrhythmic (polymorphic) delta activity:** A continuous pattern of irregular delta waves of varying amplitude and frequency, unreactive to eye opening or stimuli. May be seen in destructive white matter lesions (tumors, abscesses, herpes encephalitis). When associated with localized depression or absence of localized background activity, the likelihood of an underlying lesion is high. May be seen transiently in complicated migraine.

IV. Periodic patterns
   A. **Periodic lateralized epileptiform discharges (PLEDS):** PLEDS consist of sharp waves, sharp and slow waves, spikes, or multiple spikes with amplitude of 50-100 µV occurring every one to several seconds. May be seen for several weeks following cerebral infarction. Also seen in other lesions, including brain tumors and herpes encephalitis. Bilateral PLEDS suggest herpes. PLEDS are often associated with epilepsia partialis continua or focal motor seizures.

B. <u>Subacute sclerosing panencephalitis:</u> Bursts of stereotyped, symmetrically bisynchronous slow and sharp wave complexes with a periodicity of 3-10 seconds, amplitude around 500 μV, and often associated with myoclonic jerks. Appears early in the disease process and is virtually pathognomonic.

C. <u>Creutzfeldt-Jacob disease:</u> Early disorganization and slowing is followed by bi- or tri-phasic sharp waves, 200-500 ms in duration, amplitude up to 300 μV, occurring every 0.5-1.6 seconds. Usually bisynchronous, but may be lateralized. They appear within 12 weeks of onset of symptoms and may be associated with myoclonic jerks. Startle may be activating.

Ref: Klass DW, Daly DD. Current Practice of Clinical Electroencephalography. New York: Raven Press, 1979.

EKG

Disease of the CNS, particularly infarction and subarachnoid hemorrhage, can produce changes in both EKG rhythm and morphology. Dysrhythmias include ventricular tachycardia, premature ventricular contractions, sinus tachycardia, wandering atrial pacemaker, and paroxysmal atrial tachycardia. Morphologic changes include Q waves (may simulate MI), QT prolongation, ST elevation or depression, T wave abnormalities (including inversion) and U waves. These changes appear related to altered sympathetic tone, which prolongs the myocardial refractory period. If this occurs in a nonuniform manner, re-entrant dysrhythmias can be propagated. Treatment with conventional antidysrhythmic agents may be unsuccessful. In such cases, drugs (propranolol) or procedures (stellate ganglion block) to alter sympathetic tone may prove beneficial.

Ref: Arch Int Med 142:232, 1982.

ELECTROLYTE DISORDERS (see also Calcium, Magnesium, Potassium, SIADH, Sodium)

<u>Metabolic acidosis</u> is associated with predominantly cardiovascular manifestations. Neurological manifestations of lethargy and coma are due to CSF acidosis. CSF acidosis is usually less than the accompanying systemic acidosis due to active retention of bicarbonate by the blood brain barrier. The relative impermeability of the blood brain barrier to ions results in "paradoxical"

transient alkalosis of the CSF due to loss of diffusable CO_2 with compensatory hyperventilation. Acute acidosis is more likely to cause symptoms than is chronic acidosis. The treatment of systemic acidosis with bicarbonate may cause paradoxical CNS acidosis and worsening level of consciousness for similar reasons: the hyperventilation that had been compensating for systemic acidosis ceases, and CO_2 begins to accumulate, both systemically and centrally; however, the administered bicarbonate does not reach the CSF acutely, so the rise in CO_2 is not buffered.

Respiratory acidosis is associated with confusion and lethargy as pCO_2 rises above 70 mm Hg. Chronic hypercapnea is less likely to be symptomatic. Vasodilation may manifest as headaches, increased intracranial pressure, and papilledema.

Metabolic alkalosis may cause lethargy and confusion; tetany may appear if serum calcium is borderline before alkalosis supervenes.

Respiratory alkalosis (see Hyperventilation).

EMG (ELECTROMYOGRAPHY)

Though strictly referring to studies of muscle, this term is used more generally to include both nerve conduction studies and the needle exam.

Nerve conduction studies 1) provide objective evidence of motor unit dysfunction in questions of weakness, 2) localize and characterize (axonal, demyelinating) lesions of peripheral nerves, 3) differentiate peripheral neuropathies from myopathies and motor neuron disease, 4) detect peripheral neuropathy in patients presenting clinically with a mononeuropathy, 5) provide early detection of peripheral nerve disease (e.g., in familial disorders), and 6) identify and characterize patterns of anomalous innervation.

Motor nerve conduction studies are done by stimulating a peripheral nerve and recording from a muscle innervated by that nerve. Sensory nerve conduction studies are done by stimulating a mixed nerve and recording from a cutaneous nerve, or by stimulating a cutaneous nerve and recording from a mixed or cutaneous nerve. The amplitude, duration, shape, and latency of compound muscle action potentials and sensory nerve action potentials are noted. Responses at 2 or more recording sites are compared and distal latencies and conduction velocities determined. The effect of repetitive stimulation, exercise and rest, and drugs (edrophonium) may also be studied. Nerve conduction studies vary with temperature and the age of the patient as well as other factors.

The F wave is a low amplitude muscle action potential which is seen following the initial compound muscle action potential (M wave). It results from an antidromic motor impulse traveling proximally to and synapsing in the spinal cord and traveling down the motor nerve orthodromically to activate the muscle fiber (F wave). It is a means of evaluating proximal motor fibers. The F wave latency is prolonged in neuropathies with proximal involvement such as diabetic neuropathy and Guillain-Barre syndrome. It is also prolonged in radiculopathy, motor neuron disease, and some hereditary neuropathies.

The H reflex is a muscle action potential obtainable after submaximal stimulation of certain nerves such as the tibial. It results from an orthodromic sensory potential traveling to the spinal cord, synapsing with a motor unit, and then an orthodromic motor impulse travels to the muscle to produce the H reflex. It is a means of measuring proximal conduction in sensory and motor fibers. It is prolonged in S1 radiculopathy, diabetic and uremic neuropathy, and nutritional neuropathies.

Repetitive stimulation is used to differentiate defects of neuromuscular transmission. In myasthenia gravis there is a decrement in the amplitude of repetitively evoked responses with the muscle at rest. The decrement is repaired seconds after exercise (post-tetanic or postactivation facilitation) and worsened 2-4 minutes after exercise (postactivation exhaustion). In the myasthenic syndrome the evoked responses at rest are of low amplitude with a small decrement. Prominent postactivation facilitation occurs seconds after exercise with postactivation exhaustion 2-4 minutes after exercise. In botulism, very low amplitude evoked responses with minimal decrement are associated with minimal postactivation facilitation and exhaustion.

The <u>needle exam</u> records electrical activity in muscle, yielding information on the nature and location of disorders of motor units. Insertional, spontaneous, and voluntary activity are outlined below. Localization depends on a knowledge of peripheral nervous system anatomy (see Myotomes).

<u>Insertional activity</u>, associated with needle movement, is increased in denervated muscle, myotonic disorders, and some myopathies, especially inflammatory myopathies. It is decreased in periodic paralysis during paralysis and when normal muscle tissue is replaced by other tissue.

<u>Spontaneous activity</u> is recorded while the muscle is completely relaxed.

Fibrillation potentials are seen in denervation (after 2-3 weeks), lower motor neuron disease (anterior horn cell, root, plexus, nerve - especially axonal), defects of neuromuscular transmission (myasthenia gravis, botulism), myositis, certain dystrophies and myopathies, hyperkalemic periodic paralysis, acid maltase deficiency, rhabdomyolysis, trichonosis, and muscle trauma.

Positive sharp waves are usually seen with fibrillation potentials, i.e., in denervation and various muscle disorders.

Fasciculation potentials are most common in chronic neurogenic disorders (ALS, Creutzfeldt-Jakob disease, root compression, peripheral neuropathy). Also seen in normals with fatigue or cramps and in many other disorders including tetany, thyrotoxicosis, and use of cholinesterase inhibitors.

Myotonic discharges are seen in myotonic disorders, hyperkalemic periodic paralysis, polymyositis, acid maltase deficiency, and diazocholesterol toxicity.

Bizarre repetitive (high frequency) potentials are seen in a wide variety of chronic neuropathic disorders (poliomyelitis, ALS, spinal muscular atrophy, chronic radiculopathies, chronic neuropathies) and chronic myopathic disorders (Duchenne and limb-girdle dystrophy, polymyositis, hypothyroidism, Schwartz-Jampel syndrome). These should be distinguished from other repetitive discharges.

Myokymic discharges may be recorded in facial muscle in MS, brainstem neoplasms, polyradiculopathy, or facial palsy or in appendicular muscles in radiation plexopathy or chronic nerve compression.

Neuromyotonia occurs in syndromes of continuous muscle fiber activity, anticholinesterase toxicity, tetany, and chronic spinal muscular atrophy.

Cramp potentials occur commonly in normals and in a variety of disorders including salt depletion, chronic neurogenic atrophy, hypothyroidism, pregnancy, uremia, and benign nocturnal cramps.

Voluntary motor unit potentials are evaluated for duration, amplitude, number of phases, recruitment, and pattern of firing.

Short duration motor unit potentials occur in disorders with atrophy or loss of muscle fibers in the motor unit. They may be seen in all the muscular dystrophies, many congenital myopathies, toxic myopathies, polymyositis, periodic paralysis, disorders of neuromuscular transmission, early reinnervation after nerve injury, and late neurogenic atrophy.

Long duration potentials occur in disorders with an increased number or density of fibers or a loss of synchrony of firing of fibers in a motor unit. They may be seen in motor neuron disease, chronic radiculopathies, chronic neuropathies, axonal neuropathies with sprouting or polymyositis.

NERVE CONDUCTION STUDIES, NORMAL VALUES
(<65 years, University Hospitals of Cleveland)

NERVE	AMPLITUDE	DISTAL LATENCY	CONDUCTION VELOCITY
Median			
Sensory			
Orthodromic	10–45 μV	2.2–3.5 ms	–
Palmar	50–180 μV	1.5–2.2 ms	56–73 m/s
Antidromic	25–86 μV	2.5–3.5 ms	77–71 m/s
Motor	4–18 mV	2.4–4.4 ms (F–Latency 22–31 ms)	48–70 m/s
Ulnar			
Sensory			
Orthodromic	0–15 μV	2.1–3.0 ms	– –
Palmar	12 μV	1.5–2.2 ms	55–71 m/s
Antidromic	10–15 μV	2.1–3.0 ms	55–71 m/s
Motor	5–16 mV	1.9–3.5 ms (F–Latency 21–32 ms)	49–71 m/s
Radial			
Sensory	10–22 μV	1.9–2.8 ms	48–68 m/s
Motor		1.0–3.0 ms	68–89 m/s
Musculocutaneous			
Motor	4–16 mV	1.5–3.3 ms	53–85 m/s
Peroneal			
Motor	2–12 mV	3.3–6.5 ms (F–Latency 38–57 ms)	40–57 m/s
Posterior tibial			
Motor	4–19 mV	3.0–5.8 ms (F–Latency 41–56 ms, H–Latency 33 ms)	40–58 m/s
Sural			
Sensory	6–47 μV	3.2–4.6 ms	38–59 m/s

NERVE CONDUCTION STUDIES IN NEUROMUSCULAR DISORDERS

Disorder	Amplitude	Distal Latency	Conduction Velocity	F-, H- Latency
Polyneuropathy				
Axonal	↓	NL	>70%	Mild ↑
Demyelinating	NL or ↓	NL or ↑	<50%	↑
Upper motor neuron disease	NL	NL	NL	NL
Motor neuron disease	↓ motor NL sensory	NL	>70%	NL or Mild ↑
Radiculopathy	NL or ↓	NL	>80%	↑
Neuromuscular transmission defect	Variable	NL	NL	NL
Myopathy	NL or ↓	NL	NL	NL

Polyphasic motor unit potentials (five or more phases) may be seen in myopathy and neurogenic atrophy.

Fluctuations of amplitude, duration, or shape of a given motor unit potential from moment to moment are usually due to blocking of individual muscle fiber action potentials in the motor unit and may be seen in disorders of neuromuscular transmission, myositis, muscle trauma, reinnervation after nerve injury, and rapidly progressive neurogenic atrophy.

Recruitment (the relation of firing rate of individual potentials to the total number of potentials firing) is decreased (firing rate excessive for number firing) in disorders in which there is a loss of whole motor units such as any neurogenic disorder or severe muscle disease. Increased recruitment refers to an excessive activation of motor units for a given force exerted (relation of firing rate to number is normal) and is seen in myopathies in which the force generated by individual motor units is decreased.

Abnormalities on needle exam may occur in any combination. No single abnormality is specific for any single disease process.

Myopathic disorders are generally associated with increased insertional and spontaneous activity, especially if inflammatory. Motor unit potential amplitude and duration are decreased, and there is an increased percentage of polyphasic potentials. Recruitment may be increased. In some endocrine and metabolic myopathies, EMG abnormalities may be minimal. Recruitment may be decreased in severe myopathies.

Acute neurogenic lesions are associated with normal insertional and spontaneous activity. Motor unit potentials are reduced in number (or absent) but have a normal appearance. Recruitment is decreased. Following denervation for several days (usually by 2-3 weeks) insertional activity, and then spontaneous activity, increase. With reinnervation, spontaneous activity decreases, short duration polyphasic motor unit potentials appear, and recruitment improves; variation of motor unit potentials may be noted. In progressing or chronic neurogenic atrophy, motor unit potential amplitude and duration are increased and there is an increased percentage of polyphasic potentials. In the progressive process there may be variation of the potentials.

Ref: Kimura J. Electrodiagnosis of Diseases of Nerve and Muscle: Principles and Practice. Philadelphia: FA Davis, 1983.

ENCEPHALITIS (see also Abscess, Meningitis)

Inflammation of the brain associated with infectious, postinfectious, or demyelinating states. Encephalitis is usually heralded by headache, fever, nuchal rigidity, and alteration of consciousness (lethargy, confusion, coma). In addition, ataxia, myoclonus, ocular motor palsies, nystagmus, and facial weakness may be present. Involvement of meninges or spinal cord may occur (meningoencephalitis, encephalomyelitis). Death from viral encephalitis occurs in 5-20%, and a further 20% are left with cognitive deficits, memory defects, personality changes, hemiparesis, or seizures.

Viral

Herpes simplex encephalitis (HSV Type I): Fever, headache, and malaise may be followed by behavior changes, hallucinations, focal seizures, focal signs, and progression to stupor and coma. CT may show temporal or insular low densities and focal hemorrhage or enhancement. EEG is typically abnormal, showing PLEDs or other focal abnormalities. Spinal fluid contains 0-1100 WBCs (usually <100), protein around 80, and a normal glucose (early). Hypoglycorrhachia can occur but should suggest other causes. Greater than 50 RBCs are present in 40%, but this is nonspecific. Brain biopsy results in a positive culture in 59%. A 4-fold rise in CSF titer of HSV antibody is 90% sensitive and 81% specific, peaking at 4-6 weeks. Serum to CSF ratio of HSV antibody of ≤ 20 is diagnostic but is usually not positive until day 4. The mortality from untreated HSV encephalitis is at least 70%. A recent study demonstrated lower morbidity and mortality (19%) with acyclovir (10 mg/kg IV over 1 hour q8h) than with vidarabine (40% mortality). Approximately 4% of suspected HSV cases will have an alternate treatable diagnosis, such as TB, cryptococcosis, toxoplasmosis, tumor, or stroke. Serious morbidity or mortality from brain biopsy is between 0.5%-2%. Performance of a brain biopsy is controversial, but should at least be performed in cases of hypoglycorrhachia or failure to respond to acyclovir. Outcome is related to level of consciousness at onset of treatment.

Rabies: Carriers include skunks, foxes, dogs, bats, and raccoons. Incubation is from days to months. Fever and agitation may precede confusion, seizures, dysphagia (hydrophobia), dysarthria, facial numbness, and spasm. The medullary tegmentum is intensely involved and paralysis may be secondary to spinal cord involvement.

antibody is 90% sensitive and 81% specific, peaking at 4-6 weeks. Serum to CSF ratio of HSV antibody of ≤20 is diagnostic but is usually not positive until day 4. The mortality from untreated HSV encephalitis is at least 70%. A recent study demonstrated lower morbidity and mortality (19%) with acyclovir (10 mg/kg IV over 1 hour q8h) than with vidarabine (40% mortality). Approximately 4% of suspected HSV cases will have an alternate treatable diagnosis, such as TB, cryptococcosis, toxoplasmosis, tumor, or stroke. Serious morbidity or mortality from brain biopsy is between 0.5%-2%. Performance of a brain biopsy is controversial, but should at least be performed in cases of hypoglycorrhachia or failure to respond to acyclovir. Outcome is related to level of consciousness at onset of treatment.

Rabies: Carriers include skunks, foxes, dogs, bats, and raccoons. Incubation is from days to months. Fever and agitation may precede confusion, seizures, dysphagia (hydrophobia), dysarthria, facial numbness, and spasm. The medullary tegmentum is intensely involved and paralysis may be secondary to spinal cord involvement. Death follows in 2-7 days, unless treatment is initiated before infection is established. Treatment includes cleaning of bites with soap and benzalkonium solution and administration of human rabies immune globulin and human diploid cell rabies vaccine.

Epidemic encephalitis: These are mostly arthropod transmitted viral diseases, with peak incidence in late summer and fall. St. Louis encephalitis is the most common, found in the Ohio-Mississippi River basin, with a fatality of 10-20%. Venezuelan equine encephalitis is found in the southeastern US, with a very low mortality; most infections result in flu-like illness. Eastern equine encephalitis occurs along the Gulf and Atlantic seaboard, usually affects horses and birds, is rare among humans, but has a 25-70% mortality, attacking the young and very old with a fulminant severe course. Western encephalitis occurs in the west, southwest, and central North America, and California virus encephalitis occurs in the midwestern states, both with a low incidence of overt disease and low fatality rates. Human vaccines are still experimental. Treatment is aimed at brain edema and seizures.

Nonepidemic viral encephalitis. Enteroviruses (echo, cocksackie, polio), measles, mumps, Epstein-Barr, rubella, chicken pox (varicella zoster), and lymphocytic choriomeningitis virus can all cause sporadic encephalitis without temporal lobe predilection. Treatment of disseminated varicella zoster, commonly seen in immunosuppressed patients, with acyclovir, is currently recommended though its effect on the encephalitis is unknown.

Slow latent virus infections include scrapie, Kuru, Creutzfeldt-Jakob disease, subacute sclerosing panencephalitis, progressive multifocal leukoencephalopathy, and progressive rubella panencephalitis.

Associated with immunodeficient states

Progressive multifocal leukoencephalopathy, caused by a papovavirus, usually occurs in patients with lymphoproliferative (chronic leukemia, Hodgkins, other lymphomas) or granulomatous (sarcoid) disease, or during immunosuppression. It is characterized by multifocal white matter signs, progressing to death in 1-18 months. CT may show low density nonenhancing lesions in the white matter. A brain biopsy may be necessary to rule out toxoplasmosis, especially if CSF abnormalities or CT enhancement are present. Ara-C has been used, with case reports of improvement. See also AIDS.

Nonviral encephalitis

Rickettsial: Epidemic, murine, and scrub typhus, Rocky Mountain spotted fever, and Q fever.

Bacterial: Pertussis, tularemia, brucellosis, bubonic plague, typhoid fever, dysentery, cholera, melioidosis, psittacosis, leprosy, scarlet fever, rheumatic fever, *Clostridia*.

Spirochetal: Relapsing fever, syphilis, rat-bite fever, leptospirosis.

Protozoan: *Entamoeba, Naegleria*, trypanosomiasis, leishmaniasis, malaria, toxoplasmosis.

Helminthic: Long list including ancylostomiasis, angiostrongyliasis, ascariasis, cysticercosis, echinococcosis, filariasis, schistosomiasis, toxocariasis, trichinosis.

Fungi: Including actinomycosis, aspergillosis, blastomycosis, candidiasis, coccidioidomycosis, cryptococcosis, histoplasmosis, mucormycosis, nocardiosis, and sporotrichosis.

Ref: Mandell GL, et al. Principles and Practice of Infectious Disease, 2nd ed. New York: Wiley, 1985.

ENCEPHALOPATHY, PERINATAL HYPOXIC-ISCHEMIC

This is the most important cause of neurological morbidity in full-term infants and accounts for the majority of nonprogressive deficits in children.

Selected neuronal necrosis due to hypoxia and/or related metabolic effects is associated clinically with stupor, coma, seizures, hypotonia, and abnormal suck, swallow, and eye and tongue movements in the neonate. Long-term clinical manifestations include mental retardation, spastic quadriparesis, seizure disorder, ataxia, and bulbar and pseudobulbar palsy.

Status marmoratus is due to a secondary hypermyelination along glial lesions of the corpus striatum resulting from hypoxia, acidosis and/or hypotension. Clinically there is choreoathetosis, mental retardation, and spastic quadriparesis.

Symmetrical, parasagittal "watershed" cortical infarcts are the principal ischemic lesion of the full-term infant and result from impaired cerebral perfusion or autoregulation. In the neonate there is proximal limb weakness. Long-term clinical correlation is unknown.

Periventricular leukomalacia results from white matter necrosis adjacent to the external angles of the lateral ventricles and is the principal ischemic lesion of premature infants. Hypotension or impaired cerebro-vascular autoregulation results in ischemia in periventricular arterial border zones. Clinical correlation in the neonate is unknown, but lower limb weakness might be expected. Spastic diplegia is seen long-term.

Focal or multifocal ischemic necrosis, usually within the distribution of major cerebral vessels may result from multiple etiologies including: focal and general cerebro-vascular insufficiency, postnatal cerebral hemorrhage, inflammation, infection, and pre- and postnatal trauma. Clinical manifestations in the neonate are variable, but may include hemiparesis, quadriparesis, and stereotyped, nonhabituating reflex responses. Later manifestations include spastic hemiparesis, quadriparesis, mental retardation, and seizure disorders.

Management is based on monitoring and maintaining ventilation and perfusion. Maintain blood glucose at 75-100 mg/ml. Control seizures (see Epilepsy). Avoid fluid overload and increased intracranial pressure. Do not use hyperosmolar solutions or glucocorticoids without indication. In the case of neonatal intraventricular hemorrhage, blood pressure should be maintained cautiously and factors causing cerebral hyperperfusion should be avoided.

ENDOCRINE DISORDERS (see Calcium, Glucose, Thyroid)

EPIDURAL HEMORRHAGE (see Hemorrhage)

CLASSIFICATION OF EPILEPTIC
SEIZURES (1970)

I. PARTIAL SEIZURES (seizures beginning locally)
   A. Simple partial seizures (elementary symptomatology, consciousness generally not impaired)
      1. With motor symptoms (focal motor, Jacksonian, versive, postural, aphasic, phonatory)
      2. With somatosensory or special sensory symptoms (visual, auditory, olfactory, gustatory, vertiginous)
      3. With autonomic symptoms
      4. Compound forms
   B. Complex partial seizures (generally with impairment of consciousness, may begin with elementary symptomatology)
      1. With impaired consciousness only
      2. With cognitive symptomatology (dysmnesic or ideational disturbances)
      3. With affective symptomatology
      4. With "psychosensory" symptomatology (illusions or hallucinations)
      5. With "psychomotor" symptomatology (automatisms)
      6. Compound forms
   C. Partial seizures secondarily generalized

II. GENERALIZED SEIZURES (bilaterally symmetric and without local onset)
   A. Absence ("petit mal") seizures
   B. Myoclonic seizures
   C. Clonic seizures
   D. Tonic seizures
   E. Tonic-clonic ("grand mal") seizures
   F. Atonic seizures
   G. Akinetic seizures

III. UNCLASSIFIED EPILEPTIC SEIZURES
    (due to incomplete data)

Adapted from: Gastaut H. Clinical and electro-encephalographic classification of epileptic seizures. Epilepsia 11:102-113, 1970; Merlis JK. Proposal for an international classification of the epilepsies. Epilepsia 11:114-119, 1970.

INTERNATIONAL CLASSIFICATION OF EPILEPSIES
AND EPILEPTIC SYNDROMES (1985)

I. Localization-related (focal, local, partial) epilepsies and syndromes
  A. Idiopathic with age-related onset
    1. Benign childhood epilepsy with centrotemporal spikes
    2. Childhood epilepsy with occipital paroxysms
  B. Symptomatic
    Comprises syndromes of great individual variability, mainly based on anatomical localization, clinical features, seizure types, and etiological factors (if known), for example:
    1. Frontal lobe
    2. Supplementary motor
    3. Cingulate
    4. Anterior (polar) region
    5. Orbito-frontal
    6. Dorsolateral
    7. Motor cortex
    8. Temporal lobe
      a. Hippocampal (mesiobasal limbic, primary rhinencephalic psychomotor)
      b. Amygdalar (anterior polar-amygdalar)
      c. Lateral posterior temporal
      d. Opercular (insular)
      e. Parietal lobe
      f. Occipital lobe

II. Generalized epilepsies and syndromes
  A. Idiopathic, with age-related onset
    1. Benign neonatal familial convulsions
    2. Benign neonatal convulsions
    3. Benign myoclonic epilepsy in infancy
    4. Childhood absence epilepsy (pyknolepsy)
    5. Juvenile absence epilepsy
    6. Juvenile myoclonic epilepsy (impulsive petit mal)
    7. Epilepsy with grand mal seizures (generalized tonic-clonic seizures) on awakening
    8. Other generalized idiopathic epilepsies

B. Idiopathic and/or symptomatic
  1. West syndrome (infantile spasms, Blitz-Nick-Salaam Krampfe)
  2. Lennox-Gastaut syndrome
  3. Epilepsy with myoclonic-astatic seizures
  4. Epilepsy with myoclonic absences
C. Symptomatic
  1. Nonspecific etiology
    a. Early myoclonic encephalopathy
  2. Specific syndromes
     Those diseases in which seizures are a presenting or predominant feature
    a. Malformations
      1. Aicardi syndrome
      2. Lissencephaly-pachygyria
      3. Phakomatoses
    b. Proven or suspected inborn errors of metabolism
      1. Neonate
        a. Nonketotic hyperglycinemia
        b. D-glyceracidemia
      2. Infant
        a. Phenylketonuria
        b. Phenylketonuria with biopterins
        c. Tay Sachs and Sandhoff disease
        d. Ceroid-lipofuscinosis, early infantile type
           (Santuavori-Haltia-Hagberg disease)
        e. Pyridoxine dependency
      3. Child
        a. Ceroid-lipofuscinosis, late infantile type (Jansky-Bielschowski disease)
        b. Huntington's disease, infantile type
      4. Child and Adolescent
        a. Gaucher disease, juvenile form
        b. Ceroid-lipofuscinosis, juvenile form (Spielmeyer-Vogt-Sjogren disease)
        c. Lafora disease
        d. Degenerative progressive myoclonic epilepsy (Lundborg type)
        e. Dyssynergia cerebellaris myoclonica with epilepsy (Ramsay-Hunt syndrome)
        f. Cherry red spot myoclonus syndrome
        g. Mitochondrial myopathy
      5. Adult
        a. Kuf's disease

III. Epilepsies and syndromes undetermined as to whether they are focal or generalized
   A. With both generalized and focal seizures
      1. Neonatal seizures
      2. Severe myoclonic epilepsy in infancy
      3. Epilepsy with continuous spike-waves during slow wave sleep
      4. Acquired epileptic aphasia (Landau-Kleffner syndrome)
   B. Without unequivocal generalized or focal features
      Covers all cases with generalized tonic-clonic seizures where clinical and EEG findings do not permit classification as clearly generalized or localization-related, such as in many cases of sleep grand mal

IV. Special syndromes
   A. Situation-related seizures (Gelegenheitsanfalle)
      1. Febrile convulsions
      2. Seizures related to other identifiable situations such as stress, hormonal changes, drugs, alcohol, or sleep deprivation
   B. Isolated, apparently unprovoked epileptic events
   C. Epilepsies characterized by specific modes of seizure precipitation
   D. Chronic progressive epilepsia partialis continua of childhood

Ref: Dreifuss et al. Proposal for classification of epilepsies and epileptic syndromes. Epilepsia 26:268-278, 1985.

DRUG TREATMENT OF VARIOUS SEIZURE TYPES

<u>Generalized Seizures</u>
Tonic clonic
    phenytoin
    carbamazepine
    phenobarbital
    primidone
    valproic acid
Absence
    ethosuximide
    valproic acid
    clonazepam
    oxazolidinediones
      paramethadione
      trimethadione
    other succinimides
      methsuximide
      phensuximide
      acetazolamide
Absence + tonic-clonic
    valproate
    ethosuximide + phenytoin
    ethosuximide + carbamazepine
Atypical absence (Lennox-Gastaut)
    valproate
    clonazepam
    carbamazepine
    acetazolamide
Infantile spasms
    ACTH
    prednisone
    valproic acid
    nitrazepam
    clonazepam
    ketogenic diet
Myoclonic
    clonazepam
    valproate

<u>Partial seizures</u>
    carbamazepine
    phenytoin
    phenobarbital
    primidone
    valproic acid

<u>Mixed seizures</u>
    valproic acid
    phenobarbital

<u>Febrile seizures</u>
    phenobarbital (if
    decide to treat)

MANAGEMENT OF CONVULSIVE STATUS EPILEPTICUS IN ADULTS
(after Delgado-Escueta AV and Bajorek JG, 1982)

Assess cardiac and respiratory function. Protect patient from injury to self.

Verify diagnosis of status epilepticus (continuous convulsions or repeated convulsions without return to baseline mental status interictally).

Insert oral airway. Provide O_2. Be prepared for endotracheal intubation.

Insert IV line.

Draw venous blood for glucose, electrolytes, BUN, Mg, Ca, CBC, and, if indicated, anticonvulsant levels and toxicology screen.

Draw arterial blood for pH, pO_2, pCO_2 HCO_3.

Monitor respiration, blood pressure, EKG, and, if possible, EEG.

Start IV infusion of normal saline with B vitamins (including thiamine 100 mg)

Give glucose 50%, 50 ml IV push

Infuse diazepam IV no faster than 2 mg/min until seizures stop or to total of 20 mg. Seizures should stop within 3 (33% of patients) to 5 (80% of patients) minutes. Effect lasts only 20 minutes. Be alert for respiratory suppression or hypotension, especially if patient has received drugs.

Simultaneously infuse phenytoin IV no faster than 50 mg/min to total of 18 mg/kg. Slow infusion rate if brady-cardia or hypotension develop. Effect occurs at least 10-20 (peak 20-30) minutes after starting infusion.

If seizures persist, insert endotracheal tube and treat with either phenobarbital IV infusion no faster than 100 mg/min to a loading dose of 20 mg/kg, or diazepam IV drip: diazepam 100 mg in 500 ml dextrose 5%/water infused at 40 ml/hr, but not both drugs.

If seizures persist after 20-30 minutes, general anesthesia with halothane and neuromuscular junction blockade should be instituted.

If an anesthesiologist is not immediately available, lidocaine or paraldehyde may be used. Lidocaine 50-100 mg is given IV push and if effective within 30 seconds, is given via continuous infusion at a rate of 1-2 mg/min. Paraldehyde is given as a 4% solution in normal or 0.5 normal saline and slowly injected directly from a glass syringe since it will decompose plastic. Only properly stored, freshly opened paraldehyde should be used as it may depolymerize and

oxidize to acetic acid. Paraldehyde is excreted via
the lungs and should be used with caution in patients
with pulmonary disease.

Other drugs being evaluated for use in status epilepticus
include lorazepam which may be more potent, is of
slower onset and longer duration, and is also
associated with some risk of respiratory suppression.
Valproic acid, 200-800 mg, has been given per nasogastric tube or in lipid-based suppositories prepared
by hospital pharmacies, but absorption may be erratic.

Evaluation (LP, skull films, CT scan, EEG, etc.) to
identify the cause of status epilepticus begins
promptly after the patient is stabilized, as some
causes require emergency management. Common causes
include meningitis, encephalitis, cerebral infarction
or hemorrhage, brain tumor, head trauma, cerebral
anoxia (cardiopulmonary disease), withdrawal from
anticonvulsants in chronic epileptics, and metabolic
and electrolyte disorders.

Maintenance anticonvulsant therapy should begin within 12
hours.

Persistent postictal depression of mental status may be
due to drugs rather than seizures. Drug levels may be
helpful.

Ref: Delgado-Escueta AV, et al. Management of status
       epilepticus. NEJM 306:1337-1340, 1982.

MANAGEMENT OF CONVULSIVE STATUS EPILEPTICUS IN CHILDREN

Follow the same principles outlined for adults. Drug
therapy is modified as follows:

Diazepam 0.3-0.5 mg/kg IV no faster than 1-2 mg/min. If
there is any delay in starting IV, may give diazepam
0.55-1 mg/kg per rectum via 5 French feeding catheter
flushed with saline.

Phenytoin is given simultaneously via a second IV no
faster than 25-50 mg/min to total of 18 mg/kg.

If seizures persist, intubate and infuse phenobarbital no
faster than 30 mg/min to a total of 15 mg/min.

If seizures persist, slowly infuse paraldehyde 0.15
ml/kg/hr as a 4% solution (10 ml paraldehyde in 250
ml 0.5 normal saline), i.e., 3.75 ml 4% solution/kg.

If seizures persist, general anesthesia and neuromuscular
junction blockade are instituted.

Neonatal seizures may present with tonic (usually extension of all limbs) or multifocal clonic movements, or, most commonly, with subtle manifestations such as tonic eye deviations, eyelid blinking, lip smacking, or even apnea. Jitteriness should be distinguished from seizures; it is characterized by tremulousness that is highly stimulus-sensitive. It is seen in anoxia, hypoglycemia, drug withdrawal, hypocalcemia, and otherwise normal infants.

Neonatal seizures occurring in the first 3 days after birth are most commonly due to birth injury (hypoxic-ischemic encephalopathy, intraventricular hemorrhage, etc.) but also to hypoglycemia and hypocalcemia. During days 4-7, infection, malformations and inborn errors of metabolism are more common causes. Subdural hemorrhage as well as infection may cause seizures after 10 days. Other causes of neonatal seizures include hypomagnesemia, maternal drug use, local anesthesia and pyridoxine dependency.

MANAGEMENT OF NEONATAL SEIZURES

Assess cardiac and pulmonary status.

Insert IV line.

Draw blood for glucose, electrolytes, BUN, creatinine, Ca, Mg, bilirubin.

If hypoglycemia, give glucose 25%, 2-4 mg/kg IV.

If hypocalcemia, give calcium gluconate 5%, 4 ml/kg IV with EKG monitoring; also give magnesium sulfate.

If hypomagnesemia, give magnesium sulfate 50%, 0.2 ml/kg IM.

Give phenobarbital 15-20 mg/kg IV over several minutes, may repeat dose in 10 minutes at 10 mg/kg.

If seizures persist, give phenytoin 10-20 mg/kg IV.

If seizures persist, give pyridoxine 50-100 mg IV, preferably with EEG monitoring.

If seizures persist, give paraldehyde 0.3 ml/kg per rectum in an equivalent volume of mineral oil using non-plastic materials.

Additional evaluation to determine cause.

DRUG TREATMENT OF PARTIAL AND NONCONVULSIVE
STATUS EPILEPTICUS

Simple partial status
  diazepam IV
  phenytoin
  phenobarbital

Absence status
  diazepam, lorazepam, or clonazepam IV
  valproic acid
  ethosuximide

Adult onset spikewave stupor with neurological disease
  diazepam IV
  phenytoin
  phenobarbital

Myoclonic status
  diazepam IV

Tonic status (in patients with known epilepsy)
  phenytoin
  phenobarbital
  may be exacerbated by diazepam

Unilateral status (especially in young children)
  diazepam

EYE MOVEMENTS (see Calorics, Eye Muscles, Gaze Palsy,
  Graves' Ophthalmopathy, Nystagmus, Ocular Oscil-
  lations, Ophthalmoplegia, Optokinetic Nystagmus,
  Vertigo, Vestibulo-ocular Reflex)

EYE MUSCLES

   Because of their insertional properties (see diagram
below) the six extraocular muscles affect eye movements in
three planes in primary position. In testing muscle
strength, the optical axis is aligned with a muscle's main
vector. The superior rectus, for instance, becomes a pure
elevator when abducted 23°. Despite the obliques being
abductors in primary position, their function is tested in
adduction (51°) where they contribute to elevation and
depression of the eye.

INSERTION OF OCULAR MUSCLES ON THE GLOBE
(Right Eye)

LR = lateral rectus
MR = medial rectus
SR = superior rectus
IR = inferior rectus
SO = superior oblique
IO = inferior oblique

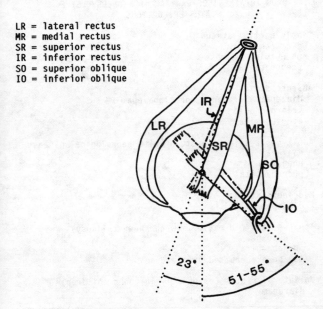

ACTIONS OF EYE MUSCLES IN PRIMARY POSITION

Muscle	Primary	Secondary	Tertiary
Lateral rectus	abduction		
Medial rectus	adduction		
Superior rectus	elevation	intorsion	adduction
Inferior rectus	depression	extorsion	adduction
Superior oblique	intorsion	depression	abduction
Inferior oblique	extorsion	elevation	abduction

124

MAIN FIELD OF ACTION OF INDIVIDUAL EYE MUSCLES

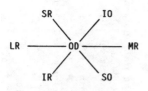
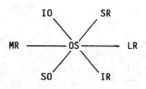

   <u>Diplopia testing in paralytic strabismus</u> begins with
identification of the paretic eye. Look for ocular
misalignment (primary deviation). When fixating with the
paretic eye (cover testing), the angle of deviation of the
eye under cover increases (secondary deviation). When
diplopia occurs in a certain direction of gaze, the red
glass or Maddox rod may help localize; the more peripheral
image is referred to the paretic eye. The Maddox rod
dissociates the images seen by both eyes and, therefore,
may produce diplopia due to a phoria which must be
distinguished from paralytic causes.

   Next identify the paretic muscle(s). Test the range
of motion of individual muscles (ductions). Perform the
cover-uncover test in primary position to demonstrate
horizontal and/or vertical deviations (tropias) and
alternate cover test in the 6 directions of gaze.
According to Hering's law of equal innervation of
synergistic muscles, the nonparetic eye will reach a more
extreme end position of gaze. Perform the Bielschowsky
head tilt test in suspected paresis of the superior
oblique.

FACIAL NERVE

   The <u>course of the facial nerve</u> (cranial nerve VII) is
diagramed below. The numbers in the diagram refer to
<u>location of the lesions</u> listed below.

1. Peripheral to chorda tympani in facial canal or
   outside stylomastoid foramen. Peripheral, upper and
   lower facial weakness (motor VII) only.
2. Facial canal (mastoid), involving chorda tympani. In
   addition to 1, patients have loss of taste over the
   anterior 2/3 of tongue and decreased salivation.
3. Facial canal, involving the stapedius nerve. As in 1
   and 2, plus hyperacusis.

FACIAL NERVE CONT.

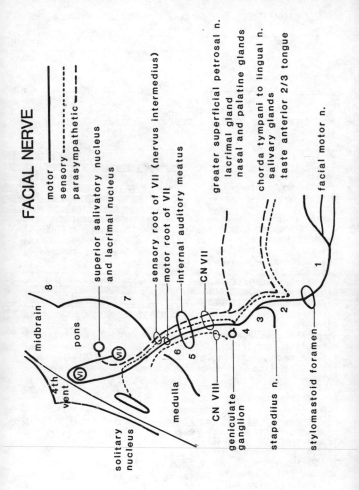

FACIAL NERVE

motor ——————
sensory ·················
parasympathetic — — —

superior salivatory nucleus and lacrimal nucleus

sensory root of VII (nervus intermedius)
motor root of VII
internal auditory meatus

CN VII

greater superficial petrosal n.
lacrimal gland
nasal and palatine glands

chorda tympani to lingual n.
salivary glands
taste anterior 2/3 tongue

facial motor n.

midbrain
pons
VII
VII
8
7
4th vent
solitary nucleus
medulla
CN VIII
geniculate ganglion
stapedius n.
stylomastoid foramen
6
5
4
3
2
1

4. Geniculate ganglion. Usually associated with pain in the ear. May have decreased lacrimation.
5. Internal auditory meatus. Complete VII (facial weakness; decreased taste, salivation, and lacrimation) plus VIII (deafness and, perhaps, vestibular symptoms).
6. Extrapontine, subarachnoid. May have other cranial nerve involvement. Hemifacial spasm is more commonly associated with more proximal lesions of VII.
7. Pontine (nuclear or infranuclear). Millard-Gubler, Fovilles' and Brissaud's syndromes (see Brainstem).
8. Supranuclear. Lesions may occur anywhere from mid pons to motor cortex and are usually associated with other findings such as hemiparesis, hemisensory deficit, language disturbance, and homonymous hemianopia, depending on location. Taste, salivation, and lacrimation are not involved. Lower facial weakness is much more prominent than upper due to ipsilateral, as well as contralateral, input to the portions of the facial nucleus controlling the upper face; input for the lower face is from contralateral cortex. Mild weakness may appear only as slight drooping of the angle of the mouth, slight widening of the palpebral fissure, or flattening of the nasolabial fold.

   Etiologies of facial nerve palsies are many. Although "idiopathic", Bell's palsy (probably herpes simplex) is most common. Other treatable and potentially serious causes should be excluded by careful history, exam, and, where indicated, neuroradiological and electrodiagnostic studies.

   Bell's palsy is attributed to swelling of the nerve or nerve sheath in the facial canal. Seventh nerve findings are variable, depending on the site and extent of lesion. Recovery is spontaneous and complete in up to 90%. EMG evidence of denervation indicates a worse prognosis for complete recovery. Partial or incomplete recovery may be associated with contractures, synkinetic motor movements (e.g., angle of mouth and lids), or excessive tearing with salivary gland stimulation (crocodile tears). Ramsay-Hunt syndrome refers to herpes zoster of the geniculate ganglion, with herpetic lesions often visible on the tympanic membrane, external auditory canal, and pinna.

   Other causes of peripheral facial weakness include: trauma (facial, skull fracture), surgery (middle ear, mastoids, cranial nerve V), neoplasms (Schwannoma, neurofibroma, nasopharyngeal carcinoma, leukemia, lymphoma, hemangioma, glomus tumors, cholesteatoma, parotid tumors), and infections involving the subarachnoid space, petrous portion of the temporal bone, middle ear, mastoid, parotid, or the facial nerve itself. Involvement may result from granulomatous infiltration of the meninges or, as in the case of sarcoid, with parotid gland swelling. Facial weakness may be congenital, as in the Mobius syndrome with upper > lower facial diplegia, paralysis of abduction of the eye, ptosis, and, occasionally, abnormal musculature of the tongue, sternocleidomastoid, and muscles of mastication. Recurrent facial paralysis and facial swelling (Melkersson syndrome) occurs rarely and may be associated with lingua plicata (Melkersson-Rosenthal). The nerve itself may be involved in Guillain-Barre, acute intermittent porphyria, and lead poisoning. Facial weakness may also be due to myasthenia gravis or various myopathies. Other rare causes include osteopetrosis, thiamine deficiency, and hemorrhage into the facial canal.

<u>Pontine</u> involvement is most commonly vascular, but may result from infection, hemorrhage, trauma, neoplasm (most commonly pontine glioma), or demyelinating disease. <u>Supranuclear</u> causes are many, including vascular, neoplastic, traumatic, and infectious.

<u>Treatment</u> is aimed at the primary cause. Corneal exposure should be prevented with a lubricating ointment. Electrical physiotherapy may be detrimental and should not be used. Corticosteroids are widely used to treat "idiopathic" Bell's palsy with good relief of pain and decrease in the number of patients with complete denervation. Prednisone, 1 mg/kg, is given in divided doses for 5-6 days and tapered over 5 days if paralysis is incomplete, but continued for another 10 days and tapered over the subsequent 5 days if paralysis is complete. Acyclovir is undergoing evaluation for use in the treatment of herpes zoster facial paralysis.

Ref: Adour KK, Hetzler DG. Am J Otol 5:499, 1984.

FLOPPY INFANT (see Hypotonic Infant)

FONTANEL

The anterior fontanel is formed at the juncture of the sagittal and coronal sutures; the posterior, at the juncture of the sagittal and lambdoidal sutures. At birth, both fontanels are open. The cranial bones may override each other if the baby has been delivered vaginally. The anterior fontanel may be quite large at birth; this has little significance. The fontanel is tense and occasionally bulges when a baby cries, but is soft and flat at other times. A "full fontanel" is a sign of increased intracranial pressure. The posterior fontanel becomes fused in the first few months of life.

By 7 months of age, the anterior fontanel is fibrous; by 2 years of age, it is palpable as a mid-sagittal depression. Disorders associated with a persistently large anterior fontanel include achondroplasia, cleidocranial dysostosis, osteogenesis imperfecta, athyrotic hypothyroidism, prematurity, trisomies 13 and 18, hypophosphatasia, and vitamin D deficiency (rickets).

FOURTH NERVE (see Ophthalmoplegia)

FRONTAL LOBE

Bilateral frontal disease has been associated with a variety of behavioral changes including apathy, euphoria, irritability, impaired judgment, asocial behavior, lack of motivation, and a shallow affect.

GAZE PALSY (see also Ocular Motor Apraxia, Ophthalmoplegia, Progressive Supranuclear Palsy)

Horizontal gaze palsies: A unilateral gaze (saccadic and pursuit) palsy may indicate a contralateral cerebral hemispheric (fronto-parietal), contralateral midbrain, or ipsilateral pontine lesion. Except when the pontine lesion is at the level of the abducens nucleus, either involving the nucleus itself or the paramedian pontine reticular formation, the eyes can be driven towards the side of the palsy with cold caloric stimulation of the ipsilateral ear. Hemispheric lesions characteristically produce transient defects; brainstem lesions may be associated with enduring defects. An acute cerebellar hemispheric lesion can result in an ipsilateral gaze palsy which can be overcome with calorics. Unilateral saccadic palsy with intact pursuit is unusual and indicates an acute frontal lesion. Unilateral impaired pursuit with normal saccades is usually secondary to an ipsilateral deep posterior hemispheric lesion with a contralateral hemianopsia.

Vertical gaze palsies: The rostral interstitial nucleus of the medial longitudinal fasciculus (riMLF) in the upper midbrain contains the cells which generate vertical eye movements. A medially placed lesion will result in both an up and down gaze palsy. An isolated down gaze palsy is due to bilateral, lateral lesions. Isolated up gaze palsies occur with lesions of the posterior commissure, bilateral pretectal regions, and large unilateral midbrain tegmental lesions. In the dorsal midbrain (Parinaud's) syndrome the paralysis of up gaze is usually associated with convergence-retraction nystagmus, lid retraction, and light-near dissociation of the pupils. An acute bilateral pontine lesion at the level of the abducens nucleus may result in a transient up gaze paralysis in addition to an enduring bilateral horizontal gaze palsy.

Conjugate eye deviations: Horizontal deviations are associated with acute gaze palsies as described above and with irritative cerebral foci (seizure, intracerebral hemorrhage) which usually drive the eyes to the side opposite the lesion. Ipsiversive eye and head movements, however, are reported with focal seizures. Upward deviations are seen in the oculogyric crisis of post-encephalitic Parkinsonism and, more commonly, as an idiosyncratic reaction to phenothiazines. It may also be seen in coma, usually due to anoxic encephalopathy. Downward deviations may occur transiently in normal neonates, but also occur in infantile hydrocephalus and in adults with metabolic encephalopathy or bilateral thalamic infarction or hemorrhage.

Ref: Daroff RB, Troost BT. Supranuclear disorders of eye movements, in Glaser JS. Neuro-ophthalmology. Hagerstown: Harper and Row, 1978, p 201.

Leigh RJ, Zee DS. The Neurology of Eye Movements. Philadelphia: FA Davis, 1983, Chapter 9.

GERSTMANN'S SYNDROME

A combination of deficits usually associated with a dominant (or bilateral) parietal lobe disorder. The 4 major features are right-left disorientation, dyscalculia, dysgraphia, and finger agnosia.

Ref: Benton AL. JNNP 24:176, 1961.

GLUCOSE

Hypoglycemia: Symptoms arise from neuroglucopenia and endogenous release of catecholamines. Mild hypoglycemia produces hunger, weakness, dizziness, blurred vision, anxiety, tremor, tachycardia, pallor, diaphoresis, headache, and mild confusion. With more severe hypoglycemia, the preceding symptoms are followed by seizures (glucose <30 mg/100 ml) with progression to coma, pupillary dilation, hypotonia, and extensor posturing (glucose <10 mg/100 ml). The presence of paresthesias may be related to hyperventilation. Focal findings may mimic cerebrovascular disease. Symptoms, signs and residual neurological deficit depend on the rate of onset, duration, and severity of hypoglycemia. Patients with chronic hypoglycemia may have no sympathetic symptoms but may have cognitive or behavioral disturbances. Repeated severe attacks of hypoglycemia may result in dementia.

Hyperglycemia: <u>Diabetic ketoacidosis</u> is the most common cerebral complication of diabetes and is frequently accompanied by decreased levels of consciousness and, occasionally, coma. Muscle cramps, hyperesthesias, dysesthesias, and diffuse abdominal pain may occur. The neurological changes correlate best with serum osmolarity although dehydration, acidosis, and associated electrolyte disorders contribute. The treatment of diabetic keto-acidosis may lead to fatal cerebral edema if blood osmolarity is rapidly lowered relative to brain osmolarity. Treatment may also cause hypophosphatemia, hypokalemia, and hypoglycemia.

<u>Hyperglycemic nonketotic states</u> result in CNS complications due to extracellular hyperosmolarity. Neurological manifestations can be seen with blood sugars >425 mg/100 ml. These include hallucinations, depression, apathy, irritability, seizures (typically focal and resistant to anticonvulsant medication), other focal signs (either postictal or in isolation), flaccidity and diminished deep tendon reflexes, tonic spasms, myoclonus, meningeal signs, nystagmus, tonic eye deviations, and reversible loss of vestibular caloric responses. As the blood sugar rises above 600 mg/100 ml coma ensues. Thrombosis of cerebral vessels and sinuses may occur. Seizures generally improve with correction of hyperglycemia and rehydration within 24 hours.

GRAVES' OPHTHALMOPATHY

Graves' ophthalmopathy may occur without clinical or laboratory evidence of thyroid dysfunction. There is no clear relation between the endocrine disorder and orbital involvement. Treatment of endocrine status may have no effect on the course of ophthalmic disease. Since the ocular motility disorder is one of the most common causes of spontaneous diplopia in middle-aged and older individuals, the associated clinical signs, by which a diagnosis can be established, are reviewed.

Lid retraction is most common in Graves' ophthal-mopathy. Lid retraction may also be seen with lesions of the posterior third ventricle or rostral midbrain, hydrocephalus in infancy, sympathomimetic eye drops, chronic high-dose steroids, hepatic cirrhosis, anomalous synkinesis, hyperkalemic periodic paralysis, and uni-lateral ptosis with overaction of the contralateral levator. Lid lag, best demonstrated with rapid following

movements downward, and decreased blinking, are also
characteristic. Restricted ocular motility is typically
associated with a positive forced duction test indicating
mechanical resistance. Conjunctival vascular engorgement
over the horizontal recti muscle insertions, which may be
hypertrophic, is a helpful clinical sign. Other orbital
signs include proptosis, lid edema, chemosis, and
conjunctival vascular engorgement. Proptosis may also be
seen with orbital neoplasms, inflammatory orbital
syndromes, vascular anomalies, axial myopia, and orbital
encephaloceles. Optic neuropathy occurs in less than 5%
of patients with Graves' ophthalmopathy, but it is a
treatable cause of potentially serious visual loss.

Treatment of the optic neuropathy, motility
disturbance, or significantly uncomfortable orbital signs
usually begins with prednisone 60-100 mg PO qd. Maximal
improvement of the motility disturbance usually occurs
within 4-12 weeks. Maximal improvement of vision usually
occurs within 6-8 weeks, with improvement beginning within
the first week. Longer term steroid therapy is usually
not indicated. If vision does not improve with steroids,
radiation therapy to the orbital apex or surgical decompression may be necessary. Steroids are not indicated for
otherwise asymptomatic proptosis.

Ref: Sergott RC, Glaser JS. Surv Ophthalmol 26:1, 1981.

HALLUCINATIONS

Sensory percepts which are erroneous and have no basis
in reality. They may involve single or multiple sensory
modalities.

Olfactory hallucinations are most frequently organic
(see Olfaction).

Gustatory hallucinations are not strongly localizing,
except that they usually denote temporal lobe or parietal
opercular lesions. They may be manifestations of partial
seizures.

Auditory hallucinations, particularly when present in
isolation, usually indicate a functional psychosis rather
than structural cerebral disease.

Visual hallucinations may be unformed or formed. They
may be due to irritative phenomena or due to release
phenomena resulting from interruption of normal visual
information at any level in the visual pathways.
Classically, unformed hallucinations (such as the aura of
classic migraine) were regarded as arising from the
occipital lobe whereas formed visual hallucinations were
felt to be temporal lobe in origin. However, formed
visual hallucinations can occur in individuals with visual

loss due to ocular or CNS disease as well as in drug intoxications or psychosis. Palinopsia is a form of visual hallucination in which a previously observed object is reperceived, usually in a hemianopic field.

HEADACHE

Classification (modified from Ad Hoc Committee)

Common migraine is an episodic, paroxysmal (lasting hours), throbbing, usually unilateral, headache often associated with nausea, vomiting, or anorexia. The patient seeks a quiet, dark room until symptoms resolve.

Classic migraine is similar to common migraine, but with sharply defined, transient sensory or motor prodromes, most typically, visual disturbances including fortification spectra (zig-zag lines), scintillating scotomas, or flashes of light (photopsias).

Vertebrobasilar migraine is characterized by occipital head pain with associated transient brainstem signs (diplopia, vertigo, incoordination, ataxia, dysarthria, etc.). In children, in particular, it may be associated with occipital lobe epileptiform activity on EEG.

Hemiplegic migraine is associated with unilateral sensory and motor phenomena.

Ophthalmoplegic migraine is most common with third nerve palsy (often pupil sparing). The ophthalmoplegia often outlasts the migraine. It is a diagnosis of exclusion after ruling out aneurysm, diabetes, and other causes of ophthalmoplegia.

Facial migraine ("lower-half" syndrome) consists of unilateral recurrent pain in the lower face. It may overlap with some cranial neuralgias (see below).

Cluster headache is a predomiantly unilateral, severe pain radiating into the region of the eye, usually associated with ipsilateral flushing, sweating, rhinorrhea, nasal stuffiness, lacrimation and, occasionally, ptosis and miosis (Horner's). The pain can last minutes to hours or become chronic. There is often clustering of the headaches, for example, at certain seasons or times of the month. Unlike migraine, men are affected more than women, and patients tend to pace the floor rather than lie quietly.

Cluster headache variants, unlike true cluster, are much briefer and occur more often in women. Variants include chronic paroxysomal hemicrania, multiple "jabs" or "ice-pick headaches". Often there is an underlying vascular type headache. These headaches are remarkable for their response to indomethacin (see below).

Tension/muscle contraction headaches are attributed to stress and "muscle contraction." They are described as tightness, pressure, or band-like constriction around the head or neck.

Combined headaches, including features of vascular and muscle contraction headaches, are very common.

Headaches of nasal vasomotor reaction ("vasomotor rhinitis" include headache and nasal discomfort from congestion and edema of nasal and paranasal mucous membranes not attributed to allergy, infection or mass lesion. They are attributed to stress.

Headaches of delusional, conversion or hypochondriacal states

Nonmigrainous vascular headaches due to dilation of cranial arteries are seen with infections (usually with fever), hypoxia, CO poisoning, vasodilating chemicals (nitrates, nitrites), caffeine-withdrawal, postconcussion syndromes, postconvulsive states, foreign-protein reactions, hypoglycemia, hypercapnea, and sudden elevations of blood pressure.

Traction headaches result from increased intracranial pressure or local traction on intracranial structures. Causes include tumors, hematomas, abscesses, CSF leakage following lumbar puncture, and brain swelling (including pseudotumor cerebri). Any acute severe headache ("worse headache of my life") associated with changes in mental status or other neurological deficit warrants emergency head CT and, possibly, lumbar puncture. Any progressive headache should be evaluated.

Headache due to overt cranial inflammation includes causes of meningeal (septic, aseptic) and vascular (intracranial, extracranial) inflammation. For temporal arteritis, see Vasculitis.

Headache due to disease of ocular, aural, sinus, dental or other cranial or neck structures.

Cranial neuritides

Cranial neuralgias include trigeminal (tic douloureux), and glossopharyngeal neuralgias. There is brief, lancinating pain, often with a "trigger point" (see also Neuralgia, Zoster).

Chronic post-traumatic headaches may result from muscle contraction, vasodilation, or local injury but are increasingly functional the longer the duration.

Treatment

A. Prophylactic treatment of migraine
   1. Avoid any precipitants such as drinking, smoking, or sleep deprivation.

2. Avoid inciting dietary factors such as red wine, aged cheese, chicken liver, pickled herring, chocolate, and foods with monosodium glutamate or nitrates.
3. Trial off oral contraceptives and nitrates, if possible.
4. Medication for those with frequent or disabling attacks.
   a. Methysergide (Sansert) 2 mg PO tid or qid. Need drug holiday every 4-6 months for 1-2 months to prevent fibrotic retroperitoneal or mediastinal changes
   b. Propranolol (Inderal) starting at 20 mg PO tid and gradually increasing as needed to 80 mg tid. Has been used in children.
   c. Amitriptyline (Elavil) starting at 25 mg PO qhs and increasing to 50-100 mg qhs
   d. Indocin 25-50 mg PO tid for cluster headache variants.
   e. Calcium channel blockers: nifedipine 10 mg PO tid or verapamil 80 mg PO tid starting doses.
   f. Cyproheptadine (Periactin) 2-4 mg PO qid.
   g. Ergotamine (Gynergen) 1 mg PO bid (up to 10 mg weekly, skipping 2 days).
   h. Ergotamine/belladonna/phenobarbital (Bellergal) 2-4 tabs PO qd.
   i. Anticonvulsants (phenytoin) in children with seizures.

B. Symptomatic or abortive therapy
   1. Routine analgesics (aspirin, acetaminophen)
   2. Narcotic analgesics should be avoided. They can be useful for occasional severe headaches.
   3. Ergotamine preparations are available for administration orally, sublingually, rectally and by inhalation:
      a. Ergotamine (Gynergen) 1 mg PO q1/2h up to 5 mg/attack.
      b. Ergotamine 1 mg/caffeine 100 mg (Cafergot), 1-2 tabs PO q1/2h up to 5/attack.
      c. Ergotamine (Ergomar) 2 mg SL q1/2h up to 3/day.
      d. Ergotamine/caffeine (Cafergot) suppository, 1 PR, may repeat in 1 hr prn.
   4. Isometheptene (Midrin) 2 capsules at onset and 1 q 1 hour prn up to 5 capsules per headache
   5. Ibuprofen (Motrin) 400-800 mg PO at onset and repeat q4h prn
   6. Metoclopramide (Reglan) 10 mg IM, IV or PO 15 minutes prior to other analgesic agents has proven useful

7. Prednisone 40-60 mg PO qd over a short course may break "status migrainosus"
8. Biofeedback

C. Treatment of cluster headache
   1. Treat as for migraine (ergotamine, methysergide)
   2. 100% O_2 by mask at 6 l/min
   3. Prednisone 40-60 mg PO qd over short course; rebound headaches can occur after discontinuation.
   4. Lithium carbonate 300 mg PO bid-qid with lithium levels (0.6-1.2mEq/l) is especially useful for chronic cluster headaches

Ref: Ad Hoc Committee on Classification of Headache. JAMA 179:717, 1962.

HEAD CIRCUMFERENCE (see Child Neurology)

HEARING

SELECTED CAUSES OF HEARING LOSS

LOCATION	TREATMENT
External ear	
Impacted cerumen	Irrigation
Foreign body	Remove
External otitis	Antibiotics
Middle ear (conductive)	
Effusion from infection or eustachian tube obstruction	Tympanotomy tube; unblock eustachian tube
Tympanomastoiditis and tympanosclerosis	Antibiotics; surgery; hearing aid
Tumors (cholesteatoma, glomus tumors)	Surgery
Middle and/or inner ear	
Otosclerosis	Sodium fluoride, calcium gluconate, and vitamin D; stapedectomy; hearing aid
Paget's disease	Hearing aid; etidronate

LOCATION	TREATMENT
Inner ear (cochlear, sensorineural)	
Presbycusis	Hearing aid
Ototoxic drugs (aspirin, aminoglycosides, diuretics)	Discontinue or reduce dose; monitor drug levels
Viral infections	
Meningitis	Antibiotics
Syphilis	Antibiotics
Trauma	
Waldenstrom's macro-globulinemia	Plasmapharesis
Meniere's disease	Low Na diet; diuretics
Eighth nerve and CNS (retrocochlear)	
Cerebellopontine angle tumors (schwannoma, meningioma, arachnoid cysts)	Surgery
Paget's disease	As above
Brainstem lesions	
Psychogenic	Psychotherapy

Bedside testing of hearing includes whispering into each ear while closing the other and comparing the distance from the ear that the patient and examiner can hear a watch ticking. Various tuning fork tests are commonly used. In Weber's, a tuning fork is placed at the midline vertex of the skull; sound referred to an ear with decreased acuity indicates conductive hearing loss. In Rinne's, a tuning fork placed on the mastoid and held in front of the ear are compared; if bone conduction is greater, conductive loss is implied. In Schwabach's, a tuning fork is placed on the mastoid until the patient no longer hears it and then transferred to examiner's mastoid for comparison.

Audiologic tests are used collectively to quantitate and localize (conductive, sensorineural, cochlear, retrocochlear) hearing loss. Pure tone threshold determines auditory threshold for tones over various frequencies and intensities for both air and bone conduction. Impairment of both air and bone conduction, especially at high frequencies, indicates sensorineural hearing loss. Bone conduction > air conduction indicates conductive hearing loss. Recruitment (alternate binaural loudness balance) measures perceived loudness of tone increases compared to their actual intensity. It is present in cochlear and absent in retrocochlear disease. Short increment sensitivity index (SISI) measures the ability to perceive small incremental increases in sound intensity superimposed on a steady background tone. It is increased in cochlear and decreased in retrocochlear hearing loss. Bekesy testing determines the auditory threshold for both continuous and intermittent tones over various frequencies and intensities. Specific types of curves distinguish cochlear from retrocochlear involvement. Tone decay tests measure the decrease in audibility of a long steady tone. It is slight in cochlear, prominent in retrocochlear disease. Speech discrimination tests evaluate perception of spoken words. They are abnormal in retrocochlear hearing loss. The stapedius reflex measures tympanic membrane impedance which is dependent on pathways from cochlea to acoustic nerve to facial nerve branch to stapedius muscle. It is often absent in retrocochlear disease. Brainstem auditory evoked responses (BAER's) evaluate auditory pathways from ear to cortex by recording computer-averaged electrical responses evoked by multiple discrete auditory stimuli.

HEMORRHAGE

Primary intraparenchymal (intracerebral) hemorrhage, due to hypertension, occurs (in order of decreasing incidence) in the basal ganglia (especially putamen), thalamus, cerebellum, and pons. It is usually due to rupture of Charcot-Bouchard hypertensive microaneurysms. Symptoms are of abrupt onset with evolution over minutes to hours. Headache is present in 50-60% of cases. Usually there are no prodromal symptoms. Specific symptoms and signs depend on location and size of the hemorrhage.

Putamenal hemorrhage is associated with contralateral hemiparesis, hemianesthesia, and homonymous hemianopia with aphasia or neglect (depending on dominant or non-dominant hemispheric involvement). There is also decreased level of consciousness, ipsilateral eye deviation, and normal pupils.

Thalamic hemorrhage produces contralateral hemisensory loss with variable hemiparesis, contralateral homonymous hemianopia, vertical and/or lateral gaze palsies (including "wrong way" deviation), and, occasionally, nystagmus.

Cerebellar hemorrhage is associated with severe occipital headache, sudden nausea and vomiting, and truncal ataxia (appendicular ataxia and nystagmus in some). Brainstem compression is not uncommon and may result in a variety of signs (ipsilateral V, VI, horizontal gaze palsy, and/or VII). Prompt diagnosis is extremely important since surgical evacuation may be lifesaving.

Pontine hemorrhage causes coma, pinpoint pupils (reactive to light), bilateral extensor posturing, impaired ocular motility, and impaired caloric testing.

Acute mortality in intracerebral hemorrhage is usually due to mass effect with herniation or brainstem compression. Acute mortality is high, especially in posterior fossa hemorrhage. The long-term prognosis for recovery of function may be better than in infarction since there is usually displacement of tissue instead of primary infarction and necrosis.

Diagnosis is confirmed with CT; blood appears as a hyperdensity. Angiography may be necessary to exclude causes such as vascular malformations or tumors.

Management is carried out in an intensive care setting with frequent neurological evaluation. Maintain adequate ventilation and pulmonary/pharyngeal toilet. Maintain adequate fluid and electrolyte balance. Antiedema agents may be used; it is not certain that they are effective. Blood pressure management is controversial; induced hypotension is contraindicated. Neurosurgical evaluation should be obtained for superficially located cerebral hemorrhages and all cerebellar hemorrhages.

Other causes of intraparenchymal hemorrhage:
1. Trauma.
2. Ruptured arteriovenous malformation (see also Angiomas). Chronic unilateral headaches or seizures occur in 1/3 of cases before rupture. Most patients survive the first hemorrhage, after which there is a 4%/year risk of rebleeding, with a high mortality. Treatment depends on size, location and other characteristics of the lesion. Treatment includes surgical excision, embolization, high energy therapy (proton beam, x-ray), or a combination of these.
3. Ruptured aneurysm with parenchymal extension (see below).

4. Metastatic carcinoma, especially lung, chorio-carcinoma, melanoma, and renal adenocarcinoma.
5. Primary neoplasm.
6. Embolic infarction with secondary hemorrhage (up to 1/3 of embolic infarcts).
7. Hematologic disorders, including leukemia, lymphoma, thrombocytopenic purpura, aplastic anemia, sickle cell anemia, hemophilia, hypoprothrombinemia (especially anticoagulant therapy), afibrinogenemia, Waldenstrom's macroglobulinemia.
8. Cerebral amyloid angiopathy usually presents as multiple, recurrent hemorrhages in white matter or cortical gray matter, sparing deep gray (as opposed to hypertensive hemorrhages). It usually occurs in elderly women with dementia. Amyloid angiopathy has been suggested as the cause in 5-10% of the cases of sporadic intracerebral hemorrhage. Attempts at surgical evacuation are usually futile since the vessels are very fragile, bleeding is very difficult to control, and there is a high incidence of recurrent hemorrhages.
9. Vasculopathies such as lupus, polyarteritis nodosa, and granulomatous arteritis.
10. Cortical vein thrombosis with secondary hemorrhage.

Subarachnoid hemorrhage (SAH) occurs with an incidence of 15/100,000, with peak incidence at 55-60 years of age. Clinical presentation is characterized by sudden severe headache ("worst headache of my life"). Changes in level of consciousness range from lethargy to coma, depending on location and extent of hemorrhage and presence or absence of intraparenchymal and ventricular extension. Such extension is associated with a significantly higher mortality. Sudden loss of consciousness is the presenting feature in 20%. Meningeal signs, papilledema (or retinal hemorrhages), and seizures are common. Focal signs present in the first 24 hours usually indicate parenchymal dissection, cerebral edema, or hypoperfusion distal to the ruptured aneurysm. After the first 48-72 hours, focal signs may be due to vasospasm.

The Hunt-Hess grading scale is commonly used for prognosis and timing of aneurysm surgery.

0	Unruptured aneurysm
1	Asymptomatic or minimal headache and mild nuchal rigidity
1a	No acute meningeal or brain reaction but fixed neurological deficit present.

2   Moderate to severe headache, nuchal rigidity, no neurological deficit other than cranial nerve palsy

3   Drowsiness, confusion or mild focal neurological deficit

4   Stupor, moderate to severe hemiparesis, possible early decerebrate rigidity and vegetative disturbances

5   Deep coma, decerebrate rigidity, moribund appearance

Causes of SAH include rupture of aneurysm (80% of nontraumatic SAH, see also Aneurysm), extension from intraparenchymal hemorrhage, rupture of AVM, trauma, hematologic disorders, and neoplasms (see also Pregnancy).

Diagnostic evaluation includes CT which may allow diagnosis in the majority of cases, although it may be negative in up to 15%. LP is necessary if the CT is negative. Angiography is done to locate and define the cause of SAH (aneurysm, AVM), and generally should be repeated in 5-15 days if it is initially negative.

Treatment consists of bed rest in an ICU with continuous monitoring and frequent neurological evaluation. Correct systemic complications. CT should be repeated if there is any significant neurological deterioration after the initial event or if a rebleed is suspected. Give phenytoin for seizure prophylaxis.

Prevention of rebleeding is aided by monitoring blood pressure and treating hypertension. Blood pressure should be kept within the normal range. There is a trend away from induced hypotension due to the significant risk of ischemic complications. Antifibrinolytic agents are used in some centers; epsilon aminocaproic acid (Amicar), at least 36 gm/day, is given by continuous IV infusion for up to 3 weeks and gradually tapered. Recent evidence suggests that the decreased mortality from rebleeding is offset by an increased mortality from vasospasm in the antifibrinolytic group. Side effects of epsilon aminocaproic acid include diarrhea (frequent), reversible myopathy, and thrombroembolic disease.

Prevention of vasospasm is a goal of the use of calcium channel blockers such as nimodipine, 0.7 mg/kg po initially followed by 0.35 mg/kg q4h for 21 days. A recent controlled, double blind study revealed that it did not prevent the occurrence of neurological deficits due to vasospasm but there was a reduction in the severe neurological complications (death, coma, permanent major motor deficit). Further study is needed. Other agents have been used with variable results, including aminophylline, dopamine, and isoproterenol. Their use cannot be recommended.

Surgical therapy consists of clipping the aneurysm under good neuroanesthesia with intraoperative induced hypotension and controlled ventilation. Recent evidence suggests that surgery may be done earlier than the conventional waiting period of 1-2 weeks without increased morbidity. Of major importance is the early risk of rebleeding (greater than 20% in the first 2 weeks). The later occurrence of hydrocephalus may require shunting.

Complications and sequelae result from systemic disorders, vasospasm, rebleeding, herniation, and hydrocephalus. Systemic complications include hyponatremia secondary to SIADH, cardiac dysrhythmias, diabetes insipidus, pulmonary embolism, gastrointestinal bleeding, and respiratory depression and arrest. Arterial vasospasm occurs frequently 4-14 days after the initial hemorrhage and may cause cerebral ischemia or infarction. The amount of subarachnoid blood is related to the rate of occurrence of vasospasm. Rebleeding is usually attributed to lysis of the clot that tamponades the aneurysm after the initial bleed. The risk of rebleeding has been considered to peak between days 5-9, although recent evidence suggests the peak occurs on the first day. Slightly more than 20% rebleed in the first 2 weeks, while 33% rebleed in the first month with a mortality rate of 42% (higher than the mortality from the initial bleed). The annual rate of rebleeding after the first 6 months is 3-6% (series variability) which carries a 1-3% annual mortality. The occurrence of apnea correlates well with a rebleed. Overall, 42% survive 30 days, 39% survive 6 months.

<u>Subdural hemorrhage</u> (SDH) may be acute or chronic. Acute SDH is usually due to trauma with tearing of bridging veins. There is initial loss of consciousness with regaining of consciousness (lucid interval) followed in several hours by progressive deterioration of mental status, confusion and headache. This pattern is variable. Lateralizing signs may be present. Diagnosis is based on clinical course, emergency CT (increased density of lesion), skull x-rays and, if necessary, angiography. The treatment is emergency neurosurgical evacuation.

Chronic SDH is less clearly related to trauma, and may be seen following minor head trauma in elderly alcoholics and in patients on anticoagulants. Symptoms and signs resemble those in acute SDH but they develop gradually over several days to weeks. Lateralizing signs are common. Mental status changes may suggest dementia. Diagnosis is as for acute SDH. The lesion on CT is usually hypodense. The treatment is neurosurgical evacuation with or without intraoperative brain expansion or postoperative drainage. The prognosis for survival and recovery in surgically treated patients is generally good.

<u>Acute epidural hemorrhage</u> results from skull fracture with laceration of the middle meningeal artery and vein. The clinical course is similar to acute SDH but is more rapidly progressive. Rapid herniation, respiratory depression, and death may ensue. The diagnosis is established emergently as for acute SDH. The treatment, like acute SDH, is a neurosurgical emergency, requiring drainage and ligation of the bleeding vessel and repair of the skull fracture.

Ref: Drake CG. Management of cerebral aneurysms. Stroke 12:273, 1981.

Kassel NF, Torner JC. Aneurysmal rebleeding: A preliminary report from the cooperative aneurysm study. Neurosurgery 13:479, 1983.

Robinson RG. Chronic subdural hematoma: Surgical management in 133 patients. J Neurosurg 61:263, 1984.

Winn HR, et al. The long term prognosis in untreated cerebral aneurysms: I. The incidence of late hemorrhage in cerebral aneurysm: A 10 year evaluation of 364 patients. Ann Neurol 1:358, 1977.

HERNIATION

Displacement of cerebral or cerebellar structures from one compartment to another, invariably due to a mass lesion or extremely focal cerebral edema. Diffuse elevations of intracranial pressure, as in pseudotumor cerebri, rarely produce herniation. The involved structures and clinical signs in the four most common herniation syndromes are summarized below.

HERNIATION SYNDROMES

Syndrome	Anatomy	Signs
Lateral tentorial (uncal)	Oculomotor nerve, cerebral peduncle, posterior cerebral artery	Oculomotor palsy, hemiparesis, hemianopsia
Central tentorial (axial brainstem)	Reticular formation Corticospinal tracts, midbrain	Altered consciousness, extensor posturing, dilated pupils, oculomotor palsies
Foramenal (tonsillar)	Medulla	Apnea
Subfalcine (cingulate)	Cingulate gyrus, anterior cerebral arteries	Leg weakness

HERPES SIMPLEX (see Encephalitis)

HERPES ZOSTER (see Zoster)

HICCUPS (SINGULTUS, HICCOUGHS)

A recurrent reflex myoclonic contraction of the diaphragm with a forceful inspiration, associated with laryngeal spasm and closure of glottis producing a characteristic sound. It is mediated by the phrenic nerve (afferent) and vagus and thoracic nerves (efferent). Gastrointestinal, pulmonary and cardiovascular symptoms and signs may be present. Carcinoma, achalasia, and hiatal hernia are common pathological causes. Intrathoracic structural causes include esophageal irritation, gastric distention, pulmonary or pleural irritation, pericarditis, mediastinitis or mediastinal mass, intrathoracic abscesses or tumors, and aortic aneurysm. CNS causes are many, including metabolic (acetonemia, uremia), drugs (sulfonamides), infection (encephalitis), hypothalamic disease (also associated with yawning), fourth ventricular tumors, and cerebrovascular disease (vertebrobasilar insufficiency). Idiopathic and psychogenic hiccups are common.

Treatment is usually not required as hiccups, which occur commonly in normal subjects, are usually self limited. They may be intractable, especially if there is a primary cause, in which case the underlying cause is treated. Drug therapies for intractable hiccups include phenothiazines (prochlorperazine, chlorpromazine), phenytoin, carbamazepine, benzodiazepines (clonazepam, diazepam), and baclofen. Surgical sectioning of the phrenic nerve or selective vagotomy are occasionally done.

HORNER'S SYNDROME (see also Ptosis, Pupil)

Results from damage to the oculosympathetic pathways (see page 146) and consists of unilateral ptosis, miosis and anhidrosis. Narrowing of the palpebral fissure is secondary to ptosis of the upper lid and slight elevation of the lower lid (paresis of Muller's muscles). Isolated "upside down ptosis" of the lower lid may occur. The anisocoria increases in darkness. Occasionally pupillary involvement can only be demonstrated on pharmacological testing. Anhidrosis occurs in 5%, usually with pre-ganglionic lesions (fibers travel with external carotid artery branches). Vascular dilation (face and conjunctiva) is transient. Iris heterochromia may be seen in congenital Horner's. Enophthalmos is not a feature of oculosympathetic palsy.

Cause of Horner's syndrome can be determined in approximately 60%. Causes include tumors 13% (lung, mediastinum, thyroid, pharynx, lymphoma, spinal cord), cluster headache 12%, iatrogenic 10%, Raeder's syndrome 4%, trauma 4%, cervical disc 3%, congenital 3%, vascular 5%+, meningitis, Wallenberg syndrome, syringomyelia, polio, ALS, cervical rib, pneumothorax, migraine, and Romberg's syndrome (unilateral facial soft tissue atrophy, uveitis, cranial nerve dysfunction, seizures). Alternating Horner's has been described in lesions of the lower cervical and upper thoracic cord and in Shy-Drager syndrome. Diabetes mellitus and hypertension occur frequently in the undiagnosed group suggesting a vascular cause.

Raeder's syndrome (paratrigeminal neuralgia) consists of hemicrania and ipsilateral postganglionic oculosympathetic palsy with or without cranial nerve (III, IV, V, VI) dysfunction. Associated cranial nerve involvement indicates disease in the middle cranial fossa and work-up is indicated. Hemicrania and postganglionic oculosympathetic palsy alone is most commonly caused by a cluster headache variant, and neuroradiological evaluation is usually not necessary. Persistent facial pain, however, may be seen with various carotid artery lesions and is an indication for further evaluation.

Oculosympathetic Pathways

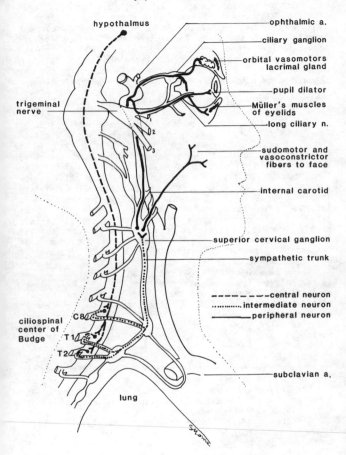

Pharmacological diagnosis of Horner's utilizes cocaine 4%-10%, which dilates normal pupils by preventing the re-uptake of norepinephrine from sympathetic nerve endings. This mydriatic effect depends on an intact sympathetic pathway. Disruption at any level will prevent norepinephrine release at the terminal endings and failure of the pupil to dilate in response to cocaine.

Hydroxyamphetamine 1%-2% is used to differentiate pre- and postganglionic lesions. It dilates normal pupils by releasing norepinephrine from nerve endings. The mydriatic effect depends on an intact third order neuron. At least 12 hours should elapse before giving hydroxy-amphetamine after cocaine. Apply 1 drop to the affected eye, repeat after 5 minutes, and determine the change in pupillary size after 30 minutes.

Prognosis in isolated, new onset postganglionic Horner's is generally benign. Preganglionic Horner's should be evaluated to exclude malignancy.

Ref: Maloney WF, et al. Am J Ophthalmol 90:394, 1980.

         Grimson BS, Thompson HS. Surv Ophthalmol 24:199, 1980.

HYDROCEPHALUS (see also Macrocephaly, Shunts)

Dilation of the ventricular system may result from atrophy or decreased volume of the cerebral parenchyma ("ex vacuo") or from a blockage of CSF flow. Blockage of CSF within the ventricular system causes non-communicating hydrocephalus. Communicating hydrocephalus is caused by blockage in the subarachnoid space, arachnoid villi or draining venous structures. Rarely, hydrocephalus may result from increased CSF production associated with choroid plexus papilloma. Sudden obstruction of CSF pathways produces an acute rise in intracranial pressure with rapid progression of clinical symptoms which may terminate in death. Gradual obstruction causes a chronic hydrocephalus with a variety of clinical symptoms depending on the underlying cause and the age of the patient; dementia is a common feature in older patients. Normal pressure hydrocephalus, a clinical syndrome of dementia, incontinence and hydrocephalus with normal CSF pressure, is of uncertain pathogenesis; response to shunting is variable.

Hydrocephalus in children is commonly congenital (aqueductal stenosis, abnormal development of the foramina of Magendie and Luschka, see Craniocervical Junction, Developmental Malformations) or secondary to hemorrhage, inflammation or pressure from intracranial masses. Causes in adults include subarachnoid hemorrhage, chronic meningeal inflammation and trauma.

CT may distinguish hydrocephalus with enlarged ventricles from cortical atrophy with associated widened sulci, increased interhemispheric fissure and increased insular cisterns (see page 149). CT may distinguish communicating from non-communicating hydrocephalus if the fourth ventricle is enlarged as well as the lateral and third ventricles. Radionuclide flow studies (isotope cisternography) and CSF pressure monitoring may yield additional information regarding CSF dynamics.

Acutely increased intracranial pressure requires emergency management (see Intracranial Pressure). Generally, management consists of surgical shunting (see Shunts). Benefit from shunting depends on acuteness of onset and duration of symptoms.

HYPERACTIVE CHILD (see also Learning Disabilities)

DSM III lists the following diagnostic criteria:

1. Excessive general activity and motor restlessness for age
2. Difficulty concentrating on and completing tasks
3. Impulsive behavior including at least two of the following:

   Sloppy work despite effort to be neat
   Speaking out of turn
   Interruption or intrusion into others' activities
   Inability to wait one's turn
   Inability to tolerate frustration
   Fighting with other children out of frustration

The etiology is unknown. There is usually no other evidence of neurological disorder. About 5% are associated with identifiable neurological disease. Evaluation should include:

1. Complete history, including perinatal, developmental, and social
2. Discussion of problem areas and corrective efforts by parents and teachers
3. Complete evaluation from the school (teachers and psychologists)
4. Neurological exam

Developmental regression or neurological findings should be assessed with appropriate tests (audiologic evaluation, metabolic screen, CT scan). If the main

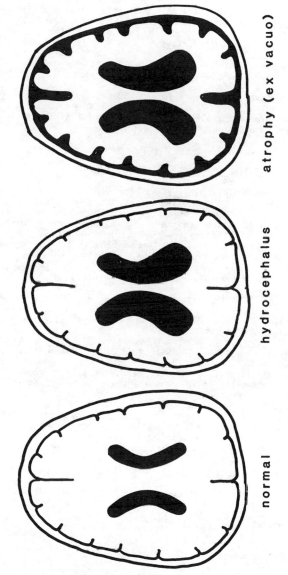

CT APPEARANCE OF NORMAL AND ENLARGED VENTRICLES

normal

hydrocephalus

atrophy (ex vacuo)

behavior problems are at school, placement in a smaller class with more individual direction may be advisable. If problems are at home and school, a trial of behavior therapy can be undertaken. Many cities and counties have residential or day-school programs using behavior therapy. Parents must be involved for this to succeed. Drug therapy (methylphenidate, dextroamphetamine, pemoline) is controversial.

Five and ten-year follow-up studies reveal that hyperactive children have continued impulsive behavior and poor performance in cognitive and visuomotor tests; adolescent drug abuse or psychotic behavior is more frequent.

Ref: Weiss G, et al. Science 205:1348, 1979.

HYPERVENTILATION (see also Respiration)

Involuntary hyperventilation due to autonomous hyperactivity of brainstem respiratory centers (central neurogenic hyperventilation) is rare in man. Before hyperventilation can be attributed to a neurological cause, it is necessary to: 1) Rule out metabolic causes of hyperventilation. There should be no hypoxemia (decreased arterial PO_2) or CSF acidosis (increased CSF $pCO2$ or decreased CSF pH). 2) Rule out cardiopulmonary causes, especially pulmonary congestion and causes of low arterial PO_2 (per above). 3) Exclude drug effects (e.g., aspirin causing an anion-gap metabolic acidosis and respiratory alkalosis). 4) Exclude voluntary hyperventilation. Tachypnea and hyperpnea should continue in sleep and/or coma.

Voluntary hyperventilation is very common and frequently associated with anxiety, including that related to organic illness or pain. Typical symptoms include acral (tips of fingers and toes) and perioral numbness and paresthesias, often with lightheadedness and occasionally with carpopedal spasm. There may be many additional symptoms, including cramps, anxiety, chest pain, dyspnea, palpitations, GI distress, insomnia, and general asthenia. Arterial blood gases revealing a respiratory alkalosis may help make the diagnosis, however, they are typically normal between attacks. Reproduction of symptoms by hyperventilation is more helpful.

Hyperventilation during exercise is hyperpneic, tachypneic normoventilation, since pCO_2 and pH generally remain normal. Alkalemia does not result, in contrast to true hyperventilation.

HYPOGLYCEMIA (see Glucose)

HYPOTONIC INFANT (See also Reflexes)

DIFFERENTIAL DIAGNOSIS OF THE FLOPPY INFANT
BY ANATOMICAL LOCALIZATION
(after Dubowitz, 1969)

LOCALIZATION AND ASSOCIATED SIGNS	CAUSE
Cerebral cortex:	
Hyperreflexia, extensor plantars; may have language or cognitive dysfunction, dysmorphic features (may become hypertonic)	Atonic cerebral palsy (most common); other encephalopathies (hypoxic-ischemic, intracranial hemorrhage, birth trauma); metabolic disorders (amino-acidurias, mucopoly-saccharidoses, lipidoses); genetic syndromes
Basal ganglia:	
Dystonia, choreoathetosis (may become hypertonic)	Athetoid cerebral palsy; kernicterus
Cerebellum:	
Ataxia	Ataxic cerebral palsy
Spinal cord:	
Hypo- or hyperreflexia, extensor plantars, sensory level, sweat level, normal cognition; may have respiratory distress or paraplegia	Birth injury (breech delivery); developmental malformations (spinal dysraphism)

LOCALIZATION AND ASSOCIATED SIGNS	CAUSE
Anterior horn cell:	
Areflexia, normal sensation normal cortical function	Infantile spinal muscular atrophy (Werdnig-Hoffman); glycogen storage disease; poliomyelitis
Root, plexus, nerve:	
Hyporeflexia, abnormal nerve conduction studies	Leukodystrophies (Metachromatic, Krabbe's)
Neuromuscular junction:	
Ocular, facial, oropharyngeal, respiratory, and/or appendicular weakness	Myasthenia gravis; hypermagnesemia; neuromuscular blocking drugs, botulism
Muscle:	
May have ptosis, ophthalmoplegia, facial weakness, sucking/swallowing difficulty, respiratory problems, contractures, arthrogryposis, dislocated hips, or dysmorphic features; abnormal EMG; or muscle biopsy	Congenital structural myopathies (nemaline, central core, myotubular), metabolic myopathies (glycogenoses); mitochondrial disease; myotonic dystrophy; polymyositis; periodic paralysis
Connective tissue:	
Normal neurological exam	Congenital laxity of ligaments; Marfan's syndrome; Ehlers-Danlos syndrome; osteogenesis imperfecta; arachnodactyly

Systemic causes of hypotonia: acute illness (infection, dehydration), hypercalcemia, renal acidosis, hypothyroidism, rickets, celiac disease. Miscellaneous causes include: Prader-Willi syndrome (hypotonia, hypomentia, hypogonadism, obesity), benign congenital hypotonia.

Ref: Dubowitz V. The floppy infant. In, Clinics in Developmental Medicine. Spastics International Medical Publications, No. 31. London: W. Heinemann, 1969.

IMMUNIZATION

Most patients receiving immunizations do not experience complications.

Influenza vaccine complications include Guillain-Barre syndrome (1/100,000 immunizations, usually within 5 weeks of immunization), encephalopathy/encephalitis (rare, usually within 4 days, accompanied by systemic signs), brachial plexopathy (usually unilateral), acute transverse myelitis, cranial neuropathies (rare, single or multiple, VII most common), and optic neuritis (rare).

Diphtheria-pertussis-tetanus (DPT) vaccine complications are almost entirely attributed to pertussis. Encephalopathy (1/310,000) may be associated with seizures and coma and a risk of permanent neurological damage. Seizures may also occur with fever unassociated with encephalopathy. Acute transverse myelitis occurs rarely after diphtheria and tetanus. Brachial plexopathy is rare after diphtheria, tetanus and DPT. Guillain-Barre syndrome is rare after tetanus. Infantile spasms, Reye's syndrome and infantile hemiplegia cannot be attributed to DPT.

Measles-mumps-rubella (MMR) vaccine complications are attributed to measles. There are no reported neurological complications after mumps vaccination. The risk of sub-acute sclerosing panencephalitis following measles vaccination is much less than following natural measles infection (5-10/1 million). A syndrome of bilateral popliteal fossa pain may occur 29-70 days post-immunization, persisting for 2-14 days. Acute transverse myelitis and optic neuropathy are rare.

Trivalent oral polio vaccination is associated with a paralytic disease reported in recipients and close contacts of vaccine recipients (1/3 million doses). It usually occurs 1 month postimmunization. Immunosuppressed individuals are at increased risk.

Ref: Fenischel GM. Ann Neurol 12:119, 1982.

IMPOTENCE

Male sexual dysfunction results from a complex interaction of psychological, neurological, vascular, endocrine, and physical factors. Reflex erection is mediated by the sacral plexus, pudendal nerve, and nerve erigentes. Psychogenic erection is mediated by cerebral cortex and sympathetic thoracolumbar and parasympathetic sacral plexus. Many authors feel that the limbic system also plays an important role in erection, with neurotransmitters modulating this higher cortical response.

Causes of impotence are approximately equally divided between functional and organic. Endocrine causes include diabetes (peripheral diabetic neuropathy, abnormal cystograms) and pituitary axis dysfunction (prolactin secreting pituitary adenoma, hypogonadism). Vascular etiologies include atherosclerosis, arteritis, priapism, and thromboembolism. Impotence may follow cystectomy, radical prostatectomy, abdominal perineal resection of the rectum, abdominal aortic aneurysm repair, or external sphincterotomy. Spinal cord dysfunction (tumor, trauma) has been implicated, however, studies of these populations show a much higher incidence of sexual function than would be expected based on the anatomical involvement. Non-diabetic autonomic dysfunction (Shy-Drager, Riley-Day) as well as multiple sclerosis, Parkinson's disease, and syphilis may be associated with impotence. Inflammation (urethritis, prostatitis, cystitis) and mechanical factors (congenital malformation, Peyronie's disease, morbid obesity, malignancy, phimosis, hydrocele, ruptured urethra) may result in impotence. Sedating drugs may impair libido. Alcohol may cause malnutrition and peripheral neuropathy as well as sedation. Anticholinergic drug side effects may impair erection. Drugs that interfere with sympathetic neurotransmission may impair ejaculation.

History is aimed at distinguishing between functional and organic factors (adequacy of neurological and vascular pathways) and identification of specific causes. Inquire about:

1. Onset and progression of sexual dysfunction
2. Ejaculation and orgasm
3. Morning and nocturnal erection pattern
4. Relation to masturbation
5. Response to different sexual partners
6. Endocrine, vascular, or neurological disease
7. Previous surgery
8. Medication, alcohol.

Examination is aimed at identifying evidence of systemic or endocrine illness and peripheral vascular disease. Neurological exam should seek evidence of peripheral neuropathy, autonomic neuropathy, myelopathy or sacral radiculopathy. Urological or gynecological consultation should be obtained. Laboratory studies should include fasting blood sugars, prolactin and testosterone levels. Additional urological or neurological studies may be necessary.

Conjoint sex therapy is the mainstay of treatment for functional impotence. After remediable organic etiologies have been treated, penile prosthesis implantation can be done by a urologist in refractory cases. Pelvic revascularization is largely experimental.

Ref: Montague DK. Urology 14:545, 1979.

Ellenberg M. Ann Int Med 75:213, 1971.

INFECTION (see Abscess, Encephalitis, Meningitis)

INTRACRANIAL PRESSURE (ICP)

Normal ICP is <15-20 mm Hg. Increased ICP is seen with mass lesions (tumors, abscesses, hematomas), with or without associated focal edema, and with diffuse cerebral edema, such as from hypoxia or head trauma. A rapid elevation in ICP is a neurological emergency. In such cases, plateau waves, consisting of episodic surges of pressure exceeding 35 mm Hg, can occur several times an hour and are associated with an increased risk of herniation if a focal lesion is present.

The medical treatment of increased intracranial pressure includes elevation of the head to >30° above the horizontal, hyperventilation with maintenance of the P_{CO_2} between 25-30 mm Hg, avoiding hypotonic intravenous solutions, and fluid restriction. Dexamethasone 100 mg IV is given stat, followed by 6 mg q6h. The effect begins in 4-6 hrs and peaks in 24 hrs, and is greater for vasogenic rather than cytotoxic edema. Mannitol is also given acutely as a 20% solution IV at 1.5-2.0 gm/kg (usually 50 gm or 250 ml of 20% solution). The effect is immediate and lasts several hours. A bladder catheter should be in place. Vital signs, electrolytes, BUN, and osmolality are monitered. Serum osmolality is increased to 300-320 mOsm/l. Hypothermia (cooling blanket) is recommended by some.

Barbiturate coma should still be considered experimental and be done only in well equipped neurological intensive care units by experienced personnel.

When feasible, ICP is continuously monitored after placement of an intraventricular catheter or subdural pressure screw. Surgical decompression or shunting may be indicated in certain settings.

ISCHEMIA (see also Amaurosis Fugax, Hemorrhage, Lacunar Syndromes)

"Stroke" is a nonspecific term referring to the acute onset of neurological dysfunction due to cerebrovascular disease (hemorrhagic or ischemic) which lasts longer than 24 hours. Transient ischemic attack (TIA) refers to a vascular neurological deficit usually lasting <15-30 minutes, but which may last up to 24 hours. Reversible ischemic neurological deficits (RIND) last from 24 hours to 3 weeks. Progressing "stroke" (infarction) refers to a vascular neurological deficit with worsening symptoms and signs, usually over a time course of up to 18 hours in the carotid distribution and up to 2-3 days in the vertebro-basilar distribution. Completed "stroke" (infarct) indicates that a patient has acquired a stable neuro-logical deficit, complete or incomplete, without evidence of progression. See also Lacunar Syndromes.

Central nervous system ischemia or infarction should be described in terms of its vascular anatomy. Middle cerebral artery distribution involvement typically produces contralateral hemiparesis (face and arm greater than leg), horizontal gaze palsy, hemisensory deficits, and homonymous hemianopia, as well as various "higher cortical" deficits (aphasia, alexia, apraxia, agnosia, neglect). Anterior cerebral artery distribution lesions produce contralateral hemiparesis (leg > arm and face) and may also produce contralateral grasp reflex, Gegenhalten rigidity, abulia, gait disorder, persevera-tion, and urinary incontinence. The vascular anatomy of the anterior cerebral artery may vary, producing, for example, bilateral anterior cerebral artery signs due to involvement of a single vessel of common origin. The middle cerebral and anterior cerebral arteries are both distal to the internal carotid artery ("anterior circulation") and, thus, the above deficits may also be seen with more proximal involvement. Retinal artery distribution ischemia (see Amaurosis Fugax) may reflect internal artery disease. The posterior cerebral arteries, though usually supplied by the vertebrobasilar artery ("posterior circulation"), may be supplied from the anterior circulation. Posterior cerebral involvement characteristically produces a contralateral homonymous hemianopia (or quadrantanopia), but may also produce memory loss, dyslexia without dysgraphia, color anomia, contralateral hemisensory deficits, and mild contralateral hemiparesis. Vertebrobasilar involvement may produce a variety of unilateral or bilateral signs reflecting involvement of motor and sensory tracts, cerebellum, the various cranial nerves and/or posterior cerebral arteries (see above). See also Brainstem Syndromes. Vertebrobasilar symptoms and signs include diplopia, ipsilateral horizontal gaze palsy, internuclear ophthalmoplegia, ataxia, nystagmus, vertigo, nausea, vomiting, hearing loss, tinnitus, dysphagia, dysarthria, drop attacks, as well as motor (quadraparesis, hemiparesis) and sensory (face and body crossed) involvement. Other causes of an isolated symptom (vertigo, diplopia, dysphagia, drop attack) should be excluded before attributing it to vertebrobasilar insufficiency. Cerebellar infarction is characterized early by dizziness, nausea, vomiting, nystagmus, and ataxia. Recognition is important in order to detect brainstem compression due to swelling; neurosurgical decompression may be lifesaving.

The characteristic clinical profile of embolic infarction is that of a sudden onset maximal neurological deficit that may rapidly improve. Thrombotic infarction is often preceded by TIA's and may progress over hours or days in a stuttering fashion. Intraparenchymal and subarachnoid hemorrhages are typically of sudden onset with severe headache and, often, with changes in mental status. The advent of CT has revealed the limitations of these profiles.

In addition to the history and neurological exam, attention should be given to blood pressure (in both upper extremities and with postural changes), cardiac exam, bruits, facial pulses, funduscopy (for evidence of retinal emboli), ophthalmodynamometry, and evidence of peripheral emboli.

Initial diagnostic evaluation consists of excluding hemorrhage with a CT scan (may be negative in 10% of subarachnoid hemorrhages) and spinal fluid exam. Additional studies should include CBC, platelet count, ESR, blood chemistries, PT, PTT, VDRL, urinalysis, chest x-ray, EKG, and, in selected patients, sickle cell testing. Serial blood cultures should be obtained if there is any evidence of endocarditis. If there is any history of heart disease or abnormality on cardiac exam, cardiology consultation with echocardiography and Holter monitoring, should be obtained. Although several non-invasive methods of evaluating the vascular system are available, angiography remains the best way to study vascular anatomy. Angiography is not necessary in those cases in which no specific therapy is planned. Additional evaluation such as ANA, serum viscosity, protein electrophoresis, serum amino acids, and hematology consultation may prove useful, especially in younger patients without an obvious cause. An EEG may help exclude a focal seizure disorder with Todd paralysis as a cause for a transient neurological deficit; focal slowing, however, should be differentiated from that which may also be seen with infarction.

The natural history of ischemic cerebrovascular disease is poorly understood. Following a TIA, the incidence of stroke is 20-50% within five years, 20% in the first year, and 5%/year (5 times normal) thereafter. The major risk period in the first year is in the first two months. Mortality following a TIA is more commonly due to myocardial infarction than stroke.

Management should include treatment of any underlying conditions (cardiac, hematologic). Bed rest is recommended initially to maximize hemodynamics. Rapid lowering of blood pressure should be avoided, unless the diastolic pressure is consistently greater than 120, to minimize hypoperfusion. Much of the specific therapy of ischemic cerebrovascular disease is highly controversial.

Surgery is commonly done for carotid occlusive disease and selected cases of subclavian steal, aortic arch disease, and extracranial vertebral artery disease. Carotid endarterectomy is commonly performed, relatively safe (less than 2% mortality in good hands), and can relieve symptoms of TIA. There are no randomized, well-controlled studies which document the efficacy of carotid surgery in prevention of cerebral infarction or improvement of life span. Nevertheless, carotid endarterectomy is generally done in patients with extracranial occlusive disease who have symptoms of TIA's or RIND's referable to the involved vascular supply. In some centers, endarterectomy is performed for fluctuating or progressive neurological deficits. There is no evidence to support surgery for asymptomatic carotid occlusive disease. The extracranial-intracranial (superficial temporal artery to middle cerebral artery) bypass has recently been demonstrated to be of no benefit. Although controversial, angiography and surgery are usually deferred for 5-6 weeks after an ischemic insult.

Anticoagulation and antiplatelet therapy in cerebral ischemic disease remains a subject of great controversy. Although many studies have been done, there is a lack of good randomized, controlled trials which demonstrate a clear overall benefit. Although the value of anticoagulation is unproven and the higher hemorrhagic complication rate is well known, many clinicians recommend heparin and warfarin in the treatment of TIA, RIND, and stroke in evolution. In the specific case of rheumatic heart disease and atrial fibrillation there is good evidence that anticoagulation reduces the risk of further embolization. Since the risk of stroke in nonrheumatic atrial fibrillation and sinus node disease is 5 times greater than normal, many argue that all patients with atrial fibrillation should be anticoagulated. The Canadian Cooperative Study demonstrated reduced rates of infarction and death in males only following treatment with aspirin, 1200 mg/day for TIA's in the carotid and vertebrobasilar distributions. Some argue, on the basis of in vitro studies, that lower dose aspirin (300 mg/day) should be more effective.

As a very general guideline, patients with TIA or RIND in the carotid distribution should undergo angiography if they are considered candidates for surgery after evaluation of their general medical status. While undergoing evaluation they should be anticoagulated with heparin. If no surgical lesion is identified or surgery is not indicated, they should be treated with warfarin for 6 months, followed by aspirin indefinitely. Alternatively, they may be treated with antiplatelet agents alone. Vertebrobasilar disease may be treated with aspirin alone or warfarin for 6 months, followed by aspirin as for carotid symptoms.

Anticoagulation is usually achieved rapidly with intravenous heparin and then maintained chronically with oral warfarin. Anticoagulation is contraindicated in patients with bleeding diatheses, predisposition to hemorrhage (peptic ulcer disease, neoplasm), severe liver disease, uremia, or those at risk for frequent falling. Anticoagulation is appropriate only in compliant patients who can be followed closely. Treatment of cerebral ischemia depends upon exclusion of hemorrhage by CT and spinal fluid examination.

Heparin is administered IV, beginning with a bolus of 5,000-10,000 units, followed by a continuous infusion of 1,000-2,000 units/hr. Alternatively, the initial bolus may be followed by 5,000-10,000 unit boluses q4h. Hemorrhagic complications are said to be less with continuous infusion. The heparin infusion rate is adjusted to maintain the Lee-White clotting time at 2x control or the activated partial thromboplastin time (PTT) at 2-2.5x control (60-90 seconds). Patients should be clinically monitored for evidence of excessive anticoagulation (petechiae, microscopic hematuria). Heparin anticoagulation can be reversed in minutes with protamine sulfate. Protamine is given slowly IV over 1-3 minutes in doses not to exceed 50 mg in a 10 minute period. Facilities for treatment of anaphylactoid shock should be readily available. Each 1 mg of protamine sulfate neutralizes approximately 90-115 USP units of heparin, depending upon the preparation. By 30 minutes after the dose of heparin, the protamine dose required for neutralization will be reduced by approximately one-half. Due to the anticoagulant effect of protamine, no more than 100 mg should be given in any single period unless a larger requirement is clearly established. If more than 4 hours have elapsed since the last heparin dose, protamine is generally not given. Side effects of protamine include hypotension, bradycardia, dyspnea, and flushing.

Warfarin loading is unnecessary. Warfarin is initiated with a maintenance of 10-15 mg/day. The prothrombin time (PT) is determined daily and the dosage adjusted to maintain the PT at 0.5-2x control (18-24 seconds). Greater degrees of anticoagulation are associated with a greater incidence of hemorrhagic complications. Numerous factors, including many drugs, may influence the response to warfarin, requiring great care in using this drug. Heparin may affect the PT; patients receiving heparin and warfarin should have PT's drawn just prior to the next heparin dose, or at least 5 hours after the last IV injection. After satisfactory anticoagulation is attained with warfarin, the PT should be determined at least every 2 weeks. Excessive prolongation of the PT can be corrected with the parenteral administration of vitamin K with initial doses of 2.5-10 mg or up to 25 mg, depending on the need for continued anticoagulation. If the PT has not been adequately shortened after 6-8 hours, the dose should be repeated. Up to 50 mg may be required. Rapid reversal, in the event of excessive blood loss, may require fresh frozen plasma, beginning with 15-20 ml/kg IV, then 1/3 that dose q8-12h as needed.

Antiplatelet therapies include aspirin, 300 mg PO qd and/or dipyridamole 50 mg PO tid or sulfinpyrazone 200 mg PO tid. The most common side effects of aspirin are gastrointestinal irritation and exacerbation of peptic ulcer disease. Dipyridamole should be used cautiously in patients with hypotension; adverse reactions are usually minimal and transient, but include headache, dizziness, nausea, flushing, weakness, syncope, mild gastrointestinal distress and skin rash. Sulfinpyrazone is contraindicated in patients with ulcerative or inflammatory gastrointestinal disorders or blood dyscrasias. As a potent uricosuric agent, sulfinpyrazone may precipitate urolithiasis and renal colic. It may accentuate the action of coumarin anticoagulants and should be used with caution in patients taking sulfa drugs, sulfonylurea hypoglycemic agents, and insulin.

The role of antiedema agents in the control of increased intracranial pressure in ischemic cerebrovascular disease is not well established (see also Intracranial Pressure). Steroids are of no clear benefit, though they may be used if there are signs of increased intracranial pressure. Use of anticonvulsants is usually reserved until there is evidence of a seizure disorder. Vasodilators are of no proven benefit and may even reduce perfusion in areas of ischemia.

Occupational, physical and speech therapy should be instituted early for optimal rehabilitation.

Ref: Millikan CH, McDowell FH. Treatment of transient ischemic attacks. Stroke 9:299, 1978.

McDowell FH, et al. Treatment of impending stroke. Stroke 11:1, 1980.

Canadian Cooperative Study Group. A randomized trial of aspirin and sulfinpyrazone in threatened stroke. NEJM 299:53, 1978.

Sandok BA, et al. Guidelines for the management of transient ischemic attacks. Mayo Clin Proc 53:665, 1978.

DIFFERENTIAL DIAGNOSIS OF CEREBRAL INFARCTION IN YOUNG ADULTS
(modified from Hart and Miller)

I.   Cerebrovascular atherosclerosis (thrombotic or embolic), hypertension is high risk factor

II. Embolism
  A. Cardiac source
    1. Valvular (mitral stenosis, prosthetic valve, infective endocarditis, marantic endocarditis, Libman-Sacks endocarditis, mitral annulus calcifications, mitral valve prolapse, calcific aortic stenosis)
    2. Atrial fibrillation, sick-sinus syndrome
    3. Acute myocardial infarction and/or left ventricular aneurysm
    4. Left atrial myxoma
    5. Cardiomyopathy
  B. Paradoxical embolism and pulmonary source
    1. Pulmonary arteriovenous malformation (including Osler-Weber-Rendu syndrome)

    2. Atrial and ventricular septal defects with shunt
    3. Patent foramen ovale with shunt
    4. Pulmonary vein thrombosis
    5. Pulmonary and mediastinal tumors
  C. Other
    1. Aortic cholesterol embolism
    2. Transient embologenic aortitis
    3. Emboli distal to unruptured aneurysm
    4. Fat embolism syndrome

III. Arteropathy
  A. Inflammatory
    1. Takayasu's disease
    2. Allergic (Churg-Strauss), granulomatous
    3. Infectious: syphilis, mucormycosis, ophthalmic zoster, TB, malaria, severe tonsillitis or lymphadenitis
    4. Associated with amphetamine use
    5. Associated with systemic disease (lupus, Wegener's, polyarteritis nodosa, rheumatoid arthritis, Sjogren's, scleroderma, Dego's, Behcet's, acute rheumatic fever, inflammatory bowel disease)
  B. Noninflammatory
    1. Spontaneous dissections
    2. Postradiation
    3. Fibromuscular dysplasia
    4. Moya-moya, progressive arterial occlusion syndrome
    5. Congophilic (amyloid) angiopathy
    6. Thromboangiitis obliterans
    7. Familial: homocystinuria, Fabry's pseudoxanthoma elasticum
    8. Neoplastic angioendotheliosis

IV. Vasospasm associated with:
  A. Migraine
  B. Subarachnoid hemorrhage
  C. Hypertensive encephalopathy
  D. Cerebral arteriography

V. Hematological disease and coagulopathies
  A. Hyperviscosity
    1. Polycythemia, myeloproliferative disorders
    2. Dysproteinemia (myeloma, Waldenstrom's, cryoglobulinemia)
  B. Coagulopathy
    1. Thrombotic thrombocytopenic purpura
    2. Diffuse intravascular coagulation

3. Paroxysmal nocturnal hemoglobinuria
4. Oral contraceptive use, peripartum, pregnancy
5. Thrombocytopenia
6. Sickle cell and hemoglobin C disease
7. Lupus anticoagulant
8. Nephrotic syndrome
9. C_2 deficiency (familial)
10. Protein C deficiency (familial)
C. Controversial associations
   1. Platelet hyperaggregability
   2. Fibrinolytic insufficiency
   3. Increased factor VIII
   4. Antithrombin III deficiency
   5. Vitamin K and antifibrinolytic therapy
   6. Acute alcohol intoxication

VI. Miscellaneous
A. Trauma (direct, indirect, rotation and extension injuries)
B. Mechanical (cervical rib, atlantoaxial subluxation)
C. Related to systemic hypotension
D. Iatrogenic (perioperative, especially cardiac surgery, and periprocedural, especially cardiac catheterization, including air and foreign particle embolism)
E. Cortical vein or sinus thrombosis

Ref: Hart RG, Miller VT. Cerebral infarction in young adults: a practical approach. Current concepts of cerebrovascular disease 17:15, 1982.

LACUNAR SYNDROMES (see also Ischemia)

Clinical manifestations of infarcts up to 20 mm (mostly 10 mm) size located in the subcortical cerebrum and in the brainstem resulting from occlusion (lipo-hyalinosis) of small arteries (40-200 μm). A small cavity, or lacune forms after healing. Lacunes are frequently associated with hypertension (60-90%) and atherosclerosis of large and middle sized intracranial arteries. Although the true incidence is unknown, lacunes are infrequently associated with embolism and extracranial carotid occlusive disease. Lacunes occur in the lenticular nuclei (37%), caudate nucleus (10%), thalamus (14%), internal capsule (10%), pons (16%), corona radiata, external capsule, pyramids, and other brainstem structures.

Clinical presentations are probably related to the size of the lesion and range from asymptomatic through the classic lacunar syndromes to more complex syndromes. Onset is often gradual overnight or stepwise. Approximately 30% are preceded by TIA's.

Head CT demonstrates up to 70% of lesions within 7 months. Multiple lacunes are present in 30%. Thirty percent of lesions on CT are asymptomatic.

Treatment consists of low dose aspirin and control of hypertension and other vascular risk factors. Cerebral angiography is not recommended in pure lacunar syndromes. Prognosis is usually favorable, but there is a high probability of recurrence.

Ref: Fisher CM. Neurology 32:871, 1982.

        Mohr JP. Stroke 13:1, 1982.

        Miller VT. Arch Neurol 40:129, 1983.

LEARNING DISABILITIES (See also Hyperactive Child)

The learning disabled child may be assessed by a battery of tests of specific skills such as reading, spelling, arithmetic, drawing/handwriting, symbol/nominal recall, listening comprehension and intelligence testing. From these tests, the psychologist will specify particular areas of difficulty. The neurologist is asked to make anatomic clinical associations and identify causative processes where possible. At present, many of these associations are speculative. Evaluation by the neurologist should include:

History: Perinatal, growth and development (including language), psychosocial, learning problems in family, educational level of family, evidence of seizures (absence).

Physical Exam: General physical and neurological examination including evaluation of vision and hearing. Assessment of writing, reading, reproduction of an auditory sequence (such as tapping out rhythms) and written sequence.

Testing: Audiologic evaluation. Consider work-up for degenerative diseases. Consider referral to a speech pathologist for further evaluation of speech, and for therapy (depending on what is available in the school system).

Treatment: Treat any underlying disease process. Reassurance if the child does not have a medical problem. Management of hyperactivity if appropriate. Refer back to school system for special classes. Refer to psychologist/psychiatrist for behavioral or psychoanalytic therapy.

Ref: Rapin I. Language disability in children. In:
        Blaw M, Rapin I, Kinsbourne M (eds). Topics in
        Child Neurology. New York: Spectrum, 1977.

        Millchamp JG (ed). Learning Disabilities and
        Related Disorders: Facts and Current Issues.
        Chicago: Year Book Medical Publishers, 1977.

LID (see Gaze Palsy, Graves' Ophthalmopathy, Ptosis))

LIMBIC SYSTEM (see Memory)

An area of the brain consisting of hippocampal
complex, fornix, mammillary bodies, anterior nucleus of
the thalamus, and cingulate cortex. It is important in
emotionality. The hippocampi and amygdala are important
in memory.

LUMBAR PUNCTURE (see Cerebrospinal Fluid)

LUMBOSACRAL PLEXUS (see diagram on page 166)

LUPUS (see Vasculitis)

MACROCEPHALY

Head circumference >2 standard deviations above the
mean for age, sex, race, gestation, and body size (see
Child Neurology). Differential diagnosis includes mass
lesions (neoplasm, arteriovenous malformation, congenital
cyst, subdural fluid), CNS structural malformations (spina
bifida, Chiari malformation, aqueductal stenosis), postinfectious (intrauterine or early life), post-traumatic,
primary CNS metabolic diseases (leukodystrophies,
lipidoses, mucopolysaccharidoses), systemic metabolic
diseases (osteogenesis imperfecta, hyperphosphatemia,
osteopetrosis, rickets), neurocutaneous syndromes (neurofibromatosis), and increased intracranial pressure (lead
poisoning, steroid withdrawal).

MAGNESIUM

Hypomagnesemia may produce neurological symptoms and
signs: irritability, depression, psychosis, apathy,
asthenia, fasciculations, carpopedal spasms, tetany,
hyperreflexia (occasionally hyporeflexia), positive
Chvostek's and Trousseau's signs, vertigo, vertical
nystagmus, ataxia, athetosis, and tremors. In addition,
anorexia, nausea, vomiting and diarrhea may occur early.

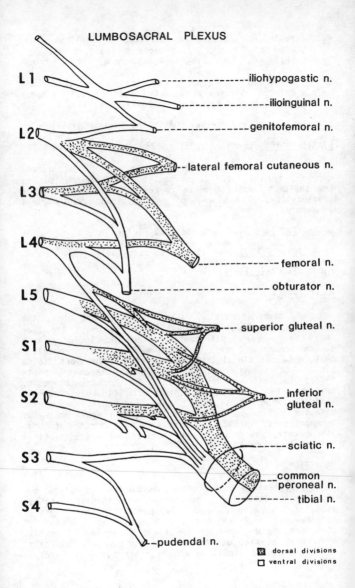

LUMBOSACRAL PLEXUS

L1 —————————————————— iliohypogastic n.
—————————————————— ilioinguinal n.

L2 ———————————————— genitofemoral n.
—— lateral femoral cutaneous n.

L3

L4
————————————— femoral n.
————————————— obturator n.

L5
——— superior gluteal n.

S1

S2
inferior
gluteal n.
————— sciatic n.

S3
common
peroneal n.
————— tibial n.

S4
—pudendal n.

▨ dorsal divisions
☐ ventral divisions

166

Most symptomatic patients have levels below 1.0 mEq/l (normal 1.5-2.5 mEq/l). EMG may show myopathic potentials. EKG may show QT prolongation along with broadening and flattening, peaking, or notching of T waves. Hypomagnesemia is seen with severe malnutrition, malabsorption, severe diarrhea, prolonged NG suctioning, excessive urinary loss (including diuretic therapy), treatment of diabetic ketoacidosis, alcoholism, hyperthyroidism, primary aldosteronism, hypo- and hyperparathyroidism, hypercalcemia, frequent transfusions of citrated blood, and therapy with aminoglycosides, carbenicillin, or cisplatin. Hypomagnesemia should be ruled out in any patient whose symptoms and signs are being attributed to hypocalcemia or hypokalemia, since alterations in these cations frequently co-exist. Serum levels may not accurately reflect body stores. Deep tendon reflexes should be followed in patients being repleted (see below).

Hypermagnesemia also produces neurological symptoms and signs. Loss of deep tendon reflexes occurs at levels of about 6 mEq/l. Alterations in consciousness and respiratory paralysis occur as levels rise from 6 towards 10 mEq/l, but an occasional patient will be stuporous with levels below 5. Renal failure, in addition to causing hypermagnesemia, may increase symptomatology at a given magnesium level. Diaphoresis, nausea, and vomiting may occur. Above a level of 5 mEq/l cardiovascular signs also occur, including hypotension, cardiac conduction abnormalities and dysrhythmias, and cardiac arrest. Neuromuscular effects are mediated by neuromuscular junction blockade which may be reversed with anticholinesterases. The EKG may show QT prolongation, widened QRS, and prolongation of the PR interval. Hypermagnesemia is most commonly seen in renal failure, but is also seen in Addison's disease, hypothyroidism, lithium therapy, hyperparathyroidism, and in babies of mothers treated with magnesium for eclampsia. Hypermagnesemia is often associated with hypocalcemia and should be considered in the setting of acidosis and shock when the anion gap is normal or low, since magnesium is an unmeasured cation. In cases of life-threatening hypermagnesemia, 20 ml of calcium gluconate 10% solution given IV can be a life-saving temporizing maneuver.

MAGNETIC RESONANCE IMAGING (MRI)

MRI makes tomographic images of the body using a combination of strong magnetic fields, controlled magnetic field gradients, and radiofrequency magnetic field pulses. In contrast to CT, the image intensity varies according to the concentration of hydrogen nuclei (protons), motion of these nuclei, nuclear relaxation parameters, and the type of "sequence" or "acquisition" that the MRI device is performing. Some useful definitions and facts are given below.

Safety - There are no known significant deleterious biological effects of exposure to strong magnetic fields under the conditions of MRI. Tissue heating due to radiofrequency (RF) energy deposition with high field strengths (1.5 T and above) is a concern. The most significant risk is from unsecured ferromagnetic objects flying into the magnet bore and striking the patient. Individuals with pacemakers and neurosurgical aneurysm clips should not be imaged. The former should stay outside the 5 gauss field strength line.

Sequence - MRI signals are elicited with a sequence of gradient and RF magnetic field pulses. There are several general types of sequence: partial saturation, spin echo (SE) and inversion spin-echo as well as special pulse sequences for flow imaging, spectroscopy, etc.

Relaxation Times - Tl and T2 are the longitudinal and transverse relaxation times. These two properties, with proton concentration and motion, determine the imaging characterisitics of each point or "voxel" of tissue.

Contrast is principally determined by Tl and T2. Areas of moving tissue or fluid may appear less intense. Cortical bone gives rise to no signal. Pathology reveals itself via a multitude of changes which are beyond the scope of this section to describe. Frequently, pathologic changes are seen only on long-echo SE images which are relatively noisy when compared to the short TE counterparts. For instance, MS lesions produce a strong signal on such long TE images.

Acquisition Matrix - MRI can acquire spatial information in different ways (single-slice, 2D multislice, 3D-isotropic) and at different resolutions (128 or 256 lines). Each such combination is the acquisition matrix.

Motion degrades MRI images. Moving patients must either be sedated or not imaged. Cardiac and respiratory motion can be compensated for by the use of physiologic gating.

Slice - MRI image planes can be made at any orientation through the body. The slice thickness is determined by magnetic gradient and RF pulses. In 2D imaging the slices can be selected to vary from >1cm to <3mm in thickness. Many slices can be imaged at once in multislice operation. 3D data acquisitions allow viewing of slices of any orientation after the scan is done.

Noise - MRI performance is determined by the amount of signal and the amount of noise that is present in the

imaging device. The noise comes mainly from the environment and the patient. Signal in a diagnostic sense is a
complex concept depending on the type of lesion, its
pattern, and other imaging considerations.

Spin-Echo - A type of MRI acquisition sequence where
the MRI signal is recalled via a "spin-echo". Either
single- or multi-echo sequences may be used. Each echo
produces its own message. A SE 30/1000 sequence has an
echo appearing at 30ms and a sequence repeated every
1000ms.

TE - The time during the imaging cycle between the
initial (90°) RF pulse and the spin-echo.

TR - The time between 90° RF pulses in an imaging
(single slice) cycle.

T1-weighted - A short TR (500ms), short TE (30ms) SE
sequence gives images where the pixel intensity or signal
is highly dependent upon T1. Areas of long T1 will have
low signal and areas of short T1 will have high signal.

T2-weighted - A long TR (greater than 1000ms), long TE
(60 to 200ms) SE sequence will show long T2 regions as
high signal intensity.

Inversion Spin-Echo (ISE) - Similar to SE pulse
sequences except that there is an initial inverting pulse
in the ISE sequence. ISE 400, 30, 1000 has an inverting
pulse preceeding the SE 30/1000 imaging cycle.

Imaging Time - The time that it takes to image a
patient with MR depends on the repetition time, the number
of lines of spatial resolution and the number of signals
averaged. In 2D multislice, a number of slices can be
imaged in the same time that 2D single slice is done. 3D
imaging may take more time than 2D multislice, but more
spatial information is obtained.

MEMORY

Disturbances of memory (the amnestic syndromes) are
either retrograde or anterograde. Retrograde amnesia
usually follows a traumatic brain injury and involves loss
of memory for a variable time prior to the event. Total
global retrograde amnesia, in which an individual loses
all prior memory, is never secondary to organic
dysfunction. Anterograde amnesia is the inability to
incorporate ongoing experience into memory stores, and is
seen in Wernicke-Korsakoff's psychosis (bilateral lesions
of the dorsal median nucleus of the thalamus) or bilateral
limbic lesions (hippocampal-amygdala complex). The latter
circumstance is usually secondary to occlusive vascular
disease or encephalitis.

In the syndrome of "transient global amnesia," an
individual behaves in an apparently automatic fashion for

minutes to hours without recollection of those events and has a retrograde amnesia which may be very spotty. It may be a manifestation of partial complex epilepsy, migraine, or transient ischemic attack. It occurs in middle-aged or elderly individuals and infrequently recurs, suggesting seizure disorder or TIA are less likely causes.

Ref: Logan W, Sherman DG.   Transient global amnesia. Stroke 14:1005, 1983.

MENINGITIS (see also Abscess, Encephalitis)

Acute meningitis (invariably associated with a cortical encephalitis and, often, with ventriculitis) is an emergency and should be suspected in any patient with the acute onset of nonlocalizing CNS signs. Fever, nuchal rigidity, headache, altered mental status, vomiting and photophobia are typically present. The absence of fever is not uncommon. Meningeal signs are not usually present in infants younger than 6 months of age. Acute signs may also be less apparent in the elderly, alcoholic, immuno-compromised, or comatose.

Acute meningitis may be bacterial or "aseptic" (negative CSF gram stain and bacterial cultures). The causative organism in acute meningitis may be suspected according to patient age and clinical setting (see page 171). The "aseptic" meningitis syndrome may result from causes (see page 173) requiring antimicrobial drugs, surgery, or both.

Immediate evaluation and treatment are essential in managing patients with suspected acute meningitis. If symptoms and signs have been present for <24 hours and are rapidly progressive, the most likely cause is bacterial. The initial physical exam should be brief and should exclude papilledema or focal neurological findings. Spinal fluid and blood cultures are obtained STAT and antibiotics (see page 174) are begun immediately (<30 min). A careful history and physical exam can then be undertaken and the CSF examined in detail. Therapy is modified as needed pending further clinical evaluation, CSF lab studies, and culture and sensitivity results. Papilledema or focal findings are indications for CT prior to LP to exclude an intracranial mass lesion because of the increased risk of herniation. In such a case, anti-biotics are begun before the CT. In cases of subacute presentation (>24 hr course), the history, physical exam, and examination of CSF can be performed with care prior to beginning antibiotics (<2 hrs), unless mental status is impaired, in which case acute therapy is instituted as above.

CAUSATIVE ORGANISMS IN ACUTE MENINGITIS
ACCORDING TO PATIENT AGE AND CLINICAL SETTING

Infants less than 8 weeks old: Group B streptococci, *E. coli* and other Gram-negative enteric bacilli, *L. monocytogenes, S. pneumoniae, Salmonella* species, *P. aeruginosa, S. aureus, H. influenzae, Herpes simplex* II

Children 2 months to 15 years old: *H. influenzae, S. pneumoniae, N. meningitidis, S. aureus,* viruses

Older children and young adults: *N. meningitidis, S. pneumoniae, H. influenzae, S. aureus,* viruses

Adults greater than 40 years old: *S. pneumoniae, N. meningitidis, S. aureus, L. monocytogenes,* Gram-negative enteric organisms

Swimming in fresh water ponds: Amebas (*Naegleria*)

Contact with water frequented by rodents or domestic animals: Leptospires

Contact with hamsters or mice: Lymphocytic choriomeningitis

Exposure to pigeons or their excreta: *Cryptococcus*

Travel in Southwestern U.S.: *Coccidioides*

Prior meningitis: *S. pneumoniae* (also see below) for causes of chronic and recurrent "aseptic" meningitis)

Sibling with meningitis: *N. meningitidis, H. influenzae*

Hospital acquired: Gram-negative bacilli, staphylococci, *Candida*

Diabetes mellitus: *S. pneumoniae,* Gram-negative bacilli, staphylococci, *Cryptococcus, Mucormycosis*

Alcoholism: *S. pneumoniae*

Upper respiratory infection: Viruses, *H. influenzae, S. pneumoniae, N. meningitidis*

Pneumonia: *S. pneumoniae, N. meningitidis*

Abnormal cellular immunity (lymphoma, steroids, organ transplantation, AIDS): *L. monocytogenes, S. pneumoniae, Cryptococcus, Coccidioides, Histoplasma, Toxoplasma, Strongyloides, Mycobacterium tuberculosis*

Abnormal neutrophils (absolute neutropenia as in aplastic anemia, acute leukemia, chemotherapy; neutrophil dysfunction as in chemotherapy, diabetes mellitus, steroids, specific neutrophil diseases): *Pseudomonas aeruginosa* and other Gram-negative bacilli, *S. aureus, Candida, Aspergillus, Mucormycosis.*

Immunoglobulin deficiency (multiple myeloma, CLL, combined radiation therapy and multi-drug chemotherapy), splenectomy (surgical, hemoglobinopathy): *S. pneumoniae, N. meningitides, H. influenza*

Penetrating head trauma, skin lesions, bacterial endo-carditis or other heart disease, severe burns, IV drug abuse: *S. aureus*, streptococci, Gram-negative bacilli

Closed head trauma, CSF leak, pericranial infections (sinusitis, otitis, infections of the face or oropharynx): *S. pneumoniae, H. influenzae*, Anaerobic and micro-aerophilic streptococci, *Bacteroides* sp. and other anaerobic bacilli, *S. aureus*

Following neurosurgical procedures: *S. aureus, S. epidermidis*, Gram-negative enteric and anaerobic bacilli

Ventricular shunt infection: *S. epidermidis, S. aureus*, Gram-negative enteric bacilli, Diphtheroids, *Bacillus* sp.

   Laboratory evaluation of CSF (see also Cerebrospinal Fluid) should begin with careful Gram staining of centrifuged CSF sediment (positive in 80-90% of those with positive cultures). If the Gram stain is negative, certain other tests may be helpful before culture and sensitivity results are available. Cell count >1,200/mm3, protein >150 mg/100 ml, and glucose <30 mg/100 ml suggest bacterial infection, though there may be overlap with ranges more typical of TB, fungal, or viral meningitis. A predominance of polymorphonuclear leukocytes in the differential count is more typical of bacterial meningitis, while a predominance of lymphocytes is more typical of nonbacterial meningitis. Greater than 80% lymphocytes may be seen, however, in as much as 10% of cases of bacterial meningitis. CSF lactic acid

>35 mg/ml suggests bacterial infection. A positive limulus lysate assay indicates infection with a Gram-negative bacteria. Counterimmunoelectrophoresis (CIE) is specific, though not highly sensitive, for pneumococci, meningococci, or H. influenza. Other organism-specific CSF studies include cryptococcal antigen, coccidioidal complement fixation, radioimmunoassay for herpes virus-specific glycoprotein, and syphilis serology. If bacterial infection has been excluded, a CSF chloride <110 mEq/l suggests tuberculous meningitis. Acid fast staining of >10 ml of spun CSF is postiive in >80% of tuberculous meningitis. India ink frequently reveals cryptococci. A wet mount or hanging drop suspension of fresh, uncentrifuged CSF may reveal motile amebas (which resemble monocytes). If the diagnosis remains in doubt, repeat LP in 8 hrs is indicated.

CAUSES OF "ASEPTIC" MENINGITIS SYNDROME, CHRONIC MENINGITIS (C) AND RECURRENT MENINGITIS (R)*

Requiring Antimicrobial Therapy

Partially treated meningitis (R)
Parameningeal Foci: sinusitis, brain abscess, cranial or spinal epidural abscess, subdural empyema, dermal sinus tract (R)
M. tuberculosis (C,R)
Fungi (C,R)
Amebas
Syphilis (C)
Herpes simplex types 1 and 2
Rickettsia
Brucella (C,R)
Listeria
Toxoplasma (C)
Mycoplasma
Cysticercus (C)
Human immunodeficiency virus (C)

Requiring Other Therapy

Leptospirosis (C,R)
Viruses (R)
Carcinomatous (C,R)
Chemical
Rupture of cyst (R)
Sarcoidosis (C,R)
Lupus erythematosus (R)
Behcet's syndrome (C,R)
Uveomeningo-encephalitis (C,R)
Mollaret's (R)
Uremia
Meningitis/migraine syndrome (R)
Drugs: ibuprofen, sulindac, sulfa-methoxizole, INH
Granulomatous angiitis (C)

*Other causes of recurrent meningitis include immuno-compromised states, foreign body (shunts) and anatomical defects which may be congenital (spinal dysraphism, neurenteric cysts) or traumatic or postoperative (sinuses, cribriform plate, petrous bone)

INITIAL CHOICE OF ANTIBIOTIC IN ACUTE MENINGITIS

Neonate <2 mos:

  Ampicillin 100 mg/kg/d IV (q6h) and
  Gentamicin 7.5 mg/kg/d IV (q8h)

Children 2 mos-6 yrs:

  Chloramphenicol 75-100 mg/kg/d IV (q6h) and
  Ampicillin 200-400 mg/kg/d IV (q4h)

Children >6 and Adults:

  Penicillin 50,000 units/kg IV q4h or
  Ampicillin 4 gm/d IV (q4h)

Children and adults with risk factors (immunosuppression, cranial injury, nosocomial infection):

  Chloramphenicol 3-4 gm/d IV (q4h)
  Gentamicin 3-5 mg/kg/d IV (q8h)
  Nafcillin 12 gm/d IV (q4h)

Ref: Mandell GL, et al. Principles and Practice of Infectious Diseases. 2nd ed. New York: Wiley, 1985.

MENTAL STATUS TESTING

Testing at the bedside is, by necessity, grossly abbreviated. The clinical neuropsychologist, on the other hand, requires hours for detailed testing. For most screening purposes, one should assess level of awareness, attentiveness, orientation, memory (remote memory is determined by informational tests and recent memory by a memory task), calculations, reversals, proverbs, judgment, and insight. In addition, aphasia and apraxia testing are usually considered part of the mental status examination. Three commonly used screening methods are referenced below.

Ref: Folstein et al. J Psychiatr Res 12:189, 1975.

  Kahn et al. Am J Psychiatr 117:326, 1960.

  Jacobs et al. Ann Int Med 86:40, 1977.

METABOLIC DISORDERS OF CHILDHOOD

The basic workup for metabolic disease includes a complete developmental history and growth data points, since developmental delay is an important feature of most metabolic diseases. The following are usually helpful: urine and serum metabolic screen, NH_4, pyruvate, lactate, electrolytes, calcium, magnesium, arterial blood gas, ophthalmologic exam, CT scan, and skeletal films. Screening for lysosomal and some lipid storage diseases involve special blood tests and tissue samples (skin, muscle, peripheral nerve, bone marrow, and, in some cases, brain). Nerve conduction studies are helpful in several degenerative disorders.

MICROCEPHALY

Head circumference <2 standard deviations below the mean for age, sex, race, gestation and body size (see Child Neurology). Except for severe cases of premature closure of the sutures (craniosynostosis), small skull size reflects small brain size. Causes of the latter are classified as primary and secondary. Primary microcephaly reflects anomalous development during the first 7 months of gestation, which may result from genetic factors, radiation (particularly during the first two trimesters of pregnancy), intrauterine infections (especially CMV, toxoplasmosis, and rubella), or chemical agents. Secondary microcephaly reflects anomalous development during the last 2 months of pregnancy, the perinatal period, or early infancy; causes include infection, trauma, or metabolic or anoxic brain damage.

MOTOR NEURON DISEASE (see also Hypotonic Infant, Muscle Disorders)

CLASSIFICATION OF MOTOR NEURON DISEASE

Inherited

Spinal muscular atrophy (SMA)

Type I	Infantile (Werdnig-Hoffman)
Type II	Late (benign) infantile
Type III	Juvenile (Kugelberg-Welander-Wohlfart)
Type IV	Adult
	Limb girdle
	Fascioscapulohumeral
	Scapuloperoneal

                        Peroneal
                        Ophthalmoplegia plus
                        Other
            Hexosaminidase deficiency
        Familial amyotrophic lateral sclerosis (ALS)
        Juvenile progressive bulbar palsy (Fazio-Londe)
        ALS-like syndrome in hexosaminidase deficiency

Acquired

Acute: Acute anterior poliomyelitis (polio,
            coxsackie, other enteroviruses)
Chronic: ALS
            Anterior horn cell degeneration in:
                Spinocerebellar degeneration
                Creutzfeldt-Jacob disease
                Huntington's disease
                Parkinsonism
                Shy-Drager syndrome
                Joseph's disease
                Paraneoplastic syndromes

Amyotrophic lateral sclerosis (ALS) is a chronic, progressive, degenerative disease of unknown etiology, characterized pathologically by progressive loss of motor neurons in the spinal cord, brainstem, and motor cortex. The neuronal loss may occur at one or several levels.

Clinically, patients present with upper or lower motor neuron symptoms and signs in bulbar and/or spinal innervated muscles.

CLASSIFICATION OF MOTOR NEURON DISEASE BY INITIAL PRESENTATION

	Spinal Cord	Brainstem
Lower motor neuron (atrophic)	Spinal muscular atrophy	Progressive bulbar palsy
Upper motor neuron (spastic)	Primary lateral sclerosis	Progressive pseudobulbar palsy

Frequently there is weakness and atrophy of one muscle group which then spreads to all extremities and to the bulbar muscles. Fasciculations are common. There is weakness of the muscles of mastication and palate with dysphagia and hypophonic dysarthria. Ophthalmoparesis is rare. Jaw jerk may be decreased (progressive bulbar palsy). Upper motor neuron findings in the form of spasticity and hyperreflexia develop. Most cases progress to the typical picture of ALS with generalized upper and lower motor neuron findings. Death usually results from recurrent aspiration pneumonia and respiratory insufficiency.

Prognosis is related to the onset of bulbar involvement. Life expectancy is usually less than 1.5-2 years after bulbar involvement, especially if mainly lower motor neuron. With predominantly spinal involvement (especially upper motor neuron), survival is longer; 20% survive for longer than 5 years. Overall survival in ALS averages 1-3 years. Most cases are sporadic. Some cases are familial, usually among the Chamorro people of Guam and in the Kii peninsula in Japan, and may be associated with dementia and Parkinsonism. Age of onset is usually between 40 and 70 years, peaking in the sixth decade.

Diagnostic evaluation includes EMG which reveals widespread denervation with fibrillation potentials, positive waves, fasciculation potentials, and, occasionally, giant motor unit potentials. Nerve conduction studies are normal. If the disease presents as primary lateral sclerosis, myelography will exclude spinal cord compression. CSF is normal. Muscle biopsy demonstrates denervation, but is usually not required.

Treatment does not exist. Thyrotropine releasing hormone is experimental. Management is centered around supportive measures, patient and family education, good pulmonary toilet, and nasogastric or gastrostomy feeding.

Acute anterior poliomyelitis is due to destruction of spinal cord and brainstem motor neurons by the polio virus. Cerebral cortex and deep gray nuclei may also be involved. The virus initially infects and multiplies in the pharynx and the gastrointestinal tract.

Clinically, the gastrointestinal infection and viremia are usually asymptomatic or only mildly symptomatic, followed in several days by fever, meningeal signs, and asymmetric paralysis. The sensory system is usually spared. Paralysis usually progresses over 3-5 days. Bulbar involvement carries a worse prognosis.

Incidence of poliomyelitis has dropped due to the attenuated and killed polio vaccines from about 50,000 cases per year in the mid 1950's to an occasional case per year, usually in persons who have not been vaccinated or were inadequately vaccinated.

Laboratory findings include peripheral leukocytosis, slightly to moderately elevated CSF protein with a lymphocytic pleocytosis, and fourfold rise between acute and convalescent viral titers. The virus may be isolated from blood, pharynx, stool, or CSF.

Treatment is supportive, with mechanical ventilation if needed.

Ref: Rowland LP. Looking for the cause of amyotrophic lateral sclerosis. NEJM 311:979, 1984.

MOVEMENT DISORDERS (see Asterixis, Athetosis, Chorea, Choreoathetosis, Dyskinesia, Dystonia, Myoclonus, Neuroleptics, Parkinson's Disease, Progressive Supranuclear Palsy, Rigidity, Tremor)

MRI (see Magnetic Resonance Imaging)

MULTIPLE SCLEROSIS (see also Demyelinating Disease)

Most common of the demyelinating diseases. By established criteria, MS can be classified as clinically definite, probable, or possible. Symptomatic attacks should last a minimum of 24 hours, occur in different locations in the CNS, and be separated by a period of at least 1 month. Onset of the disease is usually between the ages of 10 and 50. The course is typically relapsing and remitting but can become chronically progressive. Common symptoms and signs include upper motor neuron findings, spasticity, sensory disturbances, optic neuritis, ataxia, vertigo, internuclear ophthalmoplegia, diplopia, bowel and bladder dysfunction, Lhermitte's sign, and disturbance of affect. Other symptoms include limb pain, trigeminal neuralgia, dementia, facial palsy, facial myokymia, impotence, hearing loss, and seizures.

Laboratory studies may support the clinical diagnosis. CT is usually normal, but can show enlarged ventricles, cortical atrophy, and focal areas of contrast enhancement. MRI frequently demonstrates white matter lesions. CSF may reveal a mild lymphocytosis (<20 cells/mm3), oligo-clonal banding (in 80% of patients with untreated clinically definite MS), IgG/Albumin ratio >0.27, and IgG index = (CSF IgG/Albumin)/(Serum IgG/Albumin) >0.66 (false positives do occur). Myelin basic protein (>8 mg/ml is abnormal) correlates with active disease, but is present in other destructive CNS disorders. Visual, auditory, and somatosensory evoked potentials may reveal abnormalities in the respective pathways. Cystometrics (CMG) may be abnormal, most commonly revealing an uninhibited neuropathic bladder with detrusor muscle instability; CMG may also be helpful in monitoring therapy.

Incidence of MS varies regionally. Risk for development is based upon area of life prior to age 15. There is also a small familial predisposition for its development.

General management includes avoidance of heat and excessive fatigue. Hot showers, fever, and hot weather can decrease conduction and exacerbate symptoms. Uhthoff's phenomenon refers to the worsening of visual function under such circumstances.

Bladder dysfunction should be evaluated with CMG (see Bladder). Failure to store is most common, and is treated with oxybutynin or propantheline and/or imipramine. Failure to empty is treated with bethanechol and/or phenoxybenzamine; valsalva or Crede maneuvers, catheterization (intermittent, permanent), or surgery (artificial sphincters, urinary diversion) may be necessary.

Spasticity is treated with baclofen, diazepam, or dantrolene sodium (see Spasticity).

Immunosuppression and a multitude of other primary therapies have been described; none are of proven benefit. Some recommend ACTH or steroids for acute attacks. It has been suggested that high dose cytoxan and ACTH may stabilize progressive MS.

Ref: Poser CM, et al. New diagnostic criteria for
       multiple   sclerosis: guideline   for   research
       protocols. Ann Neurol 13:227, 1983.

       Hauser SL, et al. Intensive immunosuppression in
       progressive multiple sclerosis. NEJM 308:173, 1983.

MUSCLE DISORDERS (see also Hypotonic Infant, Motor
     Neuron   Disease,   Muscular   Dystrophy,   Myopathy,
     Myotonia, Periodic Paralysis)

CLASSIFICATION OF DISORDERS OF MUSCLE
(Adapted from Walton)

A. Genetically determined myopathies
    1. Muscular dystrophies
        a) X-linked (pseudohypertrophic)
            1) Sex-linked recessive, severe (Duchenne)
            2) Sex-linked recessive, mild (Becker)
        b) Facioscapulohumeral (Landouzy-Dejerine)
            1) Autosomal dominant involving face, scapu-
                lohumeral and anterior tibial muscles
            2) With inflammatory changes in muscle
            3) With Mobius' syndrome

      c) Scapuloperoneal muscular atrophy
         1) Autosomal dominant
         2) X-linked
         3) With inflammatory changes and cardiopathy
      d) Limb-girdle
         1) Autosomal recessive or sporadic
         2) Limited to quadriceps
         3) Autosomal recessive, of childhood
         4) Autosomal dominant, of late-onset
      e) Distal myopathy
         1) Autosomal dominant, late-onset
         2) Ascending distal type
         3) Juvenile distal type
      f) Ocular myopathy (progressive external ophthalmoplegia - primary myopathy)
         1) Isolated (dominant)
         2) With pigmentary retinal degeneration (dominant or sporadic)
         3) With retinal degeneration, short stature, heart block, ataxia, etc. (Kearns-Sayre-Daroff - sporadic, a mitochondrial encephalomyopathy)
      g) Oculopharyngeal muscular dystrophy
      h) Congential ophthalmoplegia in Goldenhar-Gorlin syndrome
      i) Neonatal ophthalmoplegia with microfibers
  2. Obscure congenital myopathies, unknown etiology
      a) Congenital muscular dystrophy (including some cases of arthrogryposis multiplex congenita)
      b) Benign congenital myopathy without specific features
      c) Central core disease
      d) Nemaline (rod-body) myopathy
      e) The mitochondrial myopathies (no exact classification is possible at present)
         1) Hypermetabolic
         2) Pleoconial with salt craving and periodic weakness
         3) Megaconial
         4) With fatigability and mitochondrial inclusions
         5) With growth failure and seizures
         6) With diabetes and distal myopathy
         7) With facioscapulohumeral syndrome
         8) With ophthalmoplegia and glycogen storage
         9) With cytochrome b deficiency
      f) Myotubular (centronuclear) myopathy
      g) Familial myosclerosis (myodysplasia fiberosa multiplex)
      h) Myopathy in Marfan's syndrome

    i) Familial congenital myopathy with cataract and gonadal dysgenesis
    j) Myopathies with characteristic histochemical abnormalities
        1) Type I fiber hypotrophy
        2) Reducing body myopathy
    k) Myopathy with defect in relaxing factor
    l) Cardioskeletal myopathy with polysaccharide accumulation
    m) Myopathies with disordered lipid metabolism
        1) Carnitine deficiency and lipid storage
        2) With cramps and myoglobinuria
        3) Carnitine palmityl transferase deficiency
    n) Myopathies with cytoplasmic inclusions, "finger-print" inclusions
    o) "Multi-core disease"
    p) Sarcotubular myopathy
    q) Myopathy with tubular aggregates
    r) Myopathy with crystalline intranuclear inclusions
    s) Autosomal dominant "spheroid body" myopathy
    t) Hypertrophic branchial myopathy
    u) Monomelic hypertrophic myopathy
    v) Cytoplasmic body neuromyopathy with respiratory failure and weight loss
3. Myotonic disorders
    a) Myotonic dystrophy, myotonia atrophica
        1) Adult
        2) Infantile hypotonic (congenital)
    b) Myotonia congenita (autosomal dominant, Thomsen)
    c) Myotonia congenita (autosomal recessive, Becker)
    d) Myotonia, dwarfism, diffuse bone disease and eye and face abnormality (chondrodystrophic myotonia, Schwartz-Jampel syndrome)
    e) Paramyotonia congenita (Eulenburg)
    f) Paramyotonia without paralysis on exposure to cold (de Jong)
    g) Primary hyperkalemic periodic paralysis (adynamia episodica hereditaria, Gamstorp)
    h) Secondary to diazocholesterol
    i) Associated with carcinoma of lung
4. Glycogen-storage diseases
    a) Glucose-6-phosphatase deficiency (von Gierke, hypotonia without direct muscle involvement)
    b) Amylo-1,6 glucosidase deficiency (Forbes)
    c) Amylo-1,4 glucosidase (acid maltase) deficiency (Pompe)
    d) Muscle phosphorylase deficiency (McArdle)

      e) Hereditary metabolic myopathy with myoglobinuria and abnormal glycolysis
      f) Phosphoglucomutase deficiency
      g) Myopathy with abnormal glycolytic breakdown at phosphohexoisomerase level
      h) Phosphofructokinase deficiency
      i) Multiple enzyme deficiency

5. Familial periodic paralysis and related syndromes
    a) Familial hypokalemic periodic paralysis
    b) Adynamia episodica hereditaria (hyperkalemic)
    c) Normokalemic periodic paralysis
    d) Biphasic periodic paralysis
    e) Myotonic periodic paralysis
    f) Thyrotoxic periodic paralysis

6. Generalized myositis ossificans

7. Dysproteinemic ataxias with myopathy
    a) Ataxia telangiectasia (secondary to neurogenic atrophy)
    b) Abetalipoproteinemia (acanthocytosis)

8. Myopathy in xanthinuria

9. Familial myoglobinuria, unknown cause

10. Myopathy in malignant hyperpyrexia

11. Progressive muscle spasm, alopecia, diarrhea, and malabsorption

B. Injury due to external agents
  1) Physical
    a) Crush syndrome
    b) Ischemic infarction or atrophy
      1) Peripheral vascular disease
      2) Polyarteritis nodosa, other vasculitides
      3) Diabetes mellitus
    c) Volkmann's contracture
    d) Anterior tibial syndrome
    e) Posterior compartment (tibial) syndrome
    f) Congenital torticollis
  2. Toxic
    a) Haff disease
    b) Malayan sea snake bite (Enhydrina schistosa)
    c) Saxitoxin poisoning
    d) Rhabdomyolysis caused by hornet venom
  3. Drugs
    a) Steroid myopathy
    b) Chloroquine myopathy
    c) Bretylium tosylate myopathy
    d) Emetine
    e) Vincristine
    f) Diazocholesterol
    g) Clofibrate
    h) Carbenoxolone

i) Amphotericin B (K$^+$ depletion)
j) Anodiaquine
k) Colchicine
l) Meperidine
m) Pentazocine
n) Polymyxin E
o) Triorthocresylphosphate

C. Inflammatory
1. Infections
   a) Viral (presumed)
   b) Bacterial
      1) Gas gangrene (*Claustridia welchii*)
      2) Tetanus (*Claustridia tetani*)
      3) Staphylococci and other pyogenic organisms (septic myositis)
      4) Leprous myositis
      5) Tropical myositis (usually pyogenic)
   c) Nematode
      1) Trichinosis
   d) Cestode
      1) Cysticercosis with muscle hypertrophy
      2) Cysticercosis (asymptomatic)
   e) Trypanosomiasis
   f) Toxoplasmosis
2. Other inflammatory disorders
   a) Polymyositis (possibly an organ-specific autoimmune disease)
      1) Acute polymyositis with myoglobinuria
      2) Subacute polymyositis
      3) Chronic polymyositis (including chronic myositis fibrosa)
   b) Polymyositis or dermatomyositis (as a feature of what may become a non-organ-specific autoimmune disease)
      1) Dermatomyositis
      2) Polymyositis in disseminated lupus erythematosus
      3) Polymyositis in rheumatic fever
      4) Polymyositis in rheumatoid arthritis
      5) Polymyositis in scleroderma and/or systemic sclerosis
      6) Scleroderma with myopathy
      7) Ocular myositis (orbital pseudotumor)
      8) Muscle infarction and/or polymyositis in polyarteritis nodosa
      9) Polymyopathy in Sjogren's disease
      10) Polymyopathy in Werner's disease
      11) Localized nodular myositis

      c) Polymyositis or dermatomyositis (possibly as a conditioned autoimmune response in malignant disease)

      d) Polymyositis with associated virus particles

  3. Inflammatory disorders of unknown etiology

      a) Sarcoidosis with myopathy

      b) Granulomatous polymyositis and giant cell myositis

      c) Polymyalgia rheumatica

      d) Localized myositis ossificans

      e) Fibrositis and nodular fasciitis

      f) Myopathy in relapsing panniculitis (Weber-Christian syndrome)

      g) Myositis with necrotizing fasciitis

      h) Myopathy in psoriasis

      i) Polymyositis in the hypereosinophilic syndrome

      j) Myopathy in Reye's syndrome

D. Muscle disorder associated with endocrine or metabolic diseases

  1. Thyrotoxicosis

      a) Myopathy

      b) Myasthenia gravis

      c) Periodic paralysis

  2. Myxedema

      a) Girdle myopathy

      b) Debre-Semelaigne syndrome (cretins)

      c) Hoffmann syndrome (adults)

      d) Pseudomyotonia

      e) Neuromyopathy following 131I therapy

  3. Hypopituitarism with myopathy

  4. Acromegaly with muscle hypertrophy (and/or muscular atrophy)

  5. Graves' ophthalmopathy (infiltrative ophthalmopathy)

  6. Cushing's disease myopathy (and corticosteroid myopathy)

  7. ACTH myopathy

  8. Addison's disease with myopathy

  9. Primary aldosteronism (with hypokalemic periodic paralysis)

  10. Hyperparathyroidism with myopathy

  11. Myopathy in other forms of metabolic bone disease

      a) Osteomalacia due to

          1) Idiopathic steatorrhea

          2) Malabsorption after partial gastrectomy

          3) Renal acidosis

          4) Hypophosphatemia

          5) Anticonvulsants

12. Myopathy with calcitonin-secreting medullary carcinoma of the thyroid
13. Alcoholic myopathy
    a) Acute, with rhabdomyolysis and myoglobinuria
    b) Subacute proximal
    c) Hypokalemic
14. Nutritional myopathy
    a) Protein deficiency
    b) Vitamin E deficiency
15. Myopathy in chronic renal failure
16. Myopathy in lysine-cystinuria
17. Myopathy in xanthinuria
18. Myopathy in Lafora disease

E. Myopathy associated with malignant disease
   1. Carcinomatous myopathy (other than polymyositis)
   2. Myasthenic-myopathic syndrome
   3. Carcinomatous embolic myopathy
   4. Myopathy in the carcinoid syndrome

F. Myopathy associated with myasthenia gravis

G. Myopathy in thalassemia

H. Other disorders of muscle of unknown etiology
   1. Acute muscle necrosis
      a) Of unknown cause
      b) In chronic alcoholism
      c) In carcinoma
   2. Paroxysmal myoglobinuria or rhabdomyolysis
      a) Exertional
         1) In McArdle's disease
         2) In other metabolic myopathies
      b) Nonexertional
      c) Rhabdomyolysis due to ingestion of quail
   3. Amyloid myopathy
      a) Primary familial
      b) Primary sporadic
      c) In myelomatosis
      d) With angiopathy
   4. Conditions demonstrating muscular hypertrophy
      a) Muscular hypertrophy, extrapyramidal disorders and mental deficiency
      b) Hypertrophia musculorum vera
      c) Bilateral hypertrophy of masseters
   5. Disuse atrophy
   6. Muscle cachexia (in wasting diseases and in the elderly)
   7. Muscle wasting in contralateral cerebral lesions (particularly of parietal lobe)

I. Tumors of muscle

Ref: Walton JN. Disorders of Voluntary Muscle. 4th
ed. Edinburgh: Churchill Livingstone, 1981:474-9.

MUSCLE TESTING (see also Myotome)

GRADING OF MUSCLE POWER
(Adapted from Medical Research Council, London)

0	No contraction
1	Trace of contraction, without active movement
2	Active movement with gravity eliminated (movement in a horizontal plane)
3	Active movement against gravity but not against resistance
4-	Active movement against slight resistance
4	Active movement against moderate resistance
4+	Active movement against strong resistance but not the expected full power (taking degree of fitness and age into account)
5	Normal strength

MUSCULAR DYSTROPHY

Muscular dystrophy refers to a group of genetically
determined, progressive, degenerative myopathies. Pathogenesis is unknown. Recent evidence suggests a cell
membrane defect. Clinical features of specific muscular
dystrophies are outlined below. Muscle enzymes may be
normal or elevated. EMG shows myopathic changes (see
EMG). Nerve conduction studies are normal. Muscle biopsy
is useful in distinguishing the muscular dystrophies from
other myopathies and from neurogenic diseases. It is less
useful in differentiating between the specific types of
muscular dystrophies. Generally, in muscular dystrophy
there is a reduction in the total number of fibers, fiber
splitting, increased variability in fiber size, and there
are various stages of degeneration and necrosis of fibers
with phagocytes. Early in the course there is evidence of
regeneration with fibers having basophilic cytoplasm and
enlarged vesicular sarcolemmal nuclei. As the disease
progresses there is increasing endomysial connective
tissue and adipose tissue. Histochemically there are no
detectable enzyme abnormalities or changes in ratio of
Type I and II fibers (except in myotonic dystrophy where
there is greater atrophy of Type I fibers).

Duchenne dystrophy is the most common and severe. Inheritance is X-linked recessive. Onset is from 1.5-4.5 years of age. The course is rapidly progressive with wheelchair confinement by the early teens and death by the late teens or early twenties due to chronic respiratory insufficiency and infection. Initially there is pelvic girdle weakness followed by shoulder girdle weakness; motor milestones are mildly delayed. There is a "waddling" (reverse Trendelenburg) gait, frequent falling, difficulty arising from a chair, and difficulty elevating the arms. Pseudohypertrophy is usually present early, especially in the calves, and is followed by pelvic and shoulder girdle wasting as the disease progresses. The heart is usually involved. The EKG shows right ventricular strain with tall R waves in the right precardium and deep Q waves in the left precardium. A mild static intellectual deficit is present in 30% of patients. Creatinine kinase (CPK), pyruvate kinase (PK), and aldolase are elevated as high as 200 times normal. CPK gradually declines with progression of the disease. CPK is increased in 75-90% of carriers. CPK may be falsely low during pregnancy. Muscle biopsy is as described above, although there is more necrosis and more rapid replacement by connective and adipose tissue.

Becker dystrophy, a "benign" X-linked recessive form with age of onset between 5 and 15 years, is more slowly progressive than Duchenne dystrophy. Patients become confined to a wheelchair at 20-40 years of age; 50% survive past age 40. The distribution of weakness and wasting is similar to Duchenne, but the degree of weakness is less. The face is spared. Pseudohypertrophy is less common than in Duchenne. Heart and intellectual involvement is uncommon. CPK elevation is similar to Duchenne and decreases with progression of the disease. EMG may show repetitive high frequency discharges and fibrillation potentials in addition to myopathic changes. On muscle biopsy, the pathologic changes may be less severe than Duchenne.

Benign X-linked dystrophy, with early contractures is very rare. There is very slowly progressive proximal weakness and wasting with early contractures, especially of the gastrocnemius and biceps. The deltoids and face are spared. The heart is involved. CPK is 6-7 times normal.

X-linked (recessive) scapuloperoneal dystrophy is very rare and slowly progressive with age of onset between 5 and 10 years. Proximal lower extremities are relatively spared. Contractures are common (especially posterior neck and spine). CPK is 2-20 times normal.

Facioscapulohumeral (Duchenne-Landouzy-Dejerine) dystrophy is autosomal dominant with strong penetrance but variable expressivity. Age of onset is variable, ranging from childhood to middle age, but is usually in the teens or twenties. The course is slowly progressive. The ability to walk is usually preserved and life expectancy is normal. Initially there is facial weakness, followed by shoulder girdle and upper arm weakness and wasting with preservation of the deltoids. The forearms are preserved ("Popeye arm") but the wrist extensors may be involved. Later there is downward spread to the lower extremities with involvement of both the hip flexors and the foot dorsiflexors. Mild asymmetry may be present. Relative facial sparing with greater scapuloperoneal involvement or relatively isolated facial weakness may be the only manifestation. In the former, differentiation from limb-girdle dystrophy may be difficult on clinical grounds alone. The heart is rarely involved. Intellect is normal. Differential diagnosis includes neurogenic muscular atrophies (facioscapuloperoneal or scapuloperoneal progressive spinal muscular atrophy), polymyositis, limb-girdle dystrophy, and congenital myopathies with late manifestations. CPK is normal or only minimally elevated (usually <5 times normal). EMG may be normal in early stages, even in clinically weak muscles.

Distal myopathy (adult onset) is autosomal dominant and rare except in Sweden. Age of onset is between 40 and 60 years. The course is usually benign with slow progression. There is weakness and wasting of the distal upper and lower extremities with mild spread proximally. CPK is 20-200 times normal. The major differential diagnosis is neuronal peroneal muscular atrophy (HMSN II).

Distal myopathy (juvenile onset) is autosomal dominant and very rare. Age of onset is within 2 years with very slow progression. Enzymes are 20 times normal, becoming normal later. Differential diagnosis includes progressive spinal muscular atrophy and distal congenital myopathy.

Ocular myopathy is probably a congenital mitochondrial myopathy (see Ophthalmoplegia).

Oculopharyngeal dystrophy is autosomal dominant and rare, though more common in French-Canadians. Age of onset is between 40 and 50 years. The course is slowly progressive but dysphagia may be quite severe and may shorten the life span. There is ptosis and dysphagia with relative sparing of other extraocular muscles. The severity of dysphagia is variable. Myasthenia gravis must be excluded.

Myotonic dystrophy (dystrophia myotonica, myotonia atrophica) is autosomal dominant with variable expressivity. Age of onset is usually in the teens or twenties, although there is a congenital form. Myotonia is manifest as an impaired ability to relax skeletal muscle, apparent on shaking hands or percussing the tongue, hand, forearm, or calf (see Myotonia). Weakness is usually the presenting symptom with progressive, distal > proximal limb weakness and wasting. The face is involved with ptosis and wasting of the temporalis and masseter muscles ("hatchet facies"). There is also dysphagia, nasal regurgitation, and weakness of the anterior neck and abdominal muscles. The degree of myotonia is relatively minor compared to the degree of weakness. The course is slowly progressive, of variable severity, with death in the fifties and sixties, usually secondary to cardiac dysrhythmias, respiratory insufficiency, or infection. The congenital form usually presents with respiratory insufficiency, feeding difficulty, and frequent aspirations; myotonia is usually absent and the prognosis is poor. Associated findings include early frontal balding, subcapsular cataracts (slit lamp exam), narrow high arched palate, mild intellectual impairment and apathy, cardiac conduction abnormalities, primary testicular atrophy, glucose intolerance with decreased end-organ responsiveness to insulin, and respiratory muscle weakness. There is a high risk of prolonged respiratory depression after general anesthesia, especially with thiopental. Enzymes are normal or mildly elevated. EMG is myopathic with myotonic discharges triggered by needle insertion or voluntary contractions. These discharges consist of sustained bursts of waxing and waning frequency with varying amplitude which have a characteristic sound. Muscle biopsy reveals preferential involvement of Type I fibers and absence of significant necrosis. See also Myotonia.

Limb girdle syndromes include scapulohumeral dystrophy, childhood dystrophy, and other diseases with proximal limb girdle weakness. Scapulohumeral muscular dystrophy is autosomal recessive, uncommon, with onset in teenage years, and a slowly progressive course. Shoulder girdle and proximal upper extremity weakness and wasting with facial sparing is followed in 5-20 years by proximal lower extremity weakness with sparing of the hamstrings. The heart is not involved and intelligence is normal. Enzymes are high early in the course and decrease as the disease progresses. Childhood muscular dystrophy is autosomal recessive, uncommon, with age of onset between 5 and 10 years, and has a course similar to Becker dystrophy. Weakness of the proximal upper and lower extremities is slowly progressive. Enzymes are high but not as high as in the X-linked dystrophies. Differential diagnosis includes other diseases with proximal limb girdle weakness such as Becker dystrophy, myopathies (congenital, inflammatory, carnitine deficiency), spinal muscular atrophies, and some female carriers of Duchenne dystrophy.

<u>Management of muscular dystrophy</u> is an important determinant of patient welfare, in spite of the disease being incurable. Patient and family education and social and psychological assistance are provided.

Preservation of muscle strength and ambulation is maximized through active physical therapy. Disuse wasting is prevented through performance of normal daily physical activities such as standing, walking, and swimming. Prolonged bedrest should be avoided. A closely supervised resistive exercise program helps strengthen muscles. Low resistance, high repetition exercises increase endurance. Functional performance should be assessed frequently and patients maintained at the highest level of function consistent with the disease state.

Deformities due to imbalances between agonist and antagonist muscles are avoided by passive stretching (manually, standing/walking), orthotic devices, and strengthening weaker muscles in physical therapy. Loss of just a few pounds of excess weight may make the difference between walking and wheelchair confinement. Respiratory care includes breathing exercises, postural drainage, and IPPB.

Genetic counseling and screening should be available. In X-linked recessive disorders, a carrier has a 50% chance of having a diseased son or a carrier daughter with each pregnancy. Seventy-five to ninety percent of carriers of Duchenne dystrophy have an elevated CPK. Thirty percent of new cases are sporadic. The carrier mother has several options including prevention of further pregnancies and in-utero sex determination and abortion of all male fetuses.

In autosomal dominant disorders there are no carriers. The affected person has a 50% chance of producing a diseased offspring with each conception. An option here is adoption.

In the autosomal recessive disorders, carrier detection is not possible. An affected person has a significant risk of producing an affected offspring only if the other parent is a carrier. The chances of this occurring are minimal unless the union is consanguineous.

In cases of myotonic dystrophy with disabling myotonia, phenytoin may be useful. Other medications which may be used, except when there are heart conduction abnormalities, include procainamide 250-500 mg PO q6h and quinine 5-10 mg/kg/day given q4h.

Ref: Gardner-Medwin D. Clinical features and classification of the muscular dystrophies. Br Med Bull
36:109, 1980.

Vignos PJ. Physical models of rehabilitation in
neuromuscular disease. Muscle Nerve 6:323, 1983.

Bradley WG, Keleman J. Editorial: Genetic
counseling in Duchenne muscular dystrophy. Muscle
Nerve 2:325, 1979.

MYASTHENIA GRAVIS

An autoimmune postsynaptic neuromuscular transmission
disorder which is caused by antibodies against skeletal
muscle acetylcholine receptors (AChR). There is increased
turnover and destruction of AChR (probably complement
mediated) and subsequently there is a decreased number of
AChR on the postsynaptic membrane. The degree of AChR
loss usually parallels the clinical severity of the
disease.

Myasthenia gravis (MG) may begin at any age but is
most common in young women between the ages of 10 and 40
years. Female to male ratio is 3:1 in young adults and
approaches 1:1 after age 40. MG peaks in men between the
ages of 50-70 years. Prevalence is 3/100,000.

Symptoms and signs are characterized by fatigable,
often variable, weakness which improves with rest. Ptosis
and diplopia are the most common symptoms. Other symptoms
include dysarthria, dysphagia (often nasal regurgitation
of liquids), and facial and appendicular weakness.
Appendicular weakness is usually fairly symmetric and more
pronounced proximally than distally. Weakness of neck and
trunk muscles is not uncommon. Muscle atrophy is rare.
Sensation and reflexes are normal.

At least 50% of myasthenics present with ocular
complaints (diplopia, ptosis); at least 80% develop
ocular involvement during their illness. Twenty percent
have ocular involvement only. If progression of MG occurs,
it is usually within 2 years of onset.

Thymomas are more common in MG. They may be locally
invasive but usually do not metastasize; they are more
common in older patients. Thymic hyperplasia is very
common in young myasthenics and decreases with age (occurs
in 10% of MG, 30% of patients with thymoma have MG).
MG is associated (at least 10%) with other autoimmune
disorders including thyroid disease, systemic lupus
erythematosus and rheumatoid arthritis.

Neonatal myasthenia refers to transient weakness in
infants born to myasthenic mothers (10-30%). Infants

present with weak cry, poor suck, open mouth and paucity of limb movements. Ocular involvement is rare. It resolves spontaneously within 2-3 weeks (usually 24-36 hrs) and the treatment is supportive with temporary nasogastric intubation.

Congenital myasthenia refers to generalized MG in infants whose mothers are usually not myasthenic. Ocular involvement is common. AntiAchR antibodies are absent. Congenital MG is very rare.

Differential Diagnosis of myasthenia gravis includes certain disorders of muscle, inflammatory neuropathies, and poliomyelitis, as well as other disorders of neuromuscular transmission.

Diagnosis of MG is based on the clinical history and exam and confirmed by the response to cholinesterase inhibitors. The edrophonium (Tensilon) test is useful diagnostically, as well as in differentiating myasthenic from cholinergic crisis (see below). Several variables (e.g, ptosis, strength in selected muscles, functional activity, and vital capacity) are evaluated before and after administration of an anticholinesterase. Edrophonium, 2 mg, is injected into a secure IV line. Observe for 45-60 sec for hypersensitivity or excessive muscarinic effects, particularly bradycardia. In the absence of these, infuse an additional 8.0 mg over 30-60 sec.

CLASSIFICATION OF DISORDERS OF NEUROMUSCULAR TRANSMISSION
(Adapted from Walton)

A. Genetically determined
   1. Hereditary myasthenia
      a. Congenital and juvenile
      b. Myasthenia with myopathy
   2. Pseudocholinesterase deficiency (suxamethonium paralysis)
B. Toxic/cholinergic paralysis
   1. Botulism
   2. Tick paralysis
   3. Puffer-fish paralysis (tetrodotoxin)
   4. Certain snake venoms (bungarotoxin)
   5. Magnesium
   6. Lithium
   7. Antibiotics (aminoglycoside, others)
   8. D-penicillamine
   9. Poisoning with anticholinesterase compounds (e.g., insecticide, nerve gases)

        10. Depolarizing drugs
        11. Black widow spider venom
C. Autoimmune
        1. Myasthenia gravis and its variants (per above)
D. Other myasthenic syndromes
        1. Myasthenic-myopathic syndrome (Eaton-Lambert)
            a. With malignant disease
            b. Without malignant disease
        2. Congenital myasthenic syndrome with reduced
            acetylcholine release and deficient end-plate
            acetylcholinesterase.
        3. Other congenital and juvenile myasthenic syndromes
            due to various abnormalities of postsynaptic
            acetylcholine receptors.
        4. Symptomatic disorder of neuromuscular transmission
            a. in polymyositis and systemic lupus
            b. in motor neuron disease
            c. in chronic polyneuropathy

Ref: Walton JN. Disorders of Voluntary Muscle. 4th
        ed. Edinburgh: Churchill Livingstone, 1981:473-4

Re-evaluate the patient immediately and at 1 minute
intervals for 5 min. Onset of effect may begin during or
within seconds of completing the injection and last from
2-10 min. For diagnosis, the test may be single- or
double-blinded, using saline or nicotinic acid (100 mg/10
ml saline) as a control. Atropine should be available in
a syringe in case of bradycardia and hypotension or
excessive muscarinic side effects (nausea, gastrointestinal cramping, diarrhea, diaphoresis, lacrimation or
salivation). Tracheal intubation and ventilatory support
should be immediately available for patients with
compromised respiratory or oropharyngeal function. Note
that, while myasthenic weakness may improve, other muscles
may get weaker due to cholinergic excess. If a longer
duration of effect is desired, neostigmine (Prostigmine),
0.04 mg/Kg, is given IM. Response occurs within 15-20 min
and is maximal at 1-2 hrs. Premedication with atropine
may prevent muscarinic side effects.
        Serum AChR antibody is present in 80% of
myasthenics, but there is no clear correlation between
level and severity of disease. EMG/nerve conduction
studies should include repetitive stimulation and, where
possible, single fiber EMG. In MG there is a >10%
decremental response with supramaximal repetitive

stimulation at low frequency (2-5 Hz) in at least 2 muscles. The decrement may be repaired with edrophonium. Movement artifact must be excluded as a cause of false positive tests. Postactivation facilitation should be checked (see Myasthenic Syndrome of Lambert-Eaton). Single fiber EMG reveals increased jitter and blocking. Nerve conduction studies are normal.

<u>Additional studies</u> include CBC, ESR, ANA, anti-DNA (association with SLE, RA), thyroid function tests (association with thyroid disease), chest x-ray, chest CT scan (exclude thymoma), and antistriated muscle antibodies (present in majority of patients with thymoma). Fasting blood glucose, 2 hour postprandial blood glucose, and placement of PPD should be done prior to long-term steroid therapy.

<u>Treatment</u> options in MG include anticholinesterases, steroids, immunosuppressive drugs, thymectomy and plasmapheresis. For ocular myasthenia, patching an eye will prevent diplopia. Ptosis crutches are occasionally tolerated by patients with bilateral ptosis. <u>Cholinesterase inhibitors</u> are the initial agents of choice, particularly in milder classes of MG, although in ocular myasthenia they may improve unilateral ptosis resulting in diplopia or reduce a larger angle diplopia to a more bothersome small angle diplopia. Pyridostigmine (Mestinon) is started at 30-60 mg PO q3-4 hrs and gradually increased by 30-60 mg increments up to 240 mg q3h or 120 mg q2h while awake (up to 1200 mg/day). Smaller, more frequent dosing may increase the ratio of benefit to side effects. Muscarinic side effects are described above. Nicotinic side effects include weakness, fasciculations and cramps; this cholinergic weakness may be indistinguishable from that due to MG (see Crisis below). Treatment of side effects with atropine is best avoided, if possible. Ephedrine, 25 mg PO tid, is occasionally used to supplement cholinesterase inhibitors.

<u>Steroids</u> may be used instead of cholinesterase inhibitors in severe ocular myasthenia or added in cases of generalized myasthenia refractory to cholinesterase inhibitors. In ocular myasthenia, prednisone is started at 10 mg qod and increased by 10 mg every third dose to 50-100 mg qod. This dose is continued for 2-3 months and tapered by 10 mg/month; a maintenance dose may be required. For generalized myasthenia, initiation of prednisone is done as an inpatient, starting at 60-100 mg/day. Exacerbation of symptoms may occur anywhere from day 1 to day 21 (usually around day 5) of high dose prednisone therapy. Exacerbations last 1-20 days, are mild to moderate in 50% with respiratory failure in 8%. Onset of improvement usually begins around day 13

but ranges from day 1 to day 60 of therapy. Prednisone should be continued for 60 days before declaring clinical failure. Once there is significant improvement, dosing is changed from daily to alternate days. After several months, the dose is gradually tapered by 5-10 mg/1-2 months as long as the patient remains stable; a maintenance dose may be required. Pyridostigmine may be tapered gradually after maxmimum improvement has occurred. Because of exacerbations with high dose steroids, some advocate beginning prednisone at 10 mg PO qd and increasing by 10 mg/day to 100 mg. Improvement is seen by 6-7 weeks.

Immunosuppressive therapy may be helpful in severe MG refractory to prednisone and thymectomy or in patients who have relapses following prednisone and plasma exchange. Improvement is seen over months with cyclophosphamide 50-75 mg/m2 BSA/day and azathioprine 150-200 mg/day. Complications include GI symptoms, leukopenia, increased risk of infection, hepatotoxicity, hemorrhagic cystitis, and potential teratogenicity in pregnant women. It is not generally used in ocular myasthenia.

Thymectomy is done in severe refractory MG, although there is now emphasis on doing thymectomies early in the disease course, especially in younger patients. Younger patients do better with cholinesterase inhibitors and thymectomy, whereas older patients (>50 years) do better with steroids. Some centers recommend thymectomy following the maximal response to prednisone in all patients under 55. Thymectomy is done whenever thymoma is suspected. There is little benefit from thymectomy in ocular myasthenia. Thymectomy is generally preceded by a course of higher dose steroids and/or plasmapheresis with steroids given peri-operatively to avoid adrenal insufficiency. Improvement occurs from 2 to as long as 10 years after thymectomy (life span of T-lymphocytes).

Plasmapheresis is used as intensive intervention in acutely deteriorating myasthenics and to produce rapid improvement prior to thymectomy to reduce peri-operative morbidity. It is also used in severe refractory MG in conjunction with steroids or antimetabolites. Onset of improvement may occur as early as during the first exchange, but usually occurs 24 hours later. Improvement is sustained for weeks to months. Repeat exchanges may be necessary.

Crisis in myasthenia is a medical emergency. It may be due to acute onset of the disease, poor response to treatment, or precipitation by infection (myasthenic crisis) or to excessive cholinesterase inhibitors (cholinergic crisis). It is usually difficult to distinguish the two. Any patient with acute generalized myasthenia, with or without respiratory involvement, should be managed in an intensive care setting until stabilized on therapy since respiratory decompensation occurs very rapidly and can be fatal. Elective endotracheal intubation should be considered early. Improvement of weakness with edrophonium indicates myasthenic crisis; worsening, indicates cholinergic crisis. If there is any question, all anticholinesterase drugs should be discontinued for 3 days. Meticulous attention to pulmonary status and care is essential.

Pregnancy may alter the course of MG (see Pregnancy).

Drugs impairing neuromuscular transmission or respiration in myasthenics include:

1. Antibiotics - aminoglycosides, tetracyclines, polymyxins, colistin
2. Lithium
3. Magnesium
4. Muscle relaxants - curare, succinylcholine, quinine
5. Antidysrhythmics - quinidine, procainamide.
6. Anesthetics - ether, procaine, lidocaine
7. Analgesics, sedatives - morphine, meperidine, phenothiazines
8. Anticonvulsants - phenytoin, mephenytoin, trimethadione
9. β-adrenergic blockers
10. Chloroquine

Ref: Patten BM. Myasthenia gravis: review of diagnosis and management. Muscle Nerve 1:190, 1978.

Johns TR (ed). Myasthenia gravis. Seminars in Neurology. Vol 2, No. 3, 1982.

Swift T. Disorders of neuromuscular transmission other than myasthenia gravis. Muscle Nerve 4:334, 1981.

MYASTHENIC SYNDROME OF LAMBERT-EATON

An autoimmune presynaptic neuromuscular transmission disorder believed due to antibodies directed against the active sites of the motor nerve terminal. Clinical features include proximal weakness with difficulty climbing stairs, arising from a chair, combing hair, etc. The exertional weakness relatively spares the oropharyngeal and ocular muscles, unlike myasthenia gravis (MG). Muscle testing reveals a transient increase in strength during the first few contractions (related to postactivation facilitation). Prolonged exertion produces increasing weakness. Myalgias, paresthesias, dry mouth and impotence are often present, unlike MG. Tendon reflexes may be decreased. There is strong association with carcinoma, usually oat cell carcinoma of lung, but also GI, breast and prostatic carcinomas. Successful treatment of the tumor usually results in resolution of the syndrome. The myasthenic syndrome is also associated with autoimmune disorders such as thyroid disease, pernicious anemia, rheumatoid arthritis, and Sjogren's syndrome.

Diagnosis rests on the EMG findings. The compound muscle action potential amplitude is initially low, and there is a further 10% decrement with supramaximal repetitive stimulation at low frequencies (2-3 Hz). The distinguishing feature from MG is the markedly increased incremental response after supramaximal repetitive stimulation at high frequency (20-50 Hz) or after a sustained voluntary muscle contraction (postactivation facilitation, post-tetanic potentiation). Routine nerve conduction studies are otherwise normal. EMG shows brief, small variable amplitude polyphasic motor unit potentials. Response to edrophonium or neostigmine is variable. Acetylcholine receptor antibodies are not present.

Treatment consists of resection or chemotherapeutic treatment of carcinoma. Guanidine hydrochloride, 10-50 mg/kg/day in divided doses, increases the release of acetylcholine from the presynaptic terminal and may improve strength. Side effects include bone marrow suppression, hepatic toxicity, and renal toxicity. Response to cholinesterase inhibitors is variable. Prednisone may help, particularly if the myasthenic syndrome is due to another autoimmune disease. Azathioprine may be helpful. 3,4-diaminopyridine is an experimental drug which may be useful in combination with a cholinesterase inhibitor. Side effects include transient perioral paresthesias, diarrhea and abdominal cramps. Plasmapharesis may be helpful, at least transiently.

Ref: Jablecki C. Muscle Nerve 7:250, 1984.

MYELITIS (see Spinal Cord)

MYELOGRAPHY

The two most commonly used myelographic agents are metrizamide (Amipaque) which is water soluble and iophendylate (Pantopaque) which is not water soluble. The most common adverse reactions of metrizamide are headache, nausea and vomiting, seizures (may be potentiated in the presence of neuroleptics, MAO inhibitors, tricyclic anti-depressants and stimulants), transient encephalopathy (confusion, hallucinations, asterixis, myoclonus), and chemical meningitis (CSF pleocytosis, fever, nuchal rigidity). The peak onset of adverse symptoms occurs within hours after myelography.

Adverse effects of iophendylate may be acute or chronic. Acute effects include headache, fever, meningismus, and CSF pleocytosis of variable severity. Rarer adverse effects include confusion, seizures, dizziness, cranial neuropathies, myoclonus, transverse myelopathy, and urinary retention. Chronically, adhesive arachnoiditis may occur.

Ref: Junck L, Marshall WH. Ann Neurol 13:469, 1983.

MYELOPATHY (see Spinal Cord)

MYOCLONUS

Brief contractions of muscles, usually irregular in rhythm and amplitude (occasionally regular rhythm). Movements are brief (10-30 ms). They may involve only a single muscle, but usually larger movements involving a group of muscles displace part of a limb, the whole limb, or the trunk. Distribution of affected muscles is asymmetric, and contractions are asynchronous. Myoclonus may be precipitated, in certain cases, by stimuli such as loud sounds, flashing lights, or abrupt physical contact.

Classification of myoclonus by etiology

A. Physiological myoclonus (in normal subjects)
   1. Sleep jerks (hypnic jerks) are sudden, singular jerks on falling asleep
   2. With anxiety or exercise
   3. Hiccoughs

B. Essential myoclonus (without other associated neurological deficits)
   1. Familial essential myoclonus begins in the first
      or second decade. It is a benign disease of
      dominant inheritance with variable penetrance.
      Men and women are affected equally. It can be
      generalized or focal with a predilection for the
      face, trunk, and proximal limb muscles. It is
      absent or reduced at rest, absent in sleep, and
      worse with stress and movement. EEG is normal.
   2. Sporadic essential myoclonus is similar to above
      but without familial history.
   3. Periodic movements of sleep (nocturnal myoclonus)
      refers to repetitive jerking during sleep that may
      be synchronous or asynchronous in the two limbs.
      It occurs during non-REM sleep, every 30 seconds
      for up to several hours and associated with other
      sleep disorders. It is nonprogressive, with no
      other neurological pathology.

C. Epileptic myoclonus (seizures predominate)
   1. Generalized epileptic myoclonus is more common in
      children and adolescents than adults. Types
      include benign myoclonus of infancy, infantile
      spasms, Lennox-Gastaut, cryptogenic myoclonic
      epilepsy, myoclonus in association with absence,
      photosensitive myoclonic epilepsy, and myoclonus
      in association with primary generalized epilepsy.
   2. Myoclonus associated with isolated spike dis-
      charges in the motor cortex.
      a. Idiopathic stimulus-sensitive myoclonus
      b. Isolated epileptic myoclonic jerks
      c. Epilepsia partialis continua
   3. Patients with idiopathic epilepsy may complain of
      localized myoclonic jerks, usually confined to an
      arm or leg, and occurring singly or in short
      bursts, often upon awakening. These may be more
      frequent or severe on the day or two prior to a
      generalized seizure.

D. "Symptomatic" myoclonus as part of a more widespread
   encephalopathy or other neurological disorder (with or
   without epilepsy).
   1. Posthypoxic (chronic)
      a. Myoclonic jerks in isolation or repetitively
      b. Induced by attempts at voluntary movements
         (action or intention myoclonus) or by some
         types of sensory stimuli
      c. Associated with spikes in the EEG

2. Posthypoxic (acute) myoclonus occurs as an acute effect of hypoxia while the patient is in, or recovering from, coma and is frequently transient. It is often generalized, rhythmic, and stimulus-sensitive.
3. Metabolic encephalopathies: Hepatic failure, renal failure, dialysis syndromes, hyponatremia, hypoglycemia, nonketotic hyperglycemia, and others.
4. Viral encephalopathies: subacute sclerosing panencephalitis, encephalitis lethargica, Herpes simplex encephalitis, arbo virus encephalitis, postinfectious encephalitis.
5. Dementias: Creutzfeldt-Jakob disease (common), Alzheimer's.
6. Degenerative diseases involving the basal ganglia: Wilson's disease, torsion dystonia, Hallervorden-Spatz disease, progressive supranuclear palsy, Huntington's disease.
7. Spinocerebellar degenerations: Friedreich's ataxia, ataxia telangiectasia, dyssynergia cerebellaris myoclonica (Ramsay Hunt syndrome), familial myoclonic epilepsy of Unverricht and Lundborg (Baltic myoclonus).
8. Storage diseases: Lafora body disease, lipidoses, ceroid-lipofuscinoses, sialidosis.
9. Toxic encephalopathies: Heavy metal poisons, methylbromide, bismuth, strychnine, many drugs including penicillin, levodopa, imipramine, amitriptyline, piperazine, and chloralose.
10. Focal CNS damage: Cerebrovascular disease, tumor, trauma, post-thalamotomy.

Focal and segmental myoclonus (forms of "symptomatic" myoclonus) may have special significance.

Palatal "myoclonus" (or tremor) may be bilateral or unilateral. Contractions are rhythmic, with a rate of about 1.5-5.0 Hz, and do not cease during sleep. It may be associated with contractions of external ocular muscles (ocular/palatal myoclonus, see Ocular Oscillations), larynx, neck, tongue, face, diaphragm, trunk, and limbs. The anatomic lesion is in the "Guillain-Mollaret triangle", which consists of the red nucleus, ipsilateral inferior olivary nucleus, contralateral dentate nucleus, and connecting pathways. It usually begins 10-12 months after the precipitating cause and lasts for the life of the patient. It is seen with cerebrovascular disease, multiple sclerosis, encephalitis, and in association with hereditary tremor.

Rhythmical myoclonus of the head and neck may occur following trauma, with Creutzfeldt-Jakob disease, and with porencephalic cysts.

Spinal segmental myoclonus results from spinal cord pathology, including degenerative disease, tumor, myelopathy from cervical osteoarthritis, demyelinating disease, motor neuron disease, and following spinal anesthesia, or infection.

<u>Treatment</u> is based on identifying and treating any underlying disease. Treatment of the myoclonus itself may not be necessary unless it limits the patient's daily functioning. The following drugs have been helpful:

1. Clonazepam starting with 1-1.5 mg qd in divided doses and gradually increasing.
2. 5-hydroxytryptophan starting at 100 mg qd (divided into 2 to 4 doses). Can increase by 100 mg every 2-3 days. Can go up to 1000-1500 mg qd. Can give with carbidopa, starting at 25 mg qd (in divided doses). Also, increase this every 2-3 days up to 200 mg qd.
3. Valproic acid is gradually increased up to 1600 mg per day (especially in posthypoxic cases).

Ref: Marsden CD, et al. The nosology and pathophysiology of myoclonus. In: Marsden CD, Fahn S (eds). Movement Disorders. London: Butterworth, 1982.

MYOGLOBINURIA

Myoglobin in the urine due to rhabdomyolysis, occurring within several hours of acute muscle necrosis.
Causes of myoglobinuria:
A. Extreme muscle exertion (heavy exercise in untrained persons, "march hemoglobinuria", electric shock, seizures)
B. Trauma (crush injuries)
C. Ischemia (muscle infarction)
D. Toxins (carbon monoxide, alcohol, barbiturates, amphotericin B, licorice, hornet and sea snake venom)
E. Electrolyte disorders
    1. Acidosis (diabetic ketoacidosis, renal tubular acidosis)
    2. Hypernatremia
    3. Hypokalemia
F. Hypothermia
G. Infection/sepsis (influenza, tetanus, typhus, mononucleosis, coxsackie virus)
H. Fever
I. Metabolic/hereditary
    1. Glycogenoses
    a) Phosphorylase deficiency (McArdle's disease)
    b) Phosphofructokinase deficiency

2. Carnitine palmityltransferase deficiency
3. Malignant hyperthermia
4. Idiopathic familial myoglobinuria
J. Progressive muscular disease (rarely)

Diagnosis depends on further characterization of pigmenturia (myoglobin, hemoglobin, porphyrins) by spectrophotometry, electrophoresis, or immunoprecipitation. Myalgia is often present. Serum muscle enzymes, especially creatinine kinase, are elevated.

Complications include acute tubular necrosis (treated with hydration, alkalinization of urine and osmotic diuresis), hypocalcemia, hyperkalemia, and respiratory insufficiency secondary to severe muscle necrosis.

MYOPATHY

Congenital myopathies with distinct morphological characteristics include central core disease, nemaline (rod body) myopathy, myotubular (centronuclear) myopathy, congenital fiber type disease (CFTD), fingerprint body myopathy, multicore disease, focal loss of cross striations, and sarcotubular myopathy. It is unclear whether the morphologic changes are related to pathogenesis or are epiphenomena. Pathogenesis is unknown.

Clinically, these present as floppy infants with delayed motor milestones. A sub-type of myotubular myopathy may occur in childhood or later. Inheritance is autosomal dominant, recessive, or sporadic. The course is slowly progressive or nonprogressive except for some rapidly progressive cases of myotubular or nemaline myopathy. The pattern of weakness is usually diffuse, proximal > distal, but may be distal > proximal in myotubular and in nemaline myopathy. The facial muscles are more commonly involved in myotubular and nemaline myopathy and in CFTD. The extraocular muscles are more commonly involved in myotubular myopathy. Muscle stretch reflexes are variably decreased. Commonly associated signs include facial dysmorphism (long, thin facies and high arched palate in nemaline myopathy and CFTD), kyphoscoliosis, foot deformities (pes cavus and planus), congenital or infantile hip dislocations, contractures, and usually normal intelligence. Enzymes are usually normal. EMG shows myopathic features.

Muscle biopsy/histochemistry is the basis for morphological characterization. In general, there is variable Type I fiber predominance with or without Type I fiber atrophy. Central cores are seen along the center of fibers; there is absence of oxidative enzymes and mitochondria in the cores. Nemaline rods are structures originating in the Z lines. Myotubules are fetal muscle fibers with longitudinal chains of central nuclei. CFTD has smaller type I fibers and absence of other morphologic changes.

Management is as outlined for muscular dystrophy.

Ref: Brooke MH, et al. Muscle Nerve 2:84, 1979.

Metabolic myopathy refers to muscle involvement in the glycogenoses and disorders of lipid metabolism.

Glycogenoses are mostly autosomal recessive. Muscle biopsy shows abnormal accumulation of glycogen. The specific enzyme abnormality is diagnosed by biochemical analysis of the affected tissue (muscle, leukocytes, skin, etc.). Other useful tests include EMG, creatine kinase, and determination of lactate production after ischemic forearm exercise. Some of the glycogenoses can be diagnosed in utero. There is no effective treatment of the 11 glycogenoses for which the enzyme defect is known, 7 involve muscle.

Acid maltase deficiency (Pompe) results in generalized deposition of glycogen in all tissues. Quadriparesis in these patients is due to muscle, peripheral nerve, and CNS involvement. In the infantile type, death occurs by one year of age. In the adult type, there is proximal limb girdle weakness, which is slowly progressive; life expectancy is normal or slightly decreased.

Debranching enzyme deficiency (Forbes-Cori) causes occasional proximal weakness, which may improve after puberty. Hepatomegaly is common. Life expectancy is close to normal.

Branching enzyme deficiency causes progressive weakness, cirrhosis and hepatosplenomegaly. It is usually fatal by age 5 years.

Muscle phosphorylase deficiency (McArdle) and muscle phosphofructokinase deficiency (Tarui) causes exercise intolerance with myoglobinuria and painful cramps (contractures). Proximal weakness may be only exertional or may be permanent.

Muscle phosphoglycerate mutase deficiency and muscle lactate dehydrogenase deficiency also results in exercise intolerance and myoglobinuria.

Disorders of lipid metabolism affecting muscle include carnitine deficiency and carnitine palmityl transferase deficiency. Primary carnitine deficiency occurs in two forms, myopathic and systemic. There is slowly progressive weakness, which starts in childhood or later. In the systemic form, in addition to weakness, there are recurrent episodes of hepatic encephalopathy. Muscle biopsy and histochemistry of both forms shows abnormal lipid accumulation; biochemical analysis of muscle shows decreased carnitine content. Serum concentration of carnitine is normal in the myopathic form and decreased in the systemic form. EMG shows myopathic features. Prognosis in the systemic form is poor with death in the late teens or early twenties. Most of the cases are sporadic, but there is evidence of autosomal recessive inheritance in some. Treatment with high dose oral carnitine or prednisone may be effective. Secondary carnitine deficiency may occur in malnutrition with associated liver disease and in patients on chronic hemodialysis.

Carnitine palmityltransferase (CPT) deficiency. Symptoms begin in childhood with weakness, myoglobinuria, and painful cramps (contractures) in response to prolonged exercise and/or fasting. Strength between episodes is normal. Creatine kinase rises during attacks. Biochemical analysis of muscle and leukocytes shows markedly decreased CPT activity. Glycogen metabolism is normal, therefore, the ability to perform intense exercise of short duration is not impaired. Treatment with high carbohydrate-low fat diet may reduce the frequency of attacks.

Ref: DiMauro S, et al. Muscle Nerve 3:369, 1980

Polymyositis and dermatomyositis are inflammatory, usually sporadic, myopathies probably due to an immune mediated collagen vascular disease with both cellular mediated and humoral mechanisms.

CLASSIFICATION OF POLYMYOSITIS/DERMATOMYOSITIS
(Bohan and Peter)

Group I - primary, idiopathic polymyositis (PM)
Group II - primary, idiopathic dermatomyositis (DM)
Group III - DM or PM associated with carcinoma
Group IV - childhood DM or PM associated with a
           vasculitis
Group V - DM or PM with another associated collagen
          vascular disease (Overlap Syndrome)

Clinically there is symmetric limb girdle and neck weakness, progressing over weeks to months, with or without dysphagia or respiratory muscle weakness. There may be spontaneous exacerbations and remissions. Age distribution is bimodal with peaks at 5-15 years and 50-60 years. Reflexes are normal. Muscle wasting is absent until late. The typical "heliotrope" rash of DM consists of a lavender discoloration of the eyelids. In blacks the rash is usually dusky purple. There is associated peri-orbital edema. A scaly red rash appears over the dorsum of the hand, especially the MCP and PIP joints (Goltron's sign). The rash may also involve other joints, the chest, neck, and face. In group IV there is a generalized necrotizing vasculitis which may produce multiple infarctions of the GI tract, lungs, skin, nerves, and even brain. In group V the associated collagen vascular disorders include systemic lupus, rheumatoid arthritis, polyarteritis nodosa and Sjogrens syndrome. Arthralgias, myalgias and Raynaud's phenomenon are more common than in uncomplicated PM or DM. Serologic abnormalities are usually present.

Enzymes may be normal, but serum creatine kinase is usually mildly to moderately elevated, usually correlating with degree of weakness early in the course of the disease. EMG reveals increased insertional and spontaneous activity with myopathic motor unit potentials.

Muscle biopsy demonstrates perifascicular inflammatory infiltrates, atrophy, necrosis and phagocytosis; evidence of regeneration and increased connective tissue is more apparent in later stages. Muscle histochemistry demonstrates atrophy and degeneration of both type I and II fibers (no group type atrophy). Skin biopsy shows typical inflammatory and vasculitic changes.

The differential diagnosis is extensive; the presence of fasciculations, long tract signs, sensory changes, or group type atrophy on muscle biopsy excludes the diagnosis. The diagnosis of probable DM or PM can still be made in the presence of normal enzymes or normal EMG. Steroid responsiveness should no longer be considered part of the diagnostic criteria since other myopathies may also respond, and certain cases of DM or PM are refractory to steroids.

Occult malignancy should be excluded in older patients with PM or DM.

Treatment begins with prednisone 40-80 mg PO qd or 100 mg PO qod. High dose steroids require special precautions (see Myasthenia gravis). Prednisone should be continued for at least 2-3 months before assuming steroid resistance. If there is a clinical response (not just normalization of enzymes), prednisone should be slowly reduced by 5 mg every two weeks. Total length of therapy should be 2 years. A steroid induced myopathy with increased weakness may complicate therapy; enzymes and EMG are typically normal and biopsy may show preferential involvement of type II fibers.

Immunosuppressive therapy may be used in addition to or instead of prednisone; cyclophosphamide 50-75mg/m2

BSA/day PO or methotrexate 15-20mg/m^2 BSA biweekly, initially IV, then PO. Complications include increased risk of infection (especially opportunistic), hemorrhagic cystitis with cyclophosphamide, and hepatotoxicity with methotrexate.

Generally, treatment is more effective if started early. Consider treating for toxoplasmosis with pyrimethamine and sulfa if toxoplasma titers increase and a chorioretinitis develops. The use of plasmapharesis in polymyositis/dermatomyositis is controversial.

Ref: Bohan A, Peter JB. NEJM 292:344 and 403,

Engel WK, et al. Trans Am Neurol Assoc 97:272, 1972.

Metzger AL, et al. Ann Intern Med 81:182, 1974.

MYOTOMES (see also Reflexes)

MUSCLE	NERVE	ROOT
Levator scapulae	C3,4 and dorsal scapular	C3,4,5
Rhomboids (major and minor)	Dorsal scapular	C4,5
Supraspinatus	Suprascapular	C5,6
Infraspinatus	Suprascapular	C5,6
Deltoid	Axillary	C5,6
Biceps brachii	Musculocutaneous	C5,6
Brachioradialis	Radial	C5,6
Supinator	Radial	C5,6
Flexor carpi radialis	Median	C6,7
Pronator teres	Median	C6,7
Serratus anterior	Long thoracic	C5,6,7
Latissimus dorsi	Thoracodorsal	C6,7,8
Pectoralis major:		
Clavicular	Lateral pectoral	C5,6,7
Sternal	Medial pectoral	C6,7,8, T1
Triceps brachii	Radial	C6,7,8
Extensor carpi radialis longus	Radial	C6,7
Anconeus	Radial	C7,8
Extensor digitorum	Radial	C7,8
Extensor carpi ulnaris	Radial	C7,8
Extensor indicis proprius	Radial	C7,8
Palmaris longus	Median	C7,8, T1
Flexor pollicis longus	Median	C7,8, T1

MUSCLE	NERVE	ROOT
Flexor carpi ulnaris	Ulnar	C7,8, T1
Flexor digitorum sublimis	Median	C7,8
Flexor digitorum profundus	Median	C7,8, T1
	Ulnar	
Pronator quadratus	Median	C8, T1
Abductor pollicis brevis	Median	C8, T1
Apponens pollicis	Median	C8, T1
Flexor pollicis brevis	Median	C8, T1
Lumbricals I and II	Median	C8, T1
First dorsal interosseous	Ulnar	C8, T1
Abductor digiti minimi	Ulnar	C8, T1
Iliopsoas	Femoral	L2,3,4
Adductor longus	Obturator	L2,3,4
Gracilis	Obturator	L2,3,4
Quadriceps femoris	Femoral	L2,3,4
Anterior tibial	Deep peroneal	L4,5
Extensor hallucis longus	Deep peroneal	L4,5
Extensor digitorum longus	Deep peroneal	L4,5
Extensor digitorum brevis	Deep peroneal	L4,5, S1
Peroneus longus	Superficial peroneal	L5,S1
Internal hamstrings	Sciatic	L4,5, S1
External hamstrings	Sciatic	L5, S1
Gluteus medius	Superior gluteal	L4,5, S1
Gluteus maximus	Inferior gluteal	L5, S1,2
Posterior tibial	Tibial	L5, S1
Flexor digitorum longus	Tibial	L5, S1
Abductor hallucis brevis	Tibial (medial plantar)	L5, S1,2
Abductor digiti quinti pedis	Tibial (lateral plantar)	S1,2
Gastrocnemius lateral	Tibial	L5, S1,2
Gastrocnemius medial	Tibial	S1,2
Soleus	Tibial	S1,2

MYOTONIA (see also Cramps, Muscle Disorders, Muscular Dystrophy)

Myotonic dystrophy (see Muscular Dystrophy)

Myotonia congenita is not to be confused with adult or congenital myotonic muscular dystrophy. Inheritance is autosomal dominant (Thomsen) or recessive. Myotonia presents in infancy or later; in the recessive form it is more severe, more generalized, and of later onset. Muscle hypertrophy is prominent. Weakness is usually absent in the dominant form, but there may be mild proximal and distal weakness in the recessive form. Life expectancy is usually normal. EMG shows typical myotonic discharges

usually without myopathic features. Muscle biopsy shows
diffusely large muscle fibers with rows of central nuclei.
Type IIb fibers are usually absent.

Paramyotonia congenita (Eulenberg) is autosomal
dominant. Myotonia is more common in the face and may
worsen with exercise (paradoxical myotonia). Variable
periods of weakness (similar to periodic paralysis) may
occur which may or may not be related to exposure to cold.

Hyperkalemic periodic paralysis (see Periodic Paralysis)

Drug induced myotonia may be result from monocar-
boxylic aromatic acids or diazocholesterol.

Electrical myotonia with or without clinical myotonia
may be seen in acid maltase deficiency, polymyositis,
hyperthyroidism, and malignant hyperthermia as well as the
above myotonic disorders.

Treatment of myotonia has included phenytoin,
quinidine, or procainamide (see Muscle Disease).

Ref: Dubowitz V. Muscle Disorders in Childhood. London:
        Saunders, 1978.

NERVE CONDUCTION STUDIES (see EMG)

NEURALGIA

Trigeminal neuralgia (tic douloureaux) is of unknown
pathogenesis, although degenerative, compressive and viral
causes have been suggested. It may result from a mass
lesion or multiple sclerosis ("symptomatic" neuralgia).

Clinical features include paroxysmal, severe,
lancinating, brief (<30-60 seconds), usually unilateral
facial pain in the distribution of one or more branches of
the trigeminal nerve (most commonly the third and second
divisions). Paroxysms tend to occur in clusters. Trigger
points set off by touching, chewing, talking, or swallowing are characteristic. Onset is after age 40 in
90%, and is more common in women (3:2). Neurological
exam, including trigeminal sensory and motor exam, is
normal.

Differential diagnosis consists of those causes of
"symptomatic" neuralgia. These include multiple sclerosis
(may be bilateral, more common in age <40 years) and
posterior fossa mass lesions such as tumor (meningioma,
acoustic neuroma), aneurysm, or AVM. Trigeminal neuroma
and foramenal osteoma are other causes. Secondary or
symptomatic trigeminal neuralgia should be suspected with
onset before age 40, with trigeminal sensory or motor
abnormalities on exam, or with any other findings referrable to the base of the skull or posterior fossa. In such

cases, evaluation should include basal skull radiographs, CT of the skull base and posterior fossa (without and with contrast), and arteriography if there is evidence of tumor, AVM, or aneurysm.

Treatment of secondary trigeminal neuralgia is aimed at the underlying cause. Treatment of idiopathic trigeminal neuralgia is outlined below:

Medical

1. Carbamazepine is the drug of choice and is effective in 80%. Start at 200 mg/day and increase gradually to 1-1.2 gm/day in divided doses. Therapeutic serum levels should be achieved (see Antiepileptic Drugs).
2. Imipramine or amitriptyline starting at 25-50 mg PO qhs and gradually increasing to 150 mg qhs.
3. Phenytoin 300-500 mg qd to achieve therapeutic levels (see Antiepileptic Drugs).
4. Baclofen starting at 5 mg PO tid and increasing gradually to 20 mg PO qid.
5. Clonazepam starting at 0.5 mg PO bid and increase 0.5 mg/day to 10 mg/day in 2 or 3 divided doses.
6. Combination approaches have utilized phenytoin with carbamazepine or imipramine. Baclofen has also been used with phenytoin or carbamazepine.

Surgical therapy is reserved for intractable pain.

1. Local neurolysis and nerve block is associated with a risk of painful anesthesia and persistent paresthesias as well as recurrence.
2. Percutaneous radiofrequency coagulation of the trigeminal ganglion can be done under local anesthesia. Painful anesthesia and recurrences are less common.
3. Trigeminal rhizotomy
4. Microsurgical vascular decompression of the trigeminal root entry zone is an intracranial procedure and not indicated except in the most severe and refractory cases.

Vasoglossopharyngeal neuralgia has much the same etiology and pathogenesis as trigeminal neuralgia. Clinical features, also, are similar although the pain may be more variable with longer duration and be associated with autonomic dysfunction (salivation, lacrimation, bradycardia, possibly with syncope). Distribution is to the throat, posterior 1/3 of the tongue, tonsillar pillars, eustachian tube, and ear. Trigger points are variable, most commonly associated with swallowing or touching particular areas in the distribution of the glossopharyngeal nerve. Onset is after the age of 40 with both sexes affected equally. The differential diagnosis underlies causes such as oropharyngeal carcinoma, paratonsillar abscess, enlarged styloid process, or enlarged tortuous vertebral or posterior inferior cerebellar arteries. Evaluation is as for trigeminal neuralgia and should include a thorough ENT exam. Treatment is aimed at underlying causes of "symptomatic" neuralgias. Otherwise, carbamazepine or phenytoin or both may be used, although the response to these is <50%. Surgical therapy has included microsurgical decompression of the glossopharyngeal and vagal root entry zones and section of the glossopharyngeal nerve.

Ref: Davis EH. Headache 9:77, 1969.

        Rasmussen P, Riishede J. Acta Neurol Scand 46:385, 1970.

        Sweet WH, Wepsic JG. J Neurosurg 40:143, 1974.

NEUROCUTANEOUS SYNDROMES

Clinical features of the major phakomatoses:

Neurofibromatosis (Von Recklinghausen's disease)
    Cafe-au-lait spots
    Axillary (and other intertriginous) freckling
    Multiple neurofibromas
    Pigmented iris hamartomas (Lisch nodules)
    Increased incidence of CNS tumors
        Schwannomas
        Optic gliomas
        Astrocytomas
        Meningiomas
    Increased incidence of other neoplasms
    Kyphoscoliosis
    Pseudarthrosis
    Higher incidence of intellectual impairment

Tuberous sclerosis (Bourneville's disease)
    Seizures (may present with infantile spasms)
    Angiofibromas ("adenoma sebaceum")
    Mental retardation
    Cortical tubers
    Subependymal hamartomas
    Retinal hamartoma
    Ungual fibromas
    Hypomelanotic macules ("ash leaf")
    Subepidermal fibrosis ("shagreen patch")

Multiple renal tumors
Cardiac rhabdomyoma
Other skin lesions
May see calcification of cortical and subependymal
    lesions on CT

Meningofacial angiomatosis with cerebral calcification
(Sturge-Weber syndrome)
    Cutaneous angiomatosis of face and scalp involving
        first division of CN V
    Seizures
    Mental retardation
    Hemiparesis, homonymous hemianopia contralateral to
        facial nevus
    Angiomatosis of choroid of eye with buphthalmos and/or
        glaucoma
    Intracranial calcification beneath meningeal
        angiomatosis (usually parieto-occipital) seen on
        skull films ("tramline calcification") or CT

Von Hippel-Lindau disease
    Hemangioblastoma of brain (usually cerebellum), or,
        occasionally, spinal cord (often with syringomyelia)
    Retinal angiomatosis
    Cysts of pancreas or kidney
    Tumors of kidney
    Polycythemia from erythropoietic factor from
        cerebellar tumors

Ataxia telangiectasia
    Cerebellar degeneration with ataxia
    Oculocutaneous telangiectasia
    Mental retardation (mild)
    Strabismus, ocular dysmetria, nystagmus
    Choreoathetosis
    Chronic pulmonary infections
    Decreased IgA and IgE
    Increased serum α-fetoprotein

Ref: Riccardi VM. Von Recklinghausen neurofibromatosis.
        NEJM 305:1617, 1981.

NEUROLEPTICS

Aminoalkyl phenothiazines, such as chlorpromazine
(Thorazine), are strongly sedating. Potent α-adrenergic
antagonism results in postural hypotension. Antiemetic and
anticholinergic effects are significant. Extrapyramidal
and dystonic symptoms occur with medium frequency.

Piperidinyl phenothiazines, such as thioridazine (Mellaril) and mesoridazine (Serentil), have a relative potency similar to the aminoalkyl compounds. Sedative and α-adrenergic antagonism are less. Antiemetic effects are negligible. This class has the least incidence of extrapyramidal and dystonic side effects.

Piperazinyl phenothiazines, such as prochlorperazine (Compazine), trifluoperazine (Stelazine), perphenazine (Trilafon), and fluphenazine (Prolixin), have the highest relative potency and the strongest antiemetic effects. They also have the highest incidence of extrapyramidal and dystonic symptoms. Sedation and α-adrenergic antagonism are minimal.

The butyrophenones, such as haloperidol (Haldol), closely resemble the piperazines pharmacologically. They have strong dopaminergic blocking effects and a high incidence of extrapyramidal and dystonic symptoms. There is relatively less orthostatic hypotension and sedation.

The thioxanthines resemble the phenothiazines. Thiothixene (Navane) resembles the piperazines with greater dystonic and extrapyramidal side effects. Chlorprothixene (Taractan) resembles chlorpromazine with greater sedative and autonomic effects and less extra-pyramidal and dystonic features.

The dihydroindolones, such as molindone (Moban), have relatively frequent extrapyramidal and dystonic side effects. The dibenzoxazepines, such as loxapine (Loxitane), have sedative, anticholinergic and extra-pyramidal effects.

Dystonia may occur early (1-3 weeks) in the course of neuroleptic therapy or after a single parenteral injection. It may consist of generalized torsion dystonia, opisthotonos, torticollis, retrocollis, oculogyric crisis, trismus, or focal appendicular dystonia. It is more common in younger patients, especially children or adolescents. It resolves spontaneously within 24 hours of stopping the drug, but may be terminated within minutes with benztropine (Cogentin) 1 mg IM or IV or diphenhydramine (Benadryl) 50 mg IV; oral therapy may be continued for 24-48 hours.

Extrapyramidal or Parkinsonian symptoms are dose related and may begin as early as a few days to 4 weeks after starting therapy. The neuroleptic dosage should be decreased, or an anticholinergic agent may be added. Anticholinergic agents in use include benztropin (Cogentin) 0.5-4.0 mg bid, biperiden (Akineton) 1.0-2.0 mg tid, or trihexyphenidyl (Artane) 1.5 mg tid. Anticho-linergics may partially reverse antipsychotic effects. Routine prophylactic use of anticholinergics is not recommended due to the possibly increased risk of tardive dyskinesia.

Akathisia is a subjective sensation of motor restlessness with an urge to move around that generally occurs within several weeks of starting neuroleptics. It improves on decreasing the dose of neuroleptic or adding an anticholinergic. Neuroleptic dosage should not be increased to treat this form of "agitation".

Tardive dyskinesia, consisting of oral-lingual-facial-buccal movements most commonly or of other choreoathetoid or ballistic movements, may occur following prolonged neuroleptic therapy. Its incidence may be decreased by using neuroleptics only when indicated, keeping doses as low as possible and duration of therapy as short as possible, avoiding co-administration of anticholinergics, and early detection through careful follow-up. The more advanced the dyskinesia, the less likely is resolution. Anticholinergics may increase the intensity and duration of tardive dyskinesia, as well as possibly increase its incidence. Treatment consists of tapering and withdrawing the neuroleptic or substituting thioridazine and tapering and withdrawing anticholinergics. Reserpine 0.25 mg/day, increasing by 0.25 mg/day to 1-5 mg daily in divided doses, with care to avoid orthostatic hypotension, may help. Tetrabenazine, up to 300 mg daily may work more rapidly with less hypotension but has a greater loss of efficacy over time. Neuroleptics themselves have no role in the treatment of tardive dyskinesias.

A **withdrawal syndrome**, seen particularly in children, consisting of choreic movements may occur when chronically administered neuroleptics are suddenly stopped. It usually resolves within 6-12 weeks but can be avoided by reinstituting the drug and tapering more slowly.

The **neuroleptic malignant syndrome** is rare but often (20-30%) fatal. Hyperthermia, hypertonia of skeletal muscles, fluctuating consciousness, and autonomic instability are characteristic. Laboratory findings include elevated CPK, leukocytosis, and liver function abnormalities. The differential diagnosis includes phenothiazine-related heat stroke, malignant hyperthermia associated with anesthesia, idiopathic acute lethal catatonia, drug interactions with MAO inhibitors, and central anticholinergic syndromes. Treatment begins with discontinuing the neuroleptic and providing cooling blankets, antipyretics, and IV hydration. Dantrolene sodium 0.8-10 mg/kg per day IV has been used; 2-3 mg/kg per day IV or 50-200 mg per day PO are recommended. Bromocriptine 2.5-10 mg PO tid as well as amantadine or combination levodopa/carbidopa have also been effective.

Neuroleptics lower the **seizure threshold** and may precipitate seizures. Their use in patients with epilepsy is not contraindicated unless seizure control is a significant problem.

Ref: Klawans HL, Weiner WJ. Textbook of Clinical Neuro-
       pharmacology. New York: Raven Press, 1981.

       Guze BH, Baxter LR. Neuroleptic malignant syndrome.
       NEJM 313:163, 1985.

NEUROPATHY

CLINICAL CLASSIFICATION OF NEUROPATHY

A. Acute predominantly motor neuropathy with variable
   sensory involvement.
   1. Acute inflammatory demyelinating polyradiculo-
       neuropathy (Landry-Guillain-Barre-Strohl syndrome)
   2. Polyneuropathy associated with:
       a) Hepatitis
       b) Mononucleosis
       c) Diphtheria
       d) Porphyria
       e) Triorthocresyl phosphate
       f) Thallium
B. Acute motor neuropathy
   1. Diabetic   multiple   mononeuropathy   (asymmetric
       proximal diabetic neuropathy)
C. Acute asymmetric sensorimotor polyneuropathy, multiple
   mononeuropathy
   1. Polyarteritis nodosa
   2. Wegener's granulomatosis
   3. Diabetes
   4. Other angiopathic, vasculitic
D. Sub-acute symmetric sensorimotor neuropathy
   1. Toxic
       a) Heavy metals - arsenic, mercury, thallium
       b) Drugs
          1) Antibiotics - clioquinal, ethambutal,
             isoniazide, nitrofurantoin, streptomycin
          2) Antineoplastic - vinca alkaloids,
             cisplatinum, chlorambucil, methotrexate,
             daunorubicin
          3) Cardiovascular - clofibrate, disopyramide,
             hydralazine
          4) Other - amitriptyline, gold salts,
             colchicine, phenylbutazone, endomethazine,
             methaqualone, penicillamine, chloroquine,
             disulfiram

        c) Industrial chemicals - triorthocresyl
           phosphate, acrylamide, methyl bromide,
           n-hexane, methyl-n-butyl ketone,
           β-aminopropionitrile

2. Nutritional deficiency - vitamin B12, niacin
(pellagra), thiamine (beriberi), pyridoxine,
chronic alcoholism, vitamin E (chronic biliary
cirrhosis or malabsorption syndromes)
3. Uremia
4. Initially in chronic relapsing disimmune
polyneuropathy

E. Subacute to chronic, predominantly sensory neuropathy
1. Diabetes
2. Drugs - chloramphenicol, metronidazole, PAS,
ethambutol, amitriptyline, phenytoin (chronic),
propylthiouracil, ergotamine, methysergide
3. Leprosy
4. Remote effects of carcinoma
5. Pyridoxine toxicity

F. Subacute to chronic, predominantly motor neuropathy
1. Diabetes - proximal diabetic motor neuropathy
("amyotrophy")
2. Lead neuropathy

G. Chronic sensory motor neuropathy
1. Diabetes - mixed sensory-motor-autonomic
neuropathy
2. Remote effects of multiple myeloma
3. Remote effects of carcinoma
4. Uremia
5. Leprosy
6. Other dysproteinemias - macroglobulinemia,
cryoglobulinemia, ataxia-telangiectasia
7. Amyloidosis
8. Chronic relapsing disimmune polyneuropathy
9. Sarcoidosis

H. Hereditary motor and sensory neuropathies (HMSN) Types
I-III

I. Hereditary sensory neuropathies (HSN) Types I-IV

J. Hereditary neuropathies with known or suspected
metabolic defects
1. Ceramidetrihexaside - α-galactosidase
deficiency (Fabry's disease)
2. Aryl sulfatase A deficiency (metachromatic
leukodystrophy)
3. Phytanic oxidase deficiency (Refsum's disease)
4. Adrenomyeloneuropathy
5. Hexosaminidase deficiency
6. Tangier disease

K. **Mononeuropathies**
   1. Trauma – fractures and dislocations, penetrating injuries and pressure palsies.
      a) Brachial plexus – fracture of clavicle or humerus, birth trauma
      b) Axillary nerve – as for brachial plexus, subcoracoid subluxation
      c) Radial nerve – fracture of head of humerus, compression at the radial groove ("Saturday palsy" and "bridegroom's palsy")
      d) Ulnar nerve – fracture of radius or ulna
      e) Median nerve – carpal tunnel syndrome
      f) Sciatic nerve – fracture of pelvis (S-I joint), fracture of acetabulum
      g) Femoral nerve – fracture of femur
      h) Lateral femoral cutaneous nerve – pressure palsy due to tight fitting garments (meralgia paresthetica)
      i) Tibial nerve – fracture of tibia or fibula
      j) Common peroneal nerve – pressure palsy at fibular head from crossed legs or after weight loss
   2. Entrapment (see Carpal Tunnel Syndrome, Ulnar Neuropathy)
   3. Carcinomatous infiltration
   4. Vasculitis
   5. Leprosy

Hereditary motor and sensory neuropathies (HMSN) Types I-III

I. **Hypertrophic form of Charcot-Marie-Tooth** (peroneal muscular atrophy, Roussy-Levy syndrome). Inheritance is autosomal dominant with variable penetrance, rarely autosomal recessive. Age of onset is variable, from childhood to adulthood. There is slowly progressive distal weakness and atrophy with little sensory loss. The lower extremities are more involved than the upper. Total areflexia is common. Pes cavus or planus and hammer toes are common. Life span is usually normal. Nerve conduction velocities are diffusely slow, more so in motor than sensory nerves. EMG reveals chronic denervation. Pathologically there are hypertrophic ("onion bulb") changes secondary to chronic demyelination and remyelination. There is also a loss of myelinated axons in the fasciculus gracilis.

II. **Neuronal form of Charcot-Marie-Tooth** (peroneal muscular atrophy). Inheritance is as in Type I. Age of onset is slightly later than Type I, usually in the second decade. Clinical findings are similar to Type I. Foot deformities are common. Nerve conduction velocities are less slow than Type I, but amplitudes are severely diminished. EMG reveals spontaneous activity and greater denervation changes. Pathologically there are no hypertrophic changes and demyelination is mild; axonal number is decreased in distal myelinated nerves.

   III. Dejerine-Sottas Disease (hypertrophic neuropathy of childhood, congenital hypomyelination neuropathy). Inheritance is autosomal recessive. Onset is congenital or in infancy. The congenital form is more severe. Severe progressive weakness and atrophy is initially distal but eventually affects proximal muscles. There is severe sensory loss and severe sensory ataxia. Motor development is delayed. Skeletal deformities (kyphoscoliosis, hand and foot) are more severe and frequent than in Type I or II. Motor nerve conduction velocities are extremely slow and sensory nerve action potentials are unrecordable. Pathologically, in addition to hypertrophic changes, myelin sheaths are thinner (hypomyelination) or absent (amyelination).

   The differential diagnosis of HMSN I, II and III includes Friedreich's ataxia, hereditary distal spinal muscular atrophy, Refsum's disease, and chronic inflammatory polyneuropathy.

Hereditary sensory neuropathies (HSN) Types I-IV

   I. HSN of Denny Brown. Inheritance is autosomal dominant. Onset is in the second to third decade. There is progressive distal lower extremity dissociated sensory loss with pain and temperature relatively more involved. Distal sweating is impaired. Painless ulcerations may be present. Mild distal lower extremity weakness and atrophy is a late finding. There is distal hyporeflexia. Upper extremity sensory loss is mild. Life expectancy is normal. Nerve conduction studies of the lower extremity reveal decreased sensory amplitudes and normal or mildly decreased sensory conduction velocities; motor nerve conduction studies are normal. Pathologically there is a moderately decreased number of small myelinated fibers and unmyelinated fibers. Differential diagnosis includes diabetic neuropathy, hereditary amyloidosis (prominent autonomic dysfunction), and syringomyelia.

   II. Infantile and Congenital Sensory Neuropathy (Morvan's disease). Inheritance is autosomal recessive. HSN II is clinically similar to HSN I except that sensory modalities are equally and severely involved and there is proximal involvement. Strength is normal. Painless ulcerations and fractures are common. There is distal areflexia. Sensory nerve action potentials are unrecordable; motor nerve conduction studies are normal. Pathologically, the number of myelinated axons is severely decreased with moderately decreased numbers of unmyelinated fibers and some segmental demyelination and remyelination.

III. Familial Dysautonomia (Riley-Day syndrome). Inheritance is autosomal recessive. Onset of symptoms is usually shortly after birth with episodic cyanosis, vomiting, unexplained fever, poor suck, and an increased susceptibility to infection. Autonomic symptoms include decreased lacrimation, hyperhidrosis, fluctuating body temperature and episodic hypotension, usually postural. There is a dissociated sensory loss with predominant involvement of pain and temperature with resultant corneal ulcerations, painless skin lesions and Charcot joints. Areflexia is generalized. Strength is normal. Prognosis is generally poor, but those surviving childhood experience some improvement in adult life. Sensory nerve action potentials are severely diminished; motor nerve conduction studies may be mildly abnormal.

IV. Congenital Sensory Neuropathy with anhidrosis is autosomal recessive. This very rare disorder is characterized by congenital anhidrosis, generalized insensitivity to pain and temperature, mental retardation and episodic pyrexia.

Ref: Harding AE, Thomas PK. The clinical features of hereditary motor and sensory neuropathy types I and II. Brain 103:259, 1980.

Diabetic Neuropathy

Pathogenesis is multifactorial and may include metabolic factors, chronic hyperglycemia (distal polyneuropathy, symmetrical proximal neuropathy), myoinositol deficiency, axonal transport defects, and microangiopathy and infarction (multiple mononeuropathies).

Distal symmetrical polyneuropathies include:

Mixed sensory-motor-autonomic neuropathy is the most common diabetic neuropathy. The degree of involvement of each modality is variable. Sensory abnormalities are greatest distally. There is a proximal-distal gradient of large and small fiber abnormality. Pathologically there is predominant distal axonal loss with variable degrees of segmental demyelination. Nerve conduction studies show reduced sensory action potential amplitude and variable slowing of motor nerve conduction velocity (related to degree of demyelination). EMG shows denervation.

Predominantly sensory neuropathy with variable degree of large and small fiber involvement produces the typical distal hypesthesia. Large fiber involvement produces impaired vibratory and position sense, and sensory ataxia in more severe cases. Paresthesias and dysesthesias are common. Lancinating pains, deep aching pains and cramps also occur. Spontaneous pain may coexist with hypesthesia and, probably results from increased activity of damaged small diameter fibers or from regenerating nerve fibers with a lower depolarization threshold.

Predominantly motor neuropathy is rare. Other causes such as inflammatory polyneuropathy and insulin excess should be considered.

Predominantly autonomic neuropathy is seen mostly in young insulin dependent, ketosis prone (type I) diabetics. Signs and symptoms include orthostatic hypotension, diarrhea (especially nocturnal), gastroparesis, impotence, and bladder abnormalities. Pathologically there is both axonal loss and segmental demyelination.

Proximal diabetic motor neuropathy ("amyotrophy") is attributed to dysfunction of spinal cord motor neurons, motor roots and lumbosacral plexus. Involvement of intramuscular nerve twigs in proximal muscles may explain the primarily proximal findings. Clinically there is subacute to chronic onset of progressive proximal lower extremity weakness and wasting, most severe in the hips and thighs, usually symmetrical but may be mildly asymmetrical, and usually associated with severe weight loss. There is also frequent burning thigh pain which may at times resemble radicular pain. Patellar reflexes may be decreased or absent and ankle reflexes are usually decreased. It may coexist with a distal polyneuropathy. Variable recovery usually occurs in 6-12 months, but there may be no improvement. Control of hyperglycemia may play a role in the recovery.

Nerve conduction studies of the common peroneal and posterior tibial nerves show mild to moderately reduced conduction velocity and prolonged distal latency. EMG shows chronic denervation in the affected muscles. Muscle biopsy is consistent with neurogenic atrophy.

Focal and multifocal neuropathies include:
Mononeuropathy and multiple mononeuropathy (mononeuropathy multiplex, asymmetric proximal motor neuropathy) – Clinically there is acute onset, over hours to days, of unilateral psoas and quadriceps weakness and thigh and knee pain. It may mimic a lumbar radiculopathy. Variable contralateral involvement may be present, making it difficult to distinguish from a symmetric proximal motor

neuropathy ("amyotrophy") except that it has a much more rapid onset. Whether this and "amyotrophy" are distinct clinical entities or opposite ends of a continuum is controversial.

Cranial neuropathy (see Ophthalmoplegia).

In oculomotor neuropathy there is rapid onset of painful ophthalmoplegia without pupillary involvement or with relative pupillary sparing. In the case of pupillary involvement (usually incomplete), a cavernous sinus or posterior communicating artery aneurysm or other structural lesion must be excluded. Other cranial neuropathies include trochlear, abducens, and facial. Prognosis in cranial neuropathy is variable but generally good.

Entrapment neuropathies - Diabetics with polyneuropathies are particulary at risk. Common sites are the median nerve at the wrist, the ulnar nerve at the elbow and the peroneal nerve at the fibular head.

Ref: Brown MJ, Asbury AK: Diabetic neuropathy. Ann Neurol 15:2, 1984.

Asbury AK. Proximal diabetic neuropathy (editorial). Ann Neurol 2:179, 1977.

Inflammatory Demyelinating Polyneuropathies

Landry-Guillain-Barre-Strohl Syndrome (acute inflammatory polyradiculoneuropathy) is probably immunologically mediated. Clinical features consist of progressive weakness of more than one limb, usually described ascending. Truncal, respiratory, bulbar, facial, and extraocular muscles may be involved. Facial weakness occurs in about 50%. Ataxia may be present. The clinical features may be preceded by a viral upper respiratory infection or recent surgery. There is rapid progression to maximal symmetric or mildly asymmetric weakness within four weeks. There is generalized areflexia or distal areflexia with proximal hyporeflexia. Sensory symptoms and signs may be present but are usually mild; distal paresthesias are typical. Following maximal deficit, there is a 2-4 week plateau and then recovery over weeks to several months. Autonomic dysfunction may cause cardiac dysrhythmias or abnormal blood pressure regulation with hypotension or hypertension. With improved pulmonary care and ventilatory support in intensive care units, respiratory complications are no longer the primary cause of death, having been replaced by cardiac dysrhythmias. Overall, prognosis is good, but variable deficits may persist or there may be a chronic relapsing course.

Spinal fluid shows "albuminocytologic dissociation" with elevated protein, usually after the first week, and less than 10 mononuclear cells per mm3. Rarely, CSF protein is normal or 10-50 mononuclear cells may be present. Nerve conduction studies may be normal acutely, in spite of severe clinical deficits. Nerve conduction velocities are subsequently markedly decreased (or there is conduction block), with increased distal latencies and prolonged F-wave latencies.

Clinical variants include the Fisher variant and sensory loss and areflexia. In ophthalmoplegia, ataxia, and areflexia (Fisher variant) pupils are involved, weakness is absent or less prominent and prognosis is usually good; some consider this a transitional disorder between peripheral and central demyelination processes. Sensory loss and areflexia may be difficult to differentiate from sensory neuropathies and, therefore, the clinical, spinal fluid and electrophysiological features must be similar in order to make the diagnosis. Prognosis for recovery is not as good as in the motor form or Fisher variant.

Management is based on general supportive care. Respiratory status must be carefully and frequently monitored. If the FEV_1 declines or vital capacity falls below 500-800 cc's, mechanical ventilation must be provided. Meticulous pulmonary care is essential. Blood pressure and cardiac rhythm are monitored and abnormalities treated appropriately. Thrombophlebitis is minimized with range of motion exercises, elastic support stockings, and low-dose heparin. The role of corticosteroids is unsettled. Plasmapheresis appears to be of benefit when instituted early. Differential diagnosis and further evaluation is discussed below.

Ref: Asbury AK. Diagnostic considerations in Guillain-Barre syndrome. Ann Neurol 9(suppl):1, 1981.

Chronic Relapsing Dysimmune Polyneuropathy is similar to Guillain-Barre syndrome except that progression is slower with maximum deficit reached in 6-12 months. Plateau and recovery phases are proportionately longer. Sensory involvement is usually more pronounced. The course is relapsing and remitting. Relapses may be more severe than the initial episode. Areflexia is present, but cranial nerve involvement is not as common and autonomic dysfunction is rare. Usually there is no history of preceding illness or surgery. There may be a distal upper extremity postural or action tremor. Electrodiagnostic and spinal fluid studies are similar to the acute form.

The chronic relapsing form is steroid responsive. Prednisone is started at 100 mg/QD for 4 weeks and then tapered over 10 weeks to 100 mg/QOD by reducing an alternate-day dose by 10 mg/week. Tapering to 50 mg/QOD is continued by reducing by 5 mg decrements every 3-4 weeks. Below 50 mg QOD reduced by 2.5 mg every month until a maintenance dose of 10-20 mg/QOD is reached. Side effects of chronic steroids must be sought and treated. Initial clinical improvement may lag several weeks to months behind the institution of steroids. Azathioprine or cyclophosphamide may be added if the response to prednisone is poor. Plasmapheresis may be effective. Physical therapy is beneficial, although, when overly agressive, has resulted in undue muscle trauma.

Ref: Dalakas MC, Engel K. Chronic relapsing (dysimmune) polyneuropathy: pathogenesis and treatment. Ann Neurol 9(suppl):134, 1981.

Differential Diagnosis and Further Evaluation in acute and chronic inflammatory polyradiculoneuropathies is listed below. Nerve conduction studies and EMG, done 2 weeks after the onset of signs and symptoms, should include F-waves, H-reflex and paraspinal needle exam to look for proximal root dysfunction.

1. Heavy metal toxicity - lead, arsenic, mercury, thallium
2. Infection - mycoplasma (cold agglutinin titers), mononucleosis (heterophile titer), hepatitis (HBsAg), botulism (dilated pupils, other anti-cholinergic signs), tick paralysis, poliomyelitis (particularly if asymmetric), diphtheria (throat culture).
3. Myasthenia gravis
4. Porphyria
5. Vasculitis
6. Thyroid disease
7. Acute muscle disease - polymyositis, dermatomyositis, toxic myopathies

Evaluation of Neuropathy

History should focus on symptoms, distribution, course, family history, medications, occupational history (toxic exposure), drinking habits and symptoms of diabetes or carcinoma.

In general, polyneuropathies present with variable degrees of distal sensory loss and/or weakness and atrophy, but proximal sensory loss may be more prominent in porphyria, Tangier's and leprosy. Reflexes are decreased or absent, but may be increased in neuropathies also associated with central nervous system involvement such as vitamin B_{12} deficiency, porphyria, hydrocarbon exposure (TOCP, toluene, acrylamide), nitrous oxide and adrenomyeloneuropathy. For electrodiagnostic features see EMG. Increased CSF protein and/or pleocytosis may be seen in inflammatory radicular or meningeal processes. Albuminocytologic association is characteristic of inflammatory polyradiculoneuropathies. Spinal fluid cytology may be abnormal with infiltrative radiculopathies; at least 10 cc's of CSF should be obtained for cytocentrifugation or ultrafiltration. Other laboratory studies which may prove useful include fasting blood sugar, 2 hour postprandial blood glucose, vitamin B_{12} and pyridoxine levels, serum protein electrophoresis and immunoelectrophoresis, axial skeleton radiographs, bone marrow examination, heavy metal levels, porphyrins (see Porphyria), and urinary metachromatic material. Sural nerve biopsy will help determine whether the process is axonal, demyelinating or both. Teased nerve fiber preparation may be very useful. Nerve biopsy may establish the diagnosis in several neuropathies including leprosy, primary amyloidosis, metachromatic leukodystrophy, Fabry's disease (cerebroside α-galactosidase deficiency), familial tendency to compression palsies, and vasculitic neuropathies. Generally, axonal degeneration is seen in toxic, metabolic and nutritional neuropathies with the exception of lead and perhexilene neuropathies. Segmental demyelination is more often seen in inherited and inflammatory neuropathies. Hypertrophic neuropathies ("onion bulb") are due to chronic demyelination and remyelination and are usually inherited.

General Principals of Treatment of Neuropathies

1. Patient education and counseling
2. Genetic counseling
3. Withdrawal of medications suspected of causing neuropathy
4. Withdrawal from toxic exposure
5. Correction of nutritional and vitamin deficiencies
6. Treatment of alcoholism
7. Blood glucose control in diabetic neuropathies
8. Specific drug therapies
   a) Chelating agents (EDTA) in lead neuropathy
   b) Hematin infusions in acute intermittent porphyria

c) Long term prednisone in chronic relapsing dysimmune polyneuropathy
9. Plasmapheresis in Guillain-Barre syndrome and certain
other autoimmune neuropathies
10. Pain control
   a) Improve blood glucose control in diabetic neuropathies
   b) Simple analgesics - aspirin and acetaminophen
   c) Phenytoin and carbamazepine - achieve anticonvulsant levels (see Anticonvulsants)
   d) Tricyclic drugs - amitriptyline, imipramine
   e) Transcutaneous electrical nerve stimulation
11. Meticulous foot care
12. Orthotic devices and splints
13. Surgical correction of entrapment neuropathies
14. Physical and occupational therapy

Ref: Argon Z, Mastaglia FL. Drug induced peripheral
        neuropathies. Br Med J 1:663, 1979.

NMR (see Magnetic Resonance)

NUTRITIONAL DEFICIENCY SYNDROMES (see also Alcohol)

Isolated vitamin deficiency syndromes are unusual,
except B_{12} deficiency which occurs with pernicious
anemia. More common causes of vitamin deficiency include
chronic alcoholism, fad diets, malabsorption syndromes,
improper hyperalimentation, and drugs that interfere with
vitamin absorption or metabolism. Breast-fed infants
without vitamin supplementation and those on milk-free
substitutes may develop fat soluble vitamin deficiencies.
Vitamin A deficiency is rare except in children in
whom the early symptom of night blindness may be missed.
There is keratinization of epithelium, including conjunctiva and cornea. Reported neurological manifestations
include mental retardation, facial palsy, hydrocephalus,
and increased intracranial pressure. Vitamin A in excess
of 50,000 IU daily for several weeks or months may cause
benign intracranial hypertension (see Pseudotumor Cerebri).
Thiamine (Vitamin B1). Blood transketolase activity
is decreased in deficiency states, and this decrease
precedes symptoms of deficiency. Treatment should include
a high calorie, high vitamin diet, in addition to thiamine
replacement in a dose of 5-25 mg PO tid or thiamine hydrochloride 10-25 mg IV qd. Thiamine should always be given
to alcoholics prior to intravenous glucose since the
glucose may exacerbate the deficiency state, possibly
irreversibly. Thiamine deficiency plays a role in the
following disorders:

1. Beriberi is characterized by polyneuropathy and heart disease. There is a symmetric ascending polyneuropathy with absent ankle jerks, distal lower extremity weakness, with variable sensory involvement including paresthesias and dysesthesias and distal sensory deficits. Aching and tenderness of the calves typically precede the foot drop and sensory deficits. Upper extremity involvement occurs late. Since other vitamins may play a role in the development of nutritional polyneuropathy, the following daily treatment regimen is suggested: thiamine 25 mg, niacin 75 mg, riboflavin 5 mg, pyridoxine 5 mg, and B_{12} 5 µg.

2. Strachan's syndrome is a primarily sensory, usually painful, polyneuropathy associated with spinal sensory ataxia, optic neuropathy, and nerve deafness. Dysarthria and orogenital dermatitis also occur. The dietary deficiency or toxic factors have not been identified, although sensory polyneuropathy usually responds to thiamine and other B vitamins.

3. Retrobulbar optic neuropathy

4. Other cranial nerve disorders are implicated as anosmia, trigeminal anesthesia, nerve deafness, and laryngeal paralysis have been reported.

5. Wernicke's encephalopathy is characterized by confusion, ocular motor disturbances, and truncal ataxia. Diplopia and ataxia generally precede mental changes, but symptoms may occur in any combination or order. Associated polyneuropathies and Korsakoff's psychosis are common. Confusion occurs in 90%; one-sixth of these are complicated by DT's or other alcohol withdrawal syndromes. Although apathy and lethargy are common, stupor and coma are unusual and, in such cases, other causes such as subdural hematoma or meningitis should be excluded. Ocular motor disturbances are varied, including infranuclear external ophthalmoplegias, supranuclear gaze palsies, and internuclear ophthalmoplegias. The ocular motor signs respond rapidly to thiamine. The mental changes and ataxia respond more slowly.

6. Korsakoff's psychosis consists of a profound deficit in recent memory, often with disorientation to person, place and time. Remote memory is less severely impaired. Confabulation is often present. With therapy there may be gradual improvement over months, but significant improvement is unusual.

7. Cerebellar degeneration is seen in alcoholics with nutritional deficiency. Ataxia is most prominent in the lower extremities and trunk.

8. Degeneration of the corpus callosum (Marchiafava-Bignami) is also associated with nutritional deficiency as well as addiction to red wine.
9. Leigh's syndrome (sub-acute necrotizing encephalo-myelopathy) is a less common adult form of Leigh's disease, believed due to an abnormality of thiamine metabolism. Clinical diagnosis in adults is difficult. There is usually an insidious onset, stabilization for months to years, and finally sub-acute or acute progression to death. Course may be relapsing and remitting. Common symptoms and signs include seizures, psychiatric disturbances, visual deficit, autonomic and sleep disturbances. Pathologically there is involvement of the basal ganglia, brainstem, spinal cord, and optic nerves. There may be progression despite treatment with thiamine.

Ref: Gray F, et al. JNNP 47:1211, 1984.

Nicotinic acid deficiency (pellagra) causes diarrhea, dermatitis, and dementia as well as many neurological manifestations. The latter may be encephalopathic, myelopathic, or neuropathic. Psychiatric complaints are common and highly variable, including asthenia, anxiety, depression, irritability, insomnia, apathy, confusion, and memory loss. Other neurological manifestations include optic neuropathy, vertigo, tinnitus and deafness, spastic dysarthria, corticospinal tract signs (spasticity and hyperreflexia, often without Babinski's), extrapyramidal signs, ataxia, painful peripheral neuropathy (which responds to vitamin B_1 but not nicotinic acid), posterior column deficits, and, later, atrophy and fasciculations. Treatment consists of nicotinic acid or nicotinamide 500-1500 mg daily and vitamin B_1.

Pyridoxine (vitamin B6) deficiency or dependency may develop in infants, resulting in increased irritability and startle and seizures that are often refractory to anticonvulsant therapy. Pyridoxine deficiency is usually dietary but may result from drugs such as isoniazid. After the age of 6 months when food intake is more varied, seizures resulting from deficiency are not seen. Pyridoxine dependency is due to an increased daily requirement, presumably because of a decrease in avidity of glutamic decarboxylase or pyridoxine, resulting in diminished conversion of glutamic acid to GABA. Lifelong supplementation is required in pyridoxine dependency. Initial therapy for deficiency and dependency consists of pyridoxine 20 mg IV, repeated at 5 minute intervals up to a total of 100 mg. Seizures should stop within minutes.

Maintenance dose is 25-50 mg PO qd. In pyridoxine dependency, seizures will recur within 48 hours if maintenance therapy is omitted. Pyridoxine antagonizes the action of L-dopa by stimulating peripheral dopa decarboxylase. This effect is offset by using preparations containing carbidopa.

Ref: Krishnamoorthy KS. Ann Neurol 13:103, 1983.

Crowell, Roach. Am Fam Physician 27:183, 1983.

Pyridoxine deficiency may occur in adults due to drugs such as isoniazid or hydralazine. Isoniazid toxicity is rarely seen with doses of 3-5 mg/kg and pyridoxine need not be given as it may interfere with the antituberculous action of isoniazid. Pyridoxine 50 mg daily should be given with larger doses of isoniazid (20 mg/kg) to prevent polyneuropathy and the less frequent optic neuropathy.

A sensory polyneuropathy has been reported in patients taking 2 gm/d or more of pyridoxine. The mechanism is uncertain. Numbness and sensory ataxia beginning in the lower extemities progresses to the upper extremities within months and finally to perioral numbness. Posterior column sensory modalities are involved earlier and to a greater degree than spinothalamic modalities. Weakness is minimal or absent. Lhermitte's sign is occasionally present. Resolution begins a few months after discontinuing supplementation and continues gradually over months to a few years.

Ref: Schaumburg H, et al. NEJM 309:445, 1983.

Cyanocobalamine (vitamin B$_{12}$) deficiency occurs in pernicious anemia due to gastric achlorhydria and loss of intrinsic factor with a resultant macrocytic anemia and sub-acute combined degeneration of the spinal cord. Onset is most common in the fourth to sixth decades. The anemia usually occurs before, or at least concurrently with, neurological signs and symptoms. Less frequently the neurological signs may precede the anemia. Neurological symptoms occur in 80-95%. Neurological signs and symptoms reflect involvement of the dorsal and lateral columns of the spinal cord, the peripheral nerves, and the brain. Sensory symptoms are most prominent, but vibration and position deficits predominate on exam. Gait is spastic and/or ataxic. Tendon reflexes are usually decreased, but may be increased due to corticospinal tract involvement. Plantar responses are extensor. Mild mental status changes are common and include confusion, dementia, and psychiatric disturbances. Laboratory evaluation includes

CBC, reticulocyte count, serum cobalamine level, and Schilling test. Treatment consists of B_{12} 50 µg IM qd X 2 weeks, followed by 100 µg IM monthly thereafter. Macrocytic anemias should not be treated with folate without considering B_{12} deficiency. The sooner treatment is instituted, the better the neurological prognosis. Significant improvement is seen if repletion is begun within 3 months of the onset of symptoms. Most of the neurological improvement occurs within 3-6 months.

Folic acid (vitamin B_c) deficiency may occur in infants due to congenital folate malabsorption resulting in megaloblastic anemia, mental retardation, seizures and athetosis. Low serum folate (with normal B_{12} levels) has been reported in association with a syndrome resembling sub-acute combined degeneration. Familial restless leg syndrome associated with low serum folate may improve with folate therapy. Chronic anticonvulsant (phenytoin, phenobarbital, primidone) therapy may result in low serum folate levels as well as megaloblastic anemia responsive to folate.

Vitamin D deficiency in children causes rickets with which nystagmus and head shaking may be associated. Deficiency may produce significant hypocalcemia (see Calcium). Deficiency in adults produces osteomalacia. Chronic anticonvulsant (phenytoin, phenobarbital, primidone) therapy may produce rickets and osteomalacia which is corrected with vitamin D replacement.

Vitamin E (and vitamin A) deficiency is seen in abetalipoproteinemia (Bassen-Kornzweig disease) due to impaired transport. Though there is no specific treatment, use of vitamins E and A may delay the neurological deficits. There is steatorrhea in infancy and childhood, acanthocytosis, retinitis pigmentosa, and progressive ataxia and weakness due to demyelination of the posterior lateral columns, spinocerebellar tracts and peripheral nerves.

NYSTAGMUS (see also Vertigo, Calorics, Optokinetic Nystagmus, Ocular Oscillations)

A biphasic ocular oscillation in which at least one phase is a slow phase responsible for the genesis and continuation of the oscillation. There are two general types. In jerk nystagmus the slow phase is away from the fixated target. The fast (saccadic) phase returns the eye to the target. The nystagmus direction is defined by convention as the direction of the fast component. In pendular nystagmus, the oscillations are equal in both directions. When examining a patient with nystagmus, observe the eyes in the 9 cardinal positions of gaze.

Note changes in amplitude and frequency with change in gaze direction. Also note any changes in nystagmus with convergence or with either eye viewing alone. Often the only localizing significance of nystagmus is to indicate dysfunction somewhere in the posterior fossa, that is, vestibular system, brainstem, or cerebellum.

Congenital nystagmus is present at birth or noted in early infancy at the time of development of visual fixation, and persists throughout life. It may accompany, but is not necessarily due to, primary visual defects. It is almost always binocular, of similar amplitude in both eyes, and uniplanar (usually horizontal). It increases with attempts to fixate, decreases with convergence, and disappears in sleep. There may be "inversion" of the optokinetic reflex. There may be associated head oscillations. It is not associated with oscillopsia.

Latent nystagmus is a form of congenital nystagmus. There is no nystagmus with binocular vision. When one eye is occluded, however, jerk nystagmus develops in both eyes with the fast phase toward the viewing eye. It can be elicited by the intention of viewing with one eye. Manifest latent nystagmus occurs in patients with amblyopia, strabismus, or other eye disease who fix monocularly, although they are viewing with both eyes. The fast phase is in the direction of the fixating eye.

Acquired nystagmus in infants may be due to progressive bilateral visual loss in early childhood, CNS disease, or spasmus nutans. Spasmus nutans is a rare syndrome consisting of nystagmus, head nodding and torticollis. The nystagmus is usually bilateral but can differ in each eye; it may be monocular in a horizontal, rotary or vertical direction. The nystagmus is rapid, of small amplitude, and may vary with the direction of gaze. It begins in infancy (4-18 months) and disappears by the age of 3 years.

Acquired pendular nystagmus may be horizontal, vertical, diagonal, elliptic or circular, and may be associated with head tremor. There may be marked dissociation between the two eyes. Nystagmus may decrease when the eyes are closed. It is associated with vascular or demyelinating lesions of the brainstem and/or cerebellum. In demyelinating disease it usually indicates a cerebrellar lesion. Rarely, it is associated with visual dysfunction.

Vestibular nystagmus (see also Calorics, Vertigo) results from dysfunction of the vestibular end-organ, nerve, or brainstem connections and from acute lesions of the cerebellar flocculus. It is usually present in primary position. It increases with gaze toward fast phase, and decreases (with central lesions may reverse direction) with gaze towards the slow phase. Vertigo usually co-exists. For differentiation of peripheral from central vestibular nystagmus, see Vertigo.

Gaze-evoked nystagmus is elicited by attempting to maintain an eccentric eye position. It is the most common form of nystagmus. Drugs are the most common cause of bi-directional gaze-evoked nystagmus. Offending agents include anticonvulsants, barbiturates, tranquilizers, and phenothiazines. It may be dissociated in the two eyes. The fast phase is usually in the direction of gaze, that is, to the right on right gaze, to the left on left gaze, and upbeating in upward gaze. Downgaze usually does not produce nystagmus. Gaze-evoked vertical nystagmus almost always occurs with the horizontal type. There may be a torsional component to the nystagmus. With severe intoxications, nystagmus may be horizontal pendular in primary position. If the patient is on no medications, horizontal gazed-evoked nystagmus may indicate brainstem and/or cerebellar dysfunction. More precise localization requires assessment of the associated signs and symptoms. Gaze paretic nystagmus (a form of gaze-evoked nystagmus) occurs in patients recovering from a gaze palsy who go through a phase when they are able to make gaze movements, but they cannot maintain the new eye position. The eyes drift back to primary position, this is followed by a corrective saccade to reposition the eyes in their eccentric position. Repetition of this pattern produces nystagmus.

Downbeat nystagmus is usually in primary position with the fast phase beating downwards. It increases in gaze slightly below horizontal, especially in gaze down and laterally. It is highly suggestive of a craniocervical junction disorder such as Arnold-Chiari malformation, basilar invagination, or ankylosing spondylitis. When seen in cerebellar disease, other cerebellar eye signs are usually present. It may co-exist with periodic alter-nating nystagmus. It has also been reported in drug intoxication (phenytoin, carbamazepine, lithium), brain-stem encephalitis, magnesium depletion, communicating hydrocephalus, Wernicke's encephalopathy, cerebellar degeneration, multiple sclerosis, vascular disease and as a paraneoplastic phenomenon.

Upbeat nystagmus is usually present in primary position with the fast phase beating upward. It may be congenital, but is usually acquired secondary to structural disease. A lesion of the anterior cerebellar vermis can produce a large amplitude nystagmus which increases in upgaze. Medullary disease can produce small amplitude nystagmus that decreases in upgaze. An inter-mediate form may be seen in Wernicke's encephalopathy.

Drug intoxication is an uncommon cause.

Physiological (end-point) nystagmus occurs in normal individuals in the extremes of horizontal gaze. It is a small amplitude, irregular, variably sustained, jerk nystagmus which is often dissociated (more marked in one eye, usually the abducting eye).

See-saw nystagmus consists of one eye intorting and rising while the opposite eye extorts and falls. Repetition in alternating directions produces a see-saw effect. It may occur in all fields of gaze, but may be limited to primary position or downgaze. It is believed due to diencephalic dysfunction, and is seen with parasellar tumors expanding within the third ventricle, upper brainstem vascular disease, following severe head trauma. There is also a congenital form.

Convergence-evoked nystagmus is a rare nystagmus that may be congenital or aquired, conjugate or dysjunctive. In the several cases reported there has been no definite correlation with a specific lesion.

Periodic alternating nystagmus is a persisting horizontal jerk nystagmus that periodically changes directions. Typically, it beats for 90 seconds in one direction, spends 10 seconds in a neutral phase, and then beats 90 seconds in the opposite direction. It may persist during sleep as well as while awake. It may be congenital or due to craniocervical junction abnormalities (may co-exist with downbeat nystagmus). It may also occur in association with head trauma, vascular disease, encephalitis, syphilis, multiple sclerosis, spinocerebellar degenerations, and posterior fossa tumors.

Rotary (torsional) nystagmus occurs around the globe's A-P axis. Pure rotary nystagmus occurs with medullary or diencephalic lesions and congenitally, but not in vestibular end-organ disease. In the latter, a rotational component is usually combined with a prominent horizontal or vertical component.

Dissociated nystagmus refers to a significant asymmetry in either amplitude or direction between the two eyes. It occurs in internuclear ophthalmoplegia (see also Ophthalmoplegia), pendular nystagmus in patients with multiple sclerosis, and in a variety of posterior fossa lesions.

Rebound nystagmus is a gaze-evoked horizontal nystagmus that fatigues and changes direction with prolonged eccentric gaze, or a horizontal gaze-evoked nystagmus which, after refixation in primary position, transiently beats in the opposite direction. It usually occurs in association with cerebellar disease.

Circular or elliptic nystagmus is a form of pendular nystagmus (horizontal and vertical pendular oscillations

90° out-of-phase) with a continuous oscillation in a fine, rapid, circular or elliptical pattern. Seen in multiple sclerosis or congenitally.

Diagonal (oblique) nystagmus occurs when simultaneous, pendular horizontal and vertical components are in-phase or 180° out of-phase. It is seen in multiple sclerosis and congenitally.

Nystagmus in myasthenia gravis. The neuromuscular junction disorder of this disease may cause gaze-evoked nystagmus in any direction with asymmetry between the two eyes. Such nystagmus of the abducting eye occurring with impaired adduction of the contralateral eye constitutes the "pseudo-internuclear ophthalmoplegia" of myasthenia gravis. These findings usually resolve with anticholinesterases.

Voluntary "nystagmus" consists of bursts of very rapid, conjugate, horizontal, pendular-appearing oscillations that are actually voluntarily produced back-to-back saccades. They can rarely be sustained for more than 10-30 seconds at a time.

Lid nystagmus is of three types. Upward jerking of the lids synchronous with vertical ocular nystagmus is nonlocalizing. Rapid twitching of lids synchronous with the fast phase of horizontal ocular nystagmus induced by lateral gaze may occur with the lateral medullary syndrome. Lid nystagmus induced by convergence is associated with medullary lesions.

Convergence-retraction nystagmus occurs as a part of the dorsal midbrain syndrome, especially during attempted upgaze (see Gaze Palsy).

Ref: Daroff RB, et al. Nystagmus and related ocular oscillations. In Glaser JS. Neuro-Ophthalmology. Hagerstown: Harper and Row, 1978, pp 219-40.

Leigh RJ, Zee DS. Neurology of Eye Movements, Philadelphia: FA Davis, 1983.

OCULAR OSCILLATIONS (See also Nystagmus)

Ocular bobbing consists of fast downward jerks of both eyes followed by a slowed drift to mid-position. It usually occurs in comatose patients with extensive destruction of the pons, but it occasionally occurs with extrapontine compression, obstructive hydrocephalus, or encepalophthy.

Ocular dysmetria is elicited by having the patient make a saccade to a new target. It consists of either (1) undershooting or overshooting followed by a small amplitude saccadic oscillation before the eyes reach the new fixation point, or (2) conjugate overshooting followed by saccades that bring the eyes back to the target. It is a common sign of cerebellar system disease.

Ocular "myoclonus" (see also Myoclonus) is a continuous, pendular oscillation, (1.5-5.0 cycles/second) usually in the vertical plane. The eye movements may be dissociated. They are usually associated with movements in muscles of the soft palate (ocular/palatal myoclonus), tongue, face, pharynx, larynx, and diaphragm.

Ocular flutter is a brief, intermittent, binocular, horizontal oscillation that occurs spontaneously during straight-head fixation. It consists of several back-to-back saccades. Patients with flutter almost always have dysmetria as well. Flutter is related to opsoclonus clinically and pathophysiologically.

Opsoclonus describes involuntary, usually continuous, random, conjugate, saccadic eye movements in all directions. It is seen in children with neuroblastoma (with cerebellar ataxia) and in children with limb myoclonus. In adults it occurs in a postinfectious syndrome with myoclonus, ataxia and tremulousness as well as in association with remote carcinoma. It may also be seen with drugs and toxins (lithium, chlordecone, thallium), encephalitis, hydrocephalus, trauma, tumors and intracranial hemorrhage.

Superior oblique myokymia is an intermittent, rapid (12-15/second), small amplitude, monocular, torsional movement with associated oscillopsia due to phasic contractions of the superior oblique muscle. It appears spontaneously in otherwise healthy adults and may improve with carbamazepine.

Square wave jerks are small amplitude (0.5-3 deg), conjugate, saccadic eye movements which suddenly move the eyes from the target. After a brief latency (1/5 sec), the eyes return to the target with a similar amplitude saccade. They are seen in normals and in a variety of neurological disorders.

Macro square wave jerks are essentially large amplitude square wave jerks. They may be associated with cerebellar and demyelinating disease.

Macro saccadic oscillations, as opposed to the two types of square wave jerks, occur in bursts which increase and then decrease in amplitude, crossing the point of fixation with each saccade. They are seen in cerebellar disease.

Ref: See Nystagmus.

OLFACTION

The sense of smell, is mediated by the first cranial nerve. Complaints may include anosmia, hyposmia, parosmia, or loss of appreciation of flavors in food. Smell is tested clinically, using nonirritating aromatic compounds, such as oil of wintergreen, cloves, coffee, almond oil, or lemon oil. The stimulus is presented to one nostril with the other occluded. The ability to appreciate the presence of a substance, even if not properly identified, is evidence that anosmia is not present. Unilateral anosmia is more often due to a structural lesion rather than a diffuse process. Causes of anosmia or hyposmia include:

1. Infection - rhinitis, sinusitis, basilar meningitis, frontal abscess, osteomyelitis (frontal, ethmoidal), viral hepatitis, syphilis, influenza

2. Toxic or metabolic disorders - pernicious anemia, zinc deficiency, lead and calcium intoxication, diabetes mellitus, hypothyroidism

3. Neoplasms - frontal tumor, olfactory groove or sphenoid meningioma, radiation therapy

4. Trauma to cribriform plate

5. Congenital - olfactory agenesis (Kallmann's syndrome) and septo-optic dysplasia (De Morsier's syndrome)

6. Other - hydrocephalus, amphetamine and cocaine abuse, aging, smoking, trigeminal lesions (causing mucosal atrophy), anterior cerebral artery disease, polyps, multiple sclerosis, and Parkinson's disease.

Hyperosmia is seen in hysteria, migraine, hyperemesis gravidarum, cystic fibrosis, Addison's disease and strychnine poisoning.

Olfactory hallucinations can occur with neoplasms or vascular disease involving the inferomedial temporal lobe, near the hippocampus or uncus. "Uncinate" fits are so called because of the presence of olfactory or gustatory hallucinations as part of the complex partial or simple partial seizures; these may even be arrested or triggered by olfactory stimulation. Anosmia is not present in such cases.

Ref: Shiffman, NEJM 308:1275, and 1337, 1983.

(see also Gaze Palsy, Myasthenia
   Gravis, Graves' Ophthalmopathy)

   For the clinical evaluation of diplopia, see Eye
Muscles. This section reviews differential diagnosis
(after Leigh and Zee, and Glaser). If extraocular muscle
testing reveals misalignment of the visual axes, first
determine whether this is due to a nerve palsy or some
other cause of impaired motility.

Causes of impaired ocular motility other than a nerve palsy

   Concomitant strabismus
   Graves's ophthalmopathy
   Myasthenia gravis (and other pharmacologic or toxic
      causes of neuromuscular blockade)
   Convergence spasm
   Old blow-out fracture of the orbit with entrapment
      myopathy
   Restrictive ophthalmopathy (Brown's superior oblique
      tendon sheath syndrome)
   Orbital inflammatory disease (pseudotumor)
   Orbital masses, neoplasms
   Orbital infections
   Brainstem disorders causing abnormal prenuclear inputs
      (internuclear ophthalmoplegia, skew deviation)
   Ocular myopathies
   Chronic progressive external ophthalmoplegia
      (Kearns-Sayre-Daroff)
   Congenital syndromes

Causes of abducens (VI) nerve palsies

   Nuclear (associated with ipsilateral horizontal gaze
   palsy)
      Developmental anomalies (Mobius, some Duane's
         syndromes)
      Infarction
      Tumor (pontine glioma, cerebellar tumors)
      Wernicke-Korsakoff
   Fascicular
      Infarction
      Demyelination
      Tumor
   Subarachnoid
      Aneurysm or anomalous vessels (anterior inferior
         cerebellar artery, basilar artery)
      Subarachnoid hemorrhage
      Meningitis (infectious, neoplastic)

Sarcoid
Cerebellopontine angle tumor (acoustic neuroma,
    meningioma)
Clivus tumor (chordoma, nasopharyngeal carcinoma)
Trauma
Surgical complication
Postinfectious
Petrous
    Infection or inflammation of mastoid or petrous tip
    Trauma (petrous fracture)
    Thrombosis of inferior petrosal sinus
    Increased intracranial pressure (pseudotumor
        cerebri, supratentorial mass)
    Following lumbar puncture
    Aneurysm
    Persistent trigeminal artery
    Trigeminal schwannoma
Cavernous sinus and superior orbital fissure
    Aneurysm
    Thrombosis
    Carotid cavernous fistula
    Dural arteriovenus malformation
    Tumor (pituitary adenoma, meningioma,
        nasopharyngeal carcinoma)
    Pituitary apoplexy
    Sphenoid sinusitis (mucormycosis)
    Herpes zoster
    Granulomatous inflammation (sarcoid, Tolosa-Hunt
        syndrome)
Orbital
    Tumor
Uncertain localization
    Infarction (diabetes, hypertension)
    Migraine

Causes of trochlear (IV) nerve palsies

Nuclear and fascicular
    Developmental anomalies
    Hemorrhage
    Infarction
    Trauma
    Demyelination
    Surgical complications
Subarachnoid
    Trauma
    Tumor (pineal, tentorial meningioma, trochlear
        schwannoma, ependymoma, metastases)
    Surgical complication
    Meningitis (infectious, neoplastic)
    Mastoiditis

Cavernous sinus and superior orbital fissure/
    As for VI nerve palsies
Orbital
    Trauma
    Ethmoiditis
    Ethmoidectomy
Uncertain localization
    Infarction (diabetes, hypertension)

Causes of oculomotor (III) nerve palsies

Nuclear and fascicular
    Developmental anomaly
    Infarction
    Tumor
Subarachnoid
    Aneurysm (posterior communicating artery)
    Meningitis (infectious, syphilitic, neoplastic)
    Infarction (diabetes)
    Tumor
    Surgical complication
Tentorial edge
    Increased intracranial pressure (uncal herniation,
      pseudotumor cerebri)
    Trauma
Cavernous sinus and superior orbital fissure
    As for VI nerve palsies
    Infarction (diabetes, hypertension)
Orbital
    Trauma
Uncertain localization
    Mononucleosis and other viral infections
    Following immunization
    Migraine
    Cyclic oculomotor palsy of childhood
    Guillain-Barre syndrome

    Combined ophthalmopareses, especially if bilateral,
suggest Graves' disease, myasthenia gravis, or chronic
progressive external ophthalmoplegia. Combined palsies of
cranial nerves III, IV, and VI are most commonly unilateral and are secondary to lesions of the superior
orbital fissure or cavernous sinus. Orbital lesions will
usually produce additional signs such as proptosis,
chemosis, vascular engorgement or decreased corneal
reflex. Bilateral combined palsies may be seen with
Guillain-Barre, brainstem tumor, extension of nasopharyngeal carcinoma, sarcoid, clivus chordoma, pituitary
apoplexy, and cavernous sinus thrombosis.

237

Painful ophthalmoplegias may be due to diabetes, aneurysm, tumors (primary and metastatic), granulomas (Tolosa-Hunt), herpes zoster, cavernous sinus thrombosis, carotid-cavernous fistula, migraine, arteritis, carcinomatous meningitis, or fungal infections.

Internuclear ophthalmoplegia (INO) is noted in lateral upgaze. The abducting eye develops nystagmus and adduction of the fellow eye is incomplete or slow. This is caused by a lesion of the medial longitudinal fasciculus (MLF) between the midpons and the oculomotor nucleus on the side of the eye with impaired adduction. Patients with bilateral impairment may also have nystagmus on upward gaze and a skew deviation. Subtle defects can be observed with OKN testing (see Optokinetic Nystagmus). The most frequent cause of INO in young adults (especially when bilateral) is multiple sclerosis. In older patients, the most common cause is vascular disease. Rarely, intrinsic or extra-axial brainstem tumors are the cause. Myasthenia gravis should be excluded as a cause of very similar appearing "pseudo INO".

One-and-one-half syndrome is the result of a lesion of the MLF in the more ventral ipsilateral paramedian pontine reticular formation (PPRF) which produces an INO during gaze to the opposite side and an ipsilateral gaze palsy (see Gaze Palsy). The only intact movement is abduction of the opposite eye. Acutely, the patient may appear exotropic, with nystagmus in the deviated eye. Brainstem vascular disease is the most common cause.

Chronic progressive external ophthalmoplegia is a slowly progressive, painless, symmetric ophthalmoplegia, without fluctuations or remissions. The pupils are spared. Ptosis is associated with weakness of the orbicularis oculi. There are no orbital signs. When long-standing, fibrotic changes may occur in the extraocular muscles. The external ophthalmoplegia may occur as an isolated finding, but is more commonly associated with ptosis and orbicularis weakness. The syndrome is nonspecific and may occur in a variety of ocular myopathies or degenerative diseases, such as the spinocerebellar degenerations, spinal muscular atrophies, and Bassen-Kornzweig syndrome. Kearn-Sayre-Daroff syndrome includes such features as childhood onset without a family history, retinal pigmentary degeneration, cardiac conduction defects often leading to Stokes-Adams attacks, increased cerebospinal fluid protein, spongiform changes of the cerebrum and brainstem, and muscle mitochondrial abnormalities.

Ref: Glaser JS. Neuro-ophthalmology. Hagerstown: Harper
        and Row, 1978, Chapter 12.

        Leigh RJ, Zee DS. The Neurology of Eye Movements.
        Philadelphia: FA Davis, 1983, Chapter 8.

OPTIC NERVE

Function is assessed by measuring best corrected
visual acuity, color vision, visual fields (see Visual
Fields), and pupillary responses (see Pupil), and by
comparing light or color intensity when viewing with
either eye. Other methods such as measurement of contrast
sensitivity, and visual evoked potentials may provide
additional information in certain cases. Afferent
pupillary defects are best detected in the dark.

Funduscopy may reveal obvious optic atrophy with a
pale disc or more subtle defects of the retinal nerve
fiber layer in the case of optic neuropathy. Congenital
optic disc anomalies may also be seen. Disc swelling may
or may not be associated with visual dysfunction (see
below).

Disc swelling indicates abnormal elevation of the
optic disc generally due to blocked axoplasmic flow. It
may be seen with certain optic neuropathies, which are
suggested by evidence of optic nerve dysfunction.
Papilledema refers specifically to disc swelling due to
increased intracranial pressure. Retinal evidence of
increased intracranial pressure includes opacity of the
peripapillary nerve fiber layer, disc hyperemia, elevation
of the disc, preservation of the optic cup, flame
hemorrhages on or around the disc and absent venous
pulsations. The presence of spontaneous venous pulsations
indicates that the CSF pressure is <200 mm of H_2O at
the time of observation. Absent spontaneous venous
pulsations occur in about 20% of the normal population
and are not a specific finding. As papilledema progresses,
disc elevation increases, there is engorgement of retinal
veins, capillary dilation and microaneurysm formation on
the disc, and increased blurring of the disc margins with
obscuration of vessels at the edge of the disc. Circular
retinal folds around the disc, as well as choroidal folds
may be seen. Hard exudates may occur chronically.

Papilledema generally requires at least 2-4 hours to
develop, even with acute increases in intracranial
pressure, and its absence in neurological lesions less
than several hours old does not exclude increased intracranial pressure. Peripapillary flame hemorrhages may be
seen more acutely. Papilledema may take 6-10 weeks to
resolve after intracranial pressure returns to normal.

The course of papilledema is best followed with serial visual field testing and fundus photography. Chronic, untreated papilledema can cause loss of visual function and blindness. Acutely, visual function is usually normal, although patients may complain of transient visual obscurations consisting of several second, monocular or binocular, "gray-outs", often associated with postural changes.

Optic nerve abnormalities occur with or without visual dysfunction and with or without disc swelling. Disc swelling with normal vision should suggest papilledema or congenital disc anomalies. Abnormal vision (optic neuropathy) may be associated with congenital anomalies, usually without recent visual symptoms. Abnormal vision with new visual symptoms suggests new optic nerve disease, which is said to be anterior if disc swelling is seen and posterior in the absence of disc swelling.

Optic disc anomalies include drusen, myelinated nerve fibers, persistent Bergmeister's papilla, prepapillary vascular loops, tilted discs, hypoplasia, aplasia, dysplasia, colobomas, pits, and megalopapilla. Anterior optic neuropathies may be due to ischemia (rule out temporal arteritis), central retinal artery occlusion, inflammation (optic neuritis, papillitis), compression (less common), disc infiltration (glioma, leukemia, lymphoma, metastases, sarcoid), primary optic disc tumors, disc neovascularization, or toxic causes. Posterior (retrobulbar) optic neuropathy may be due to compression (more common), ischemia (very rare), infiltration, or toxic causes. Hereditary optic neuropathies (Leber's) may have disc swelling acutely.

Ref: Miller NR.   Walsh and Hoyt's Clinical Neuro-
       Ophthalmology.   4th ed.   Baltimore: Williams and
       Wilkins, 1982.

OPTOKINETIC NYSTAGMUS (OKN)

"OKN" is elicited at the bedside by moving a series of patterned shapes horizontally or vertically in front of the patient's eyes. Nystagmus occurs consisting of a slow tracking phase and a quick, resetting phase in the opposite direction. Although true OKN represents complex ocular motor reflex evoked by the perception of moving shapes, it is useful to conceptualize the response at the bedside as smooth pursuit in the direction of target movement with corrective saccades in the opposite direction. The nature of the OKN abnormality correlates reasonably well with smooth pursuit or saccadic system dysfunction (see also Gaze Palsy).

OKN may be used as a crude measure of visual function. It should be demonstrable to some degree even in newborns. The presence of an OKN response is evidence of at least some vision in cases of "blindness" due to malingering or hysteria.

Deep parietal lobe lesions cause a contralateral homonymous hemianopsia, but saccadic function is normal and there is no tonic eye deviation. The descending system for pursuit eye movements may be impaired, resulting in saccadic pursuit to the side of the lesion. Patients, therefore, develop defective OKN when the targets move to the side of the lesion.

Frontal lobe lesions commonly produce a supranuclear gaze palsy, but leave pursuit intact bilaterally. For example, with a right frontal lesion, the patient demonstrates impaired saccades to the left, and his eyes may be deviated to the right. With the OKN target moving to the patient's right, there is difficulty generating the fast phase component of the OKN response to the left, and the eyes remain tonically deviated to the right (or there may be diminished amplitude of the fast phases to the left). With the OKN target moving to the left, there is a normal response since pursuit to the left and saccades to the right are normal.

Extensive deep hemispheric lesions may involve both pursuit and saccadic pathways causing impairment of ipsilateral pursuit and contralateral saccades. This will produce defective OKN when the target moves to the side of the lesion.

Homonymous hemianopsias caused by strictly occipital or temporal lobe or tract lesions are generally not associated with asymmetric OKN. If a patient has a homonymous field cut of occipital origin and has asymmetric OKN, there is probable extension into the parietal lobe.

To help define a muscle paresis, have the paretic muscle make a saccade by moving the target away from the field action of the paretic muscle. The saccadic component of the response will be in the direction of the field of action of the paretic muscle. Observe for asymmetric responses of the yoke muscles; the paretic eye will move more slowly, lagging behind.

To demonstrate the adduction deficiency in internuclear ophthalmoplegia (see Ophthalmoplegia), move the OKN tape away from the field of action of the medial rectus of the eye with impaired adduction, and observe for asymmetric responses of the two eyes. To induce convergence retraction nystagmus (see Nystagmus), move the OKN tape downward. In myasthenia gravis the velocity of the fast phases may increase after the administration of edrophonium (Tensilon). In congenital nystagmus one may see an apparent "inversion" of the OKN response.

ORBIT (see Graves' Ophthalmopathy, Ophthalmoplegia, Ptosis)

PAGET'S DISEASE

Bony changes of Paget's can cause neurological dysfunction of the brainstem, cranial nerves, spinal cord, and roots. Cranial nerves involved include: I (sphenoid bone hyperostosis), II (in optic canal), III, IV, VI (superior orbital fissure), V (with trigeminal neuralgia, atypical facial pain, and, rarely sensory impairment), VII (hemifacial spasm, Bell's palsy), and VIII (tinnitus, vertigo). Severe hearing loss (common) is secondary to sensorineural and conductive (fixation of stapes in the oral window) components. Lower cranial nerve dysfunction in association with cerebellar and long tract findings may result from platybasia and basilar invagination. Rarely, there may be obstructive hydrocephalus, occipital pain, vertebrobasilar ischemia, and acute tonsillar herniation.

Radiculopathy and myelopathy may result from encroachment of distorted bone, compression by vertebral fractures, and vascular steal. The lumbosacral spine is more commonly involved than the thoracic spine, with the cervical spine involved much less frequently. Compression syndromes may improve on calcitonin. Low back pain occurs frequently in patients with Paget's disease, most often due to osteoarthritic disease of the LS spine. Peripheral entrapment neuropathies also occur. Seizures, epidural hematoma and migraine are documented in scattered case reports.

Ref: Chen J-R, et al. Neurology 29:448, 1979.

Clarke CRA, Harrison MJG. J Neurol Sci 38:171, 1978.

PAIN

May be acute or chronic. Acute pain is provoked by noxious or tissue damaging stimulation and includes a constellation of unpleasant perceptual and emotional experiences and certain associated autonomic, psychological, and behavioral responses. Chronic pain is persistent, without biological function; psychological and environmental factors play a prominent role. Chronic pain is a disease state of its own. It is the most frequent cause of disability in the United States.

Types of chronic pain include low back pain, headaches, arthritis, painful polyneuropathies, postherpetic neuralgia, facial pain, visceral pain, and cancer pain. Pain syndromes in patients with cancer include those associated with direct tumor involvement, those associated with cancer therapy, and those unrelated to cancer or its therapy.

Chronic pain always decreases an individual's ability to engage in productive and meaningful vocational and social roles. Methods which are useful in the treatment of acute pain are not applicable to individuals with chronic pain. An integrated multidisciplinary treatment directed at both physical and psychological rehabilitation is most effective in helping patients regain functional living. The goal is to control pain by instructing the pain sufferer to control factors which increase pain and suffering.

The following guidelines are useful in the management of patients with chronic pain. Do not attend to symptoms unless they are changing in a positive direction. All therapies (medications, rest) should be on a time-contingent basis. Activities should be regulated to insure equal distribution throughout the day. Reinforce healthy behaviors and ignore pain behaviors. Emphasize task orientation rather than pain orientation.

__Drug therapy__ of chronic pain is most beneficial if certain basic principles are followed. Treat pain with analgesics early and prescribe medication around the clock to maintain pain at a tolerable level. Receiving medication is, thus, not pain-dependent and the patient is not rewarded for having pain. This also reduces the patient's anxiety about medication and reduces the total amount of drug required in 24 hours.

Give each drug an adequate trial. Start with simple analgesics (aspirin, acetaminophen, propoxyphene). Increase the dose and/or frequency before changing drugs. Know the pharmacology of drugs prescribed. Be aware of individual differences among patients.

Use a combination of drugs. Add aspirin, acetaminophen to other agents. Use muscle relaxants, antiemetics, and antidepressants.

Use equianalgesic drugs and doses when changing drugs. Treat side effects prophylactically; use a set bowel regimen, and antiemetics as necessary.

Avoid excessive sedation; use antidepressants at bedtime only, and decrease dose and increase frequency as necessary.

Specific drug therapy

Antidepressants (amitriptyline, doxepine, etc) are useful in the management of all chronic pain, in particular, headache, low back pain, and patients who have sleep disturbances secondary to their pain.

Anti-inflammatory agents (nonsteroidal anti-inflammatory drugs, steroids, indomethacin) are useful for a variety of chronic pain types including headaches, back pain, and neck pain. When used together with a narcotic, they have an additive effect, and the amount of narcotic can often be decreased.

Anticonvulsants (carbamazepine, phenytoin) are useful in the management of postherpetic neuralgia, peripheral neuropathies, trigeminal neuralgia, and other types of neuropathic pain.

Antipsychotic agents (haloperidol, phenothiazines) are useful in conjunction with the antidepressants in the management of postherpetic neuralgia and peripheral neuropathies.

Other agents (amphetamines, L-dopa, L-tryptophan, D-phenylalanine, cannabinoids) are useful for certain types of cancer pain.

Non-narcotic analgesics (acetaminophen, aspirin) and narcotic analgesics are useful for all pain types. In general, narcotic analgesics are not useful for chronic pain management except for certain types of cancer pain.

Adjunct therapy of pain includes transcutaneous electrical nerve stimulation (TENS; 60-80% effective in acute pain, 30-40% effective in chronic pain), biofeedback, hypnosis, and trigger point injections.

Ref: Houde RW, et al. Clin Pharmacol Ther 1:163, 1960.

Merskey H, Hester RA. The treatment of chronic pain with psychotropic drugs. Postgrad Med J 48: 594, 1972.

Fordyce WE. Behavioral Methods in Chronic Pain and Illness. St. Louis: CV Mosby, 1976.

RELATIVE POTENCIES OF ANALGESICS FOR SEVERE PAIN
(Equivalent to 10 mg IM Morphine)

Drug	IM (mg)	PO (mg)	Major Differences from Morphine
Oxymorphone (Numorphan)	1	6	None
Hydromorphone (Dilaudid)	1.5	7.5	Shorter-acting
Levophanol (Levodromoran)	2	4	High PO to IM potency
Heroin	4		Shorter acting
Methadone (Dolophine)	10	20	High PO to IM potency
Morphine	10	60	
Oxycodone	15	30	Shorter-acting, high PO to IM potency
Pentazocine (Talwin)	60	180	Narcotic antagonist analgesic
Meperidine (Demerol)	75	300	None
Codeine	130	200	High PO to IM potency, more toxic in higher doses
Propoxyphene (Darvon)	240		Similar to codeine but more toxic in higher doses

From: Houde RW, et al. Clin Pharmacol Ther 1:163-166, 1960

RELATIVE POTENCIES OF ANALGESICS (PO)
Mild to Moderate Pain Equivalent to 650 mg Aspirin

Pentazocine (Talwin)	30	Weak narcotic-narcotic antagonist, high analgesic potential*, low addiction liability
Codeine	32	Weak narcotic, high analgesic potential, low addiction liability
Meperidine (Demerol)	50	Narcotic, high analgesic potential, high addiction liability
Propoxyphene (Darvon)	65	Weak narcotic, low analgesic potential, low addiction liability
Aspirin	650	Non-narcotic, anti-inflammatory, low analgesic potential, no addiction liability or tolerance
Acetaminophen (Tylenol)	650	Similar to aspirin

*"Analgesic potential" refers to the level of analgesia attainable by increasing doses to point of limiting side effects

From: Houde RW, et al. Clin Pharmacol Ther 1:163-166, 1960.

INDICATIONS FOR NERVE BLOCKS

Celiac plexus block: Pancreatic carcinoma, chronic pancreatitis, paravertebral mets, any visceral injury, suprarenal pain

CT guided medical rhizotomy: Any localized lesion involving more than two roots; any localized lesion where motor root has to be spared

Peripheral nerve blocks: Pain restricted to intercostal, paravertebral or peripheral nerve distributions

Stellate ganglion block: Causalgia in upper extremities

Carotid sheath block and other trunk blocks: Intractable hiccoughs; neck pain

Subarachnoid and epidural blocks: Pelvic mass or inflammation

Lumbar sympathetic blocks: Causalgia lower extremities

PAPILLEDEMA (see Optic Nerve)

PARANEOPLASTIC SYNDROMES

These remote effects of carcinoma are generally of uncertain etiology. Causes may be various and include immunological, infectious, toxic, or nutritional/metabolic factors. The syndromes include encephalomyelitis, cerebellar degeneration, limbic encephalitis, brainstem encephalitis, necrotizing myelopathy, peripheral neuropathy, myasthenic syndrome, dermatomyositis, polymyositis, retinopathy, opsoclonus, uveomeningoencephalitis, and progressive multifocal leukoencephalopathy.

Patients with malignancy are prone to opportunistic infections. They also have an increased incidence of cerebral infarction, presumably secondary to hypercoagulable states as well as disseminated intravascular coagulation, marantic endocarditis, and venous sinus thrombosis.

Ref: Spence AM, et al. Current Problems in Cancer 7:3, 1983.

PARATHYROID (see Calcium)

PARATONIA (see Rigidity)

PARIETAL LOBE

Lesions of the parietal lobes result in contralateral sensory defects. Lesions of the dominant parietal lobe may result in aphasic syndromes with impaired comprehension, Gerstmann's syndrome, constructional apraxia and ideomotor apraxia. Nondominant parietal lesions are associated with constructional apraxia, dressing apraxia, various visuo-spatial abnormalities, neglect, and denial of deficit.

PARKINSON'S DISEASE

The clinical features of Parkinson's disease include a rest tremor with a frequency of 4-5 Hz, bradykinesia (with generalized motor slowing, mask facies, and decreased associated movements such as arm swing), cogwheel or lead pipe rigidity, postural instability (with general flexion of trunk and limb joints), gait disorder characterized by slow shuffling steps, mental status changes (increased incidence of depression and dementia), and miscellaneous symptoms such as sialorrhea, seborrhea, and orthostatic hypotension.

Idiopathic Parkinsonism is secondary to degeneration of the substantia nigra. A number of disorders have Parkinsonian features. These include striatonigral degeneration (indistinguishable from Parkinsonism except that therapy is rarely effective), Shy-Drager syndrome (see Autonomic Dysfunction), olivopontocerebellar degeneration, and progressive supranuclear palsy. Neuroleptic drugs characteristically induce a Parkinsonian syndrome that is reversible. Carbon monoxide poisoning and chronic manganese intoxication may be associated with irreversible Parkinsonism. A contaminant of an illicit street drug (MPTP) produces an irreversible Parkinsonian state. Other conditions in which Parkinsonian manifestations occur include hypoparathyroidism, occasional neoplasms, the juvenile form of Huntington's disease, and Wilson' disease.

Treatment of Parkinsonism may be initiated with anticholinergics or amantidine. However, most patients with more than a mild affliction, usually require L-dopa. The role of dopamine agonists is presently being considered.

The two most common anticholinergics are benztropine (Cogentin) and trihexyphenidyl (Artane). The initial dose of benztropine is 0.5 mg bid which can be increased to 4-6 mg/day. The initial dose of trihexyphenidyl should be 1 mg bid with a gradual increase to 6-10 mg/day. The side effects of anticholinergics, which usually limit the dose that can be given, include visual blurring, dry mouth, constipation, urinary retention, and confusion. Sudden withdrawal of any anticholinergic drug may acutely worsen the Parkinsonian state.

Amantadine appears to work by inhibiting the re-uptake of dopamine. About 50% of patients respond; rarely is the response for longer than 6 months. The standard dose is 200 mg bid. Side effects include confusion, nausea, and livedo reticularis.

L-dopa is generally given in combination with carbi-dopa, a dopa decarboxylase inhibitor. Sinemet is the only approved combination drug in the U.S. It comes in 3 sizes with fixed carbidopa/L-dopa ratios (10/100, 25/100, 25/250 mg). The usual starting dose is 10/100 or 25/100 bid, increasing to 25/100 tid over 1-2 weeks. The lowest dose which provides significant improvement should be used. As the disease progresses, many patients, particularly those on high doses of L-dopa, develop dyskinesias which can only be treated by lowering the dose of L-dopa with consequent worsening of the Parkinsonism. Fluctuations between Parkinsonism akinesia, known as the on-off phenomenon, may be treated by lowering the dose and giving it more frequently. The addition of a dopamine agonist may also help. Additional side effects of L-dopa include nausea, postural hypotension, confusion, hallucinations, nightmares, and cardiac dysrhythmias.

The only dopamine agonist presently approved for use in the U.S. is bromocriptine. This is given in patients who have developed L-dopa side effects, usually dyskinesia or on-off phenomena. Bromocriptine may result in extreme confusion unless it is started in a very low dose and gradually increased. Start with 1/2 of a 2.5 mg tablet/day and increase by 1/2 tablet/week to a tid regimen. A dose of 10-20 mg/day can usually be achieved without significant side effects and the L-dopa dose may be decreased. Other side effects of bromocriptine include hypotension, nausea, and dyskinesias.

A drug holiday is often used in patients who worsen when their anti-Parkinsonian drugs are either increased or decreased. A limited holiday can be performed as an outpatient with cessation of all medications over the weekend. However, a full holiday involves admission to the hospital and discontinuaton of all medications for 4-7 days during which time the patient may become profoundly rigid and require extensive physical therapy and nursing care. The patient is then restarted with a single drug at a low dose with the expectation that they would be more drug-responsive.

PEDIATRIC NEUROLOGY (see Child Neurology)

PERIODIC PARALYSIS

Remitting and relapsing episodes of flaccid weakness categorized according to the serum potassium during the attack. They may be primary familial (autosomal dominant) or secondary to other causes. See pages 251-2 for a review of primary familial kalemic periodic paralysis.

Secondary kalemic periodic paralysis may be associated with increased or decreased potassium. Hyperkalemia may be associated with transient weakness. Potassium depletion usually causes chronic weakness, but may also cause intermittent weakness.

Thyrotoxic periodic paralysis is the most common acquired periodic paralysis and is very similar to primary hypokalemic periodic paralysis. It is most prevalent among adult, Oriental males. Treatment consists of maintaining the euthyroid state. Propranolol or spironolactone may be used in those not yet euthyroid. Acetazolamide is contraindicated.

Hypokalemia may be due to a variety of GI, metabolic and renal causes (see also Potassium). Weakness is associated with other systemic signs of hypokalemia. Barium poisoning due to contamination of foodstuffs with barium carbonate or the use of table salt with large amounts of barium chloride is associated with a hypokalemic, flaccid paralysis, which may be severe and transient.

Ref: Griggs RC. Periodic paralysis. Seminars in Neurology 3:285, 1983.

PRIMARY FAMILIAL KALEMIC PERIODIC PARALYSIS

HYPOKALEMIC	HYPERKALEMIC	NORMOKALEMIC
Age of Onset:		
10-20 years, peak 20-35 years	Infancy and childhood	Childhood
Duration of Attacks:		
Hours - days	30 min - several hours	Days - weeks
Frequency of Attacks:		
Every 1-2 mos., ↓ with age	Weekly ↓ with age	Every 1-3 mos. Less improvement with age
Precipitating Factors:		
High carbohydrate intake Heavy exercise followed by rest Cold Emotion Infection Trauma Insulin Alcohol Epinephrine Hydrocortisone	High potassium intake Heavy exercise followed by rest Cold ACTH Glucocorticoids Heavy metal exposure	Prolonged rest Heavy exercise followed by rest Cold Emotion Alcohol
Evocative Tests:		
Epinephrine Glucose and insulin NaCl Fluorohydrocortisone	KCl Bicycle ergometer	KCl

HYPOKALEMIC	HYPERKALEMIC	NORMOKALEMIC

Clinical Features:

HYPOKALEMIC	HYPERKALEMIC	NORMOKALEMIC
Often occurs during sleep or prolonged inactivity	Often occurs during rest after exercise	Rare
		Often awake paralyzed
Weakness usually generalized	More common in daytime	May have pharyngeal and respiratory muscle weakness
Pharyngeal and respiratory muscles rarely involved	Weakness often focal	
	May have pharyngeal and respiratory muscle weakness	
	May have myotonia	
	Paresthesias common	
	Sore muscles after attack (up to days)	

Acute Treatment:

HYPOKALEMIC	HYPERKALEMIC	NORMOKALEMIC
KCl up to 130 mEq PO	Calcium gluconate and glucose IV	0.9% NaCl IV
	Inhalation of salbutamol aerosol	

Prophylaxis:

HYPOKALEMIC	HYPERKALEMIC	NORMOKALEMIC
Avoid cold	Avoid cold, overexertion	Avoid high K foods
"Warm down" exercise after exertion	Higher carbohydrate diet	"Warm down" exercise after exertion
High K, low Na, low carbohydrate diet,	Salbutamol 2 mg/d	Fluorohydrocortisone
K supplement	Thiazide diuretic	Acetazolamide (with mineralocorticoid)
Acetazolamide 250-1500 mg/d in divided doses	Acetazolamide	
Triamterene	Propranolol 80-320 mg/d	
Spironolactone		

PERIPHERAL NERVE (see also Brachial Plexus, Dermatomes, Lumbosacral Plexus, Myotomes, Neuropathy)

Anatomical course and distribution of individual peripheral nerves are depicted on the next 8 pages.

MUSCULOCUTANEOUS NERVE

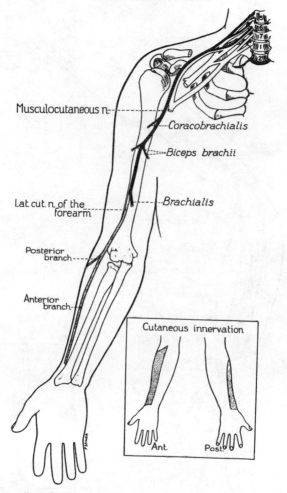

Musculocutaneous n.

Coracobrachialis

Biceps brachii

Lat. cut. n. of the forearm

Brachialis

Posterior branch

Anterior branch

Cutaneous innervation

Ant.

Post.

From: Haymaker W, Woodhall B. Peripheral Nerve Injuries: Principles of Diagnosis. Philadelphia: WB Saunders, 1953, p 238.

RADIAL NERVE

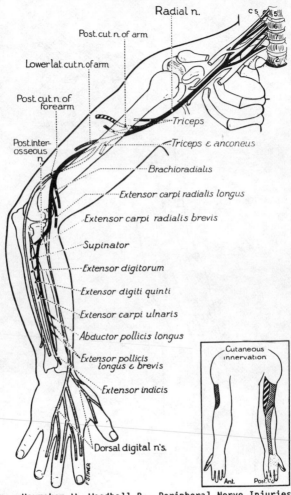

Radial n.

Post. cut. n. of arm

Lower lat. cut. n. of arm

Post. cut. n. of forearm

Post. inter-osseous n.

Triceps

Triceps & anconeus

Brachioradialis

Extensor carpi radialis longus

Extensor carpi radialis brevis

Supinator

Extensor digitorum

Extensor digiti quinti

Extensor carpi ulnaris

Abductor pollicis longus

Extensor pollicis longus & brevis

Extensor indicis

Dorsal digital n's.

Cutaneous innervation

Ant.   Post.

From: Haymaker W, Woodhall B. Peripheral Nerve Injuries: Principles of Diagnosis. Philadelphia: WB Saunders, 1953, p 265.

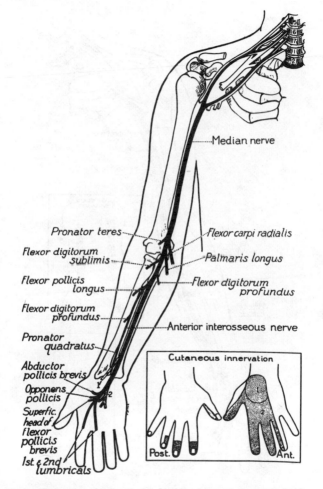

Median nerve

Pronator teres

Flexor digitorum sublimis

Flexor pollicis longus

Flexor digitorum profundus

Pronator quadratus

Abductor pollicis brevis

Opponens pollicis

Superfic. head of flexor pollicis brevis

1st & 2nd lumbricals

Flexor carpi radialis

Palmaris longus

Flexor digitorum profundus

Anterior interosseous nerve

Cutaneous innervation

Post.   Ant.

From: Haymaker W, Woodhall B. Peripheral Nerve Injuries: Principles of Diagnosis. Philadelphia: WB Saunders, 1953, p 242.

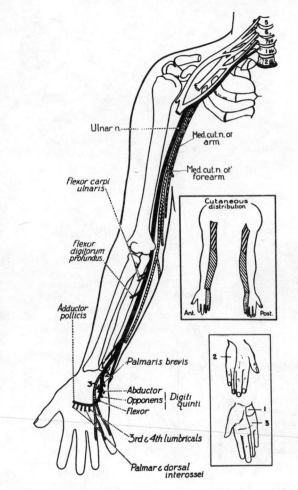

Ulnar n.

Med. cut. n. of arm

Med. cut. n. of forearm

flexor carpi ulnaris

flexor digitorum profundus

Cutaneous distribution

Ant.   Post.

Adductor pollicis

Palmaris brevis

3

Abductor
Opponens } Digiti quinti
flexor

2

1

3

3rd & 4th lumbricals

Palmar & dorsal interossei

From: Haymaker W, Woodhall B. Peripheral Nerve Injuries: Principles of Diagnosis. Philadelphia: WB Saunders, 1953, p 252.

256

FEMORAL NERVE

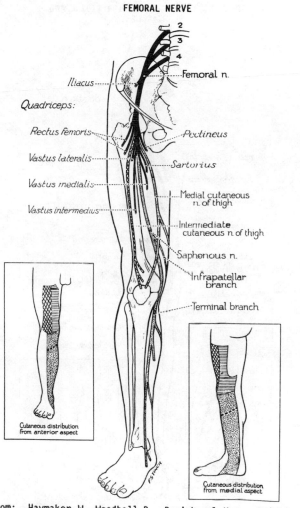

2
3
4

Femoral n.

Iliacus

Quadriceps:

Rectus femoris

Vastus lateralis

Vastus medialis

Vastus intermedius

Pectineus

Sartorius

Medial cutaneous n. of thigh

Intermediate cutaneous n. of thigh

Saphenous n.

Infrapatellar branch

Terminal branch

Cutaneous distribution from anterior aspect

Cutaneous distribution from medial aspect

From: Haymaker W, Woodhall B. Peripheral Nerve Injuries: Principles of Diagnosis. Philadelphia: WB Saunders, 1953, p 282.

SCIATIC, TIBIAL, POSTERIOR TIBIAL AND PLANTAR NERVES

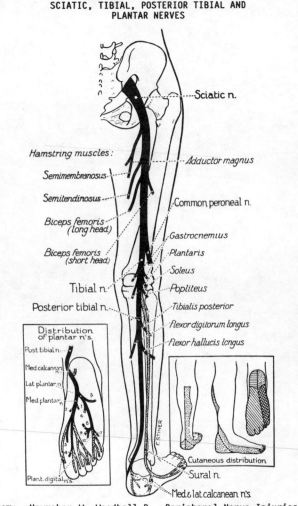

From: Haymaker W, Woodhall B. Peripheral Nerve Injuries: Principles of Diagnosis. Philadelphia: WB Saunders, 1953, p 290.

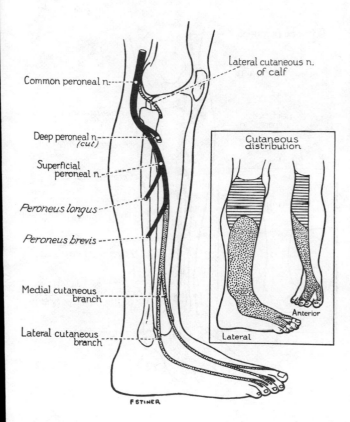

From: Haymaker W, Woodhall B. Peripheral Nerve Injuries: Principles of Diagnosis. Philadelphia: WB Saunders, 1953, p 292.

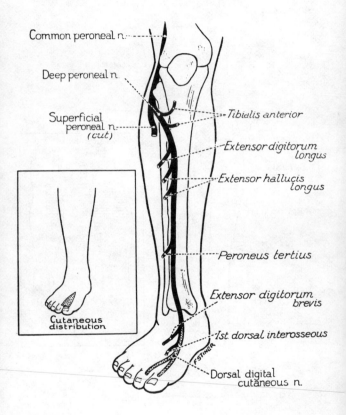

Common peroneal n.

Deep peroneal n.

Superficial peroneal n. (cut)

Tibialis anterior

Extensor digitorum longus

Extensor hallucis longus

Peroneus tertius

Extensor digitorum brevis

1st. dorsal interosseous

Dorsal digital cutaneous n.

Cutaneous distribution

From: Haymaker W, Woodhall B. Peripheral Nerve Injuries: Principles of Diagnosis. Philadelphia: WB Saunders, 1953, p 293.

PHAKOMATOSES (see Neurocutaneous Syndromes)

PHENOTHIAZINES (see Neuroleptics)

PITUITARY (see also Ophthalmoplegia, Visual Fields)

Mass lesions occurring within the sella include pituitary adenomas, arachnoid cysts, and rare tumors of the neurohypophysis. Meningiomas, metastases, dermoids, teratomas, arachnoid cysts, and cholesteatomas may occur in any of several locations around the sella. Suprasellar lesions include craniopharyngiomas, optic gliomas, chondromas, hypothalamic gliomas, supraclinoid carotid artery aneurysms, choroid plexus papillomas, and colloid cysts of the third ventricle. Parasellar lesions include cavernous carotid aneurysms, temporal lobe neoplasms, and gasserian ganglion neuromas. Cordomas and basilar artery aneurysms are seen in the retrosellar region. Infrasellar lesions include sphenoid sinus mucoceles, carcinomas, granulomas, and other nasopharyngeal tumors.

Pituitary adenomas may cause only endocrine symptoms if less than 10 mm in diameter (microadenoma). Larger tumors usually produce visual symptoms and/or headache with or without endocrine abnormalities, including variable hypopituitarism. Pituitary adenomas are usually classified histologically on the basis of immunoperoxidase stains to identify specific hormones. Prolactin-secreting and nonsecreting adenomas (usually chromophobe adenomas) are the most common. The most common of these, the prolactinomas, usually present with amenorrhea and/or galactorrhea in females and decreased libido and impotence in males. In the absence of hormonal dysfunction, the nonsecreting tumors typically present with visual disturbance, usually after having enlarged considerably. The less common growth hormone and ACTH-secreting adenomas present with acromegaly and Cushing syndrome, respectively, usually while small in size. Acromegaly may also be associated with entrapment neuropathies such as carpal tunnel syndrome. Cushing syndrome may be associated with mental status changes and myopathy. Gonadotropin and TSH-secreting adenomas are rare.

Prolactinomas may rapidly expand with subacute onset of neurological dysfunction during pregnancy. The differential diagnosis of hyperprolactinemia includes hypothalamic and infundibular lesions (loss of inhibitory control of prolactin secretion), renal failure, Chiari-Frommel syndrome, and drugs (phenothiazines, butyrophenones, benzodiazepines, reserpine, morphine, α-methyl-dopa and isoniazid). Serum prolactin levels >100 ng/ml (normal, less than 15 ng/ml) are almost

always due to tumor. Levels from 15-100 ng/ml may be due
to tumor, but are more commonly due to the other disorders
listed above, particularly drugs.

Treatment of prolactinomas and nonsecreting tumors
consists of transphenoidal microsurgical resection if
there is optic nerve or chiasmal involvement. Extension
into brain parenchyma requires an intracranial approach.
Corticosteroid coverage should be provided during surgery.
Visual and endocrine function may improve after surgery
and should be followed regularly postoperatively. Postoperative radiation therapy is often used for incomplete
resections. Bromocriptine alone may suffice for treatment
of microadenomas and may be used occasionally in
conjunction with surgery for macroadenomas, except in
pregnant women with asymmetric sellar enlargement who
should undergo surgery. Various combinations of surgery
and proton beam therapy are used in growth hormone and
ACTH-secreting tumors.

Craniopharyngiomas, which may be distinguished from
pituitary adenomas by calcifications (see below), are
treated by surgical removal and postoperative radiation
therapy. There is a fairly high recurrence rate, even if
resection seems complete. Stereotactic decompression of
recurrent fluid-filled cysts may obviate the need for
craniotomy in some cases.

Pituitary apoplexy refers to the sudden expansion of
the pituitary gland, usually from hemorrhage. There is
sudden severe headache, variable ocular motor palsies,
rapid loss of vision (chiasmal or optic nerve), evidence
of dyspituitarism (usually preexisting pituitary adenoma),
and subarachnoid hemorrhage with associated changes in
mental status. The association of subarachnoid hemorrhage
with ocular motor palsies can be distinguished from that
due to rupture of an aneurysm by the presence of mixed,
and usually, bilateral ophthalmoplegias, and the presence
of an afferent pupillary defect or chiasmal patterns of
field loss, although the latter frequently goes unnoticed
in obtunded patients. Diagnostic procedures include CT
which may show a pituitary mass containing blood, skull
films showing bony changes of the sella, angiography to
exclude an intracavernous aneurysm, and LP consistent with
subarachnoid hemorrhage. Treatment includes immediate
high-dose IV corticosteroids and prompt transphenoidal
decompression to prevent further loss of vision.

Empty sella syndrome is the major cause of asymptomatic sellar enlargement. The subarachnoid space extends
into the sella through an incompetent diaphragm with
flattening of the gland inferiorly and posteriorly. It
may also follow pseudotumor cerebri, spontaneous
regressive changes of pituitary adenomas, and surgery.

Although usually asymptomatic, symptoms may occur including headache, occasional mild endocrine abnormalities, CSF rhinorrhea, and, rarely, visual disturbances. Pituitary tumor should be excluded with endocrine and neuro-ophthalmic evaluations and CT, including metrizamide-CT cisternography if needed.

Differential diagnosis of an enlarged sella turcica in the absence of endocrinopathy includes nonsecreting adenoma, empty sella syndrome, and craniopharyngioma. Hypopituitarism, diabetes insipidus, and visual field defects are much less common in the empty sella syndrome. A ballooned-sella without erosion is more characteristic of the empty sella. Suprasellar extension and calcification is more characteristic of craniopharyngioma.

PLEXUS (see Brachial Plexus, Lumbosacral Plexus)

POLYMYOSITIS (see Muscle Disorders, Myopathy)

PORPHYRIA

The porphyrias may be divided into erythropoietic and hepatic types. The hepatic types have prominent neurological manifestations. The most common of these, acute intermittent porphyria, is autosomal dominant with onset in the second to fifth decades (rarely before puberty). It is characterized by recurrent attacks of abdominal pain and neurological dysfunction. An autonomic neuropathy causes the common symptoms of abdominal pain, vomiting and constipation (or diarrhea) as well as tachycardia, orthostatic hypotension, hypertension, diaphoresis, and urinary retention. A motor > sensory polyneuropathy or mononeuritis multiplex may occur as well as occasional ascending flaccid paralysis resembling Guillain-Barre syndrome which may result in fatal respiratory failure. Back and extremity pain is not uncommon. Cranial nerves may be involved. Cerebral symptoms include headaches, seizures, and higher cortical dysfunction as well as the very common and varied psychiatric manifestations.

Laboratory diagnosis during acute attacks and usually between attacks depends on demonstrating elevated urinary delta-aminolevulinic acid (ALA) and porphobilinogen and decreased activity of erthyrocyte uroporphyrinogen-1-synthetase. Asymptomatic family members at risk may be detected by measuring the latter. Normal lead levels help distinguish lead poisoning, which may have similar symptoms and increased urinary porphyrins and delta-ALA acid. Nerve conduction studies, EMG, and muscle biopsy typically reflect the mixed demyelinating and axonal neuropathy.

PORPHYRIA

Drugs that may precipitate an attack of acute intermittent porphyria

Alcohol	Meprobamate
Barbiturates	Methsuximide
Carisoprodol	Methyldopa
Chloramphenicol	Methylprylon
Chlordiazepoxide	Pentazocine
Chloroquine	Phenytoin
Dichloralphenazone	Progesterones
Ergots	Pyralones
Estrogens	Sulfonamides
Eucalyptol	Sylfonal
Glutethimide	Testosterones
Griseofulvin	Tolbutamide
Imipramine	Trional

Drugs that do not exacerbate acute intermittent porphyria

Ascorbic Acid	Nitrofurantoin
Atropine	Opiates
B Vitamins	Penicillins
Chloral hydrate	Phenothiazines
Corticosteroids	Promethazine
Digoxin	Rauwolfia alkaloids
Diphenhydramine	Scopolamine
Guanethidine	Streptomycin
Methenamine mandelate	Tetracyclines
Meclizine	Tetraethylammonium
Neostigmine	bromide

Treatment consists of avoiding precipitating factors such as drugs (see above) that activate delta-ALA synthetase, certain hormones, infection, and starvation and dieting. Estrogen, progesterone, and testosterone activate delta-ALA synthetase. These agents, including oral contraceptives, and pregnancy may precipitate attacks. Oral contraceptives, however, may be used to prevent the regular, cyclic attacks of acute intermittent porphyria that occur in some women just prior to their menses. Prophylactic high-carbohydrate diet and propranolol may be helpful. Acute attacks may be treated with IV glucose, 10-20 gm/hr and IV hematin, 4 mg/kg over 10-12 minutes q12h. Psychiatric disturbances may be treated with phenothiazines. Chlorpromazine is very effective for treating abdominal pain. Opiates may also be used but particular care should be taken regarding respiratory suppression. Bowel hygiene, including fecal disimpaction, may be necessary. Treatment of seizures may be problematical since many anticonvulsants precipitate attacks, although phenytoin to a lesser extent. Some new anticonvulsants (e.g., carbamazepine) have not been adequately studied. The use of benzodiazepines or bromides is suggested by some.

POTASSIUM (see also Calcium, Electrolytes, Periodic Paralysis)

Hypokalemia may result in variable weakness of the arms, legs, trunk, and, occasionally, respiratory muscles. Cranial nerve innervated muscles are usually not involved. Reflexes may be decreased. There is no sensory involvement. Hypokalemia and hypocalcemia frequently co-exist and their neuromuscular manifestations may cancel one another such that treatment of one in isolation may result in clinical worsening. Cardiac manifestations are the most dangerous, and include dysrhythmias and potentiation of digoxin toxicity. The EKG shows ST depression, T-wave flattening, or inversion, and U waves.

Hyperkalemia usually does not cause neurological symptoms or signs until it is severe. A flaccid paralysis may develop rapidly, even to the point of flaccid quadraplegia within minutes. Tendon reflexes may be absent. Respiratory muscles may be involved. Cranial nerve innervated muscles are usually spared. Subjective numbness of the hands and feet and decreased position and vibration sense may be present. Again, cardiac manifestations are the most serious. The EKG shows tall, peaked T waves without QT prolongation followed by prolonged PR intervals, T wave flattening, ST depression, and widening of the QRS.

PREGNANCY (see also individual entries)

I. Neuropathy, plexopathy
   A. Endometriosis: Endometrial implants along cauda equina, roots, lumbosacral plexus or sciatic nerve have been reported. The radiculopathy, plexopathy or neuropathy is accompanied by perimenstrual pain.

B. Bell's palsy: Incidence increases threefold during pregnancy.

C. Carpal tunnel syndrome: May occur transiently during pregnancy, regressing after delivery. Splinting of the wrist usually suffices.

D. Meralgia paresthetica: Mid-lateral thigh numbness, tingling or stinging pain, usually beginning at 30 weeks' gestation, secondary to entrapment of lateral cutaneous nerve of the thigh. Treatment involves avoidance of excessive weight gain, and, if severe or persistent, local anesthetic infiltration or nerve transposition.

E. Recurrent brachial plexus neuropathy: Familial and associated with menarche, pregnancy or early puerperium with a slow full recovery in 1-3 years.

F. Guillain-Barre syndrome: Incidence and course unaffected by pregnancy. Pregnancy is not complicated by Guillain-Barre, except possibly increased prematurity in severe third trimester cases.

G. Recurrent idiopathic polyneuropathy (chronic dysimmune neuropathy) weakness is progressive during pregnancy. Recovery, after delivery, may be incomplete.

H. Gestational distal polyneuropathy: Associated with malnutrition and has been seen with hyperemesis gravidarum when vitamins (thiamine) are not replaced parenterally. May be associated with Wernicke-Korsakoff syndrome or encephalopathy.

I. Acute intermittent porphyria: Pregnancy may induce a crisis in some patients. Most (60%) occur early, but third trimester crises are complicated by hypertension, hyperemesis, eclampsia, and renal disease, and are associated with prematurity and high maternal and fetal mortality. Treatment is primarily supportive (see Porphyria).

J. Obstetrical palsies
   1. Postpartum foot drop secondary to lumbosacral trunk compression by the infant's brow. Subsequent pregnancies should be cautiously followed and C-section considered if a large baby and difficult labor are observed.
   2. Femoral neuropathy: May be caused by self-retaining retractors during C-section and, rarely, following vaginal delivery.

3. Obturator neuropathy: Can occur with difficult labor.

II. Myasthenia gravis
      Myasthenia may improve in 1/3, be unaffected in
1/3, and worsen in 1/3, or may present during
pregnancy or postpartum. Pregnancy is minimally
affected but should be avoided in patients with
severe disease. Magnesium sulfate, scopolamine,
and large amounts of procaine are contraindicated.
Great care is necessary in the use of anesthesia
and sedating drugs. Regional anesthesia is
preferred. Newborns should be observed carefully
(e.g., difficulty feeding) for 72 hours for
neonatal myasthenia.

III. Myotonic dystrophy
      Disability remains unchanged or worsens during
pregnancy, especially the third trimester. Spontaneous abortion, premature labor, uterine inertia,
and postpartum hemorrhage may all be increased.
Regional anesthesia is preferred. Depolarizing
muscle relaxants are contraindicated, but curare
may be used. Polyhydramnios suggests fetal
myotonia.

IV. Movement disorders
      A. Chorea gravidarum: Chorea during pregnancy is
           rarer (<1/100,000 pregnancies) now than in
           the past. Most chorea occurs during the first
           trimester and abates before birth in 30%
           usually within 1-2 months. It may recur with
           subsequent pregnancies. Symptoms often
           dramatically disappear after childbirth.
           Approximately 1/3 have had Sydenham's chorea in
           the past. Rule out acute rheumatic fever,
           Wilson's disease, lupus, polycythemia, and
           hyperthyroidism, idiopathic hypoparathryoidism.
      B. Wilson's disease: Penicillamine has virtually
           eliminated excess abortions. The infants are
           healthy, although penicillamine may be
           hazardous to the fetus. Pyridoxine 50-100 mg
           daily is recommended, and a reduction in
           penicillamine dosage to 250 mg daily for the
           last 6 weeks of pregnancy is recommended if
           C-section is performed.

V. Infections
   A. Poliomyelitis: Spinal or caudal anesthetic should be avoided. Pregnancy is not a contra-indication to polio immunization.
   B. Syphilis: T. pallidum has been demonstrated in 10 week conceptuses. Treatment of maternal syphilis should be prompt, with penicillin or a cephalosporin. The IgM FTA-ABS will be elevated in congenital syphilis.

VI. Multiple sclerosis
   Gestation, labor, and delivery may be normal in MS. Relapses may or may not be more frequent during pregnancy and postpartum. Half of all pregnancy associated relapses or first attacks occur during the 3 months postpartum. Parent-child pairs wih MS occur more frequently than expected, but the parent almost always develops MS after delivery. A common exposure has been postulated.

VII. Cerebrovascular disease
   A. Subarachnoid hemorrhage accounts for 10% of maternal deaths during pregnancy and postpartum in woman under 25. Arteriovenous malformations (AVMs) are a more common cause than aneurysms. Other causes include placental abruption and DIC (rare), anticoagulants, endocarditis and mycotic aneurysm, metastatic choriocarcinoma, eclampsia, postpartum cerebral phlebothrombosis, and spinal cord AVMs. AVMs tend to bleed during the second trimester and during childbirth. The risk of aneurysmal rupture increases with each trimester. The risk of childbirth suggests that AVMs should be excised and aneurysms clipped prepartum and C-sections performed for inoperable AVMs and ruptured inoperable aneurysms. Hyperventilation, hypothermia, and steroids have been safely employed during pregnancy, but mannitol should be avoided.
   B. Arterial thrombosis: The incidence of ischemic stroke may be increased 3-4 fold; however, unusual causes should still be sought and arteriography performed to rule out venous thrombosis unless an embolic source is obvious. Emboli may also be caused by peripartum cardio-myopathy, paradoxical emboli, amniotic fluid emboli, and fat emboli.

C. Venous thrombosis: Aseptic cerebral vein thrombosis occurs in approximately 1/2500 pregnancies. Sagittal sinus thrombosis presents with headache, confusion, seizures, papilledema and focal signs. Treatment consists of anti-convulsants and steroids. Heparin is controversial as intracranial hemorrhage may result. Cortical vein thrombosis presents similarly but without papilledema unless clot propagates to the sagittal sinus. Mortality is <30% and survivors often recover with little handicap.

D. Sheehan's syndrome: Postpartum hypopituitarism secondary to pituitary infarction during severe shock at the time of delivery, usually involves the anterior pituitary. Failure to lactate is followed by amenorrhea and symptoms of low thyroid and cortisol levels.

E. Carotid cavernous sinus fistulas may present during pregnancy, usually in the second half.

VIII. Tumors: Most intracranial (primary) tumors will enlarge during pregnancy and shrink again postpartum when the natural history of the tumor asserts itself. Symptoms or signs may be apparent only during the second half of pregnancy. Although slow growing tumors can usually be followed and resected 3 weeks postpartum, malignant gliomas and many posterior fossa tumors require prompt surgery. Choriocarcinomas frequently metastasize to the brain.

IX. Pseudotumor cerebri: May begin in the third to fifth month of pregnancy and may persist until delivery. Indications for treatment (shunting) are the same as for nonpregnant women.

X. Headache: Approximately 3/4 of migraineurs will improve or be free of headaches during pregnancy, but up to 1/4 may worsen. Treatment should be limited to acetaminophen and avoidance of precipitants during pregnancy.

XI. Epilepsy: Seizures increase in approximately 50% of pregnant epileptics, remain unchanged in 42% and improve in 8%. Poor prepregnancy seizure control predicts worsening. Seizures occur more frequently in children of epileptic mothers. The amount of phenobarbital or phenytoin excreted in breast milk is not associated with adverse effects. See also section XIII below.

XII. Eclampsia: Characterized by hypertension, proteinuria, edema, hyperreflexia, convulsions, and coma
occurring in the third trimester. Preeclampsia
refers to hypertension, proteinuria, and edema; it
is considered severe if BP is greater than 160/110,
proteinuria is 4+, oliguria exists, and pulmonary
edema, hyperreflexia, and headache are present.
Cerebral manifestations of eclampsia are those of
hypertensive encephalopathy and intracerebral
hematoma. If seizures occur, subarachnoid
hemorrhage, thrombotic thrombocytopenic purpura,
amniotic fluid embolus, cerebral vein thrombosis,
water intoxication, pheochromocytoma, and toxicity
of anesthetic agents should be considered. Lumbar
puncture is safe in eclampsia. CBC, glucose, BUN,
sodium, and serum procaine or lidocaine levels may
be helpful. Treatment of hypertension includes: 1)
diazoxide 300 mg IV push or 2) hydralazine 20-40 mg,
initially, IV drip and furosemide 20-40 mg IV over
several minutes. Seizures should initially be
treated by controlling blood pressure; if unsuccessful, anticonvulsants are used (see Epilepsy) as in
status epilepticus. Control of hypertension, hyperventilation, and hypothermia (after delivery) have
been used to reduce cerebral edema. Magnesium
sulfate is commonly employed to "control" seizures.
It acts by blocking neuromuscular transmission,
preventing tonic-clonic limb movements, but with no
acute effects on the CNS. It is not recommended as
an anticonvulsant.

XIII. Anticonvulsants during pregnancy
Detrimental effects of seizures on the fetus
are well documented. Malformations are more common
in the fetuses of epileptic mothers treated with
anticonvulsants as well as those untreated.
Malformations are also more frequent in epileptics
themselves and in infants whose fathers are
epileptic. Both genetic and teratogenetic factors
appear to be important.
An increased risk of cleft palate or congenital
heart disease in offspring of epileptic mothers has
been attributed to phenytoin. A fetal hydantoin
syndrome has been described consisting of
intrauterine growth retardation, mental retardation,
developmental delay, craniofacial abnormalities
(depressed nasal bridge, ptosis, inner epicanthal
folds, ocular hypertelorism), and nail and digital
hypoplasia. Cause and effect has not been
established. Phenytoin requirement may increase
during pregnancy due to increased clearance.

Phenobarbital has not been conclusively implicated as a human teratogen although a fetal barbiturate syndrome has been reported. Fetal liver enzymes are induced, altering bilirubin, vitamin D and steroid metabolism. Withdrawal symptoms may be seen in the neonate. Dose requirements may increase during pregnancy due to increased clearance.

Carbamazepine risk during pregnancy is unknown. It is not presently recommended as a first-line seizure drug during pregnancy, but is used for severe trigeminal neuralgia. Anecdotal effects of trimethadione during pregnancy have been reported. Valproic acid has been associated with spinal dysraphic syndromes.

Vitamin K should be administered to correct coagulation defects in neonates whose mothers took anticonvulsants.

Antiepileptics should not be discontinued in patients who require them to prevent major seizures due to the high risk of precipitating status epilepticus and to attendant complications. Maternal drug requirements may change rapidly (usually decrease) postpartum, therefore, drug levels should be monitored more carefully after delivery. Many infants experience a postnatal drug withdrawal syndrome, most frequently with phenobarbital and phenytoin, which may be delayed as long as a week. It usually consists of jitteriness, irritability or a change in sleep pattern.

Ref: Donaldson. Neurology of Pregnancy. Philadelphia: FA Davis, 1978.

Stumpf DA. Anticonvulsant use during pregnancy. Clin Therapeut 7:258, 1985.

PROGRESSIVE SUPRANUCLEAR PALSY

A progressive degenerative disease with onset usually in the sixth or seventh decade. Clinical features include supranuclear ophthalmoplegia (usually beginning with paresis of downward gaze, later involving upward gaze, and ultimately horizontal gaze), axial rigidity, pseudobulbar palsy, marked bradykinesia, gait disturbance resembling Parkinsonism and/or spasticity, Parkinsonian facies with infrequent blinking, and sub-cortical dementia. Patients are often diagnosed as having Parkinson's disease until the ophthalmoparesis develops. The course is usually progressive, leading to immobility and anarthria.

CT is usually unremarkable but may occasionally show midbrain atrophy. CSF and EEG are not helpful.

Some patients have a lessening of rigidity, but not ophthalmoparesis, with anti-Parkinsonian drugs. Methysurgide is said to improve dysphagia.

Ref: Jackson JA, et al. Ann Neurol 13:273, 1983.

PSEUDOBULBAR PALSY

Most lower brainstem nuclei are bilaterally inner-vated. Unilateral involvement of supranuclear pathways, therefore, may not produce symptoms. Bilateral involve-ment of corticobulbar fibers, which pass through the genu of the internal capsule and the medial cerebral peduncles, and frontal efferents subserving emotional expression, also passing near the genu, results in pseudobulbar palsy. This should be distinguished from infranuclear involvement (see Bulbar Palsy). In pseudobulbar palsy there is decreased voluntary movement and spastic hyperreflexia of the involved muscles. Thus, gag and jaw jerk reflexes may be hyperactive, even though the patient is unable to swallow or chew. Frequently, there is a spontaneous release of emotional responses such as crying or, less frequently, laughing with little or no provocation. Although a variety of lesions (demyelinating disease, motor neuron disease) can interrupt the corticobulbar and anterior fronto-pontomedullary fibers, infarction is most common.

Frontal release signs (grasp, palmomental, suck, snout, rooting and glabellar reflexes) may be prominent. These should be interpreted with caution as many normal elderly people exhibit palmomental and snout reflexes without neurological disease.

Pseudobulbar palsy may occur with unilateral involve-ment of the opercular cortex, producing the operculum syndrome. It is usually caused by infarction in the distribution of the sylvian branches of the middle cerebral artery although other causes such as tumor and meningitis have been reported. It differs from classical pseudobulbar palsy in that it may improve over several days and the emotional symptoms are rare. It is often associated with contralateral hemiplegia and, occasion-ally, contralateral hemianesthesia.

PSEUDOTUMOR CEREBRI

A clinical syndrome, also called "benign" or idiopathic intracranial hypertension, consisting of increased intracranial pressure, papilledema, normal spinal fluid formula, and normal ventricles on CT. It is most common in young obese women. Symptoms include headache (90%) which is often increased with valsalva, transient visual obscurations of <10 seconds (35-70%), diplopia due to unilateral or bilateral VI nerve palsy (a nonspecific sign of increased intracranial pressure), and visual loss in some. There should be no other neurological signs. The CT scan is normal although an occasional empty sella or enlarged optic nerve sheaths may be seen. Lumbar puncture opening pressure is >200 mm H2O.

Increased intracranial pressure may be associated with certain drugs, endocrine and metabolic disorders, and systemic illnesses. Endocrine factors include menstrual disorders, pregnancy, menarche, Addison's disease, Turner's syndrome, and hypoparathyroidism. Systemic illnesses include lead toxicity, iron deficiency anemia, blood dyscrasias, and chronic pulmonary hypoventilation. Drugs which can cause pseudotumor cerebri include chronic steroids, steroid withdrawal, oral contraceptives, tetracycline, nitrofurantoin, nalidixic acid, excess vitamin A, and various psychiatric drugs and anti-inflammatory agents.

Management begins with removing or correcting any associated factors. Weight loss should be vigorously encouraged in obese patients. Furosemide or acetazolamide may be helpful. Steroids (prednisone 20-50 mg qd x 2 weeks, then tapered) may help, however, the benefits probably do not outweigh the side effects. Repeated lumbar punctures are not recommended since they decrease intracranial pressure only transiently and they tend to discourage follow-up. Regardless of medical therapy, regular evaluation, including quantitative perimetry and fundus exam, is necessary since visual loss may occur early or late in the disease. If there is any evidence of visual loss, optic nerve sheath decompression or lumbo-peritoneal shunt placement should be done.

Ref: Corbett JJ, et al. Arch Neurol 39:461, 1982.

PTOSIS

Deficiency of levator tonus.

I.   Congenital ptosis
     A. Isolated
     B. With double elevator palsy
     C. Anomalous synkinesis (including Gunn jaw winking)
     D. Lid or orbital tumor (hemangioma, dermoid)
     E. Neurofibromatosis
     F. Blepharophimosis syndromes
     G. First branchial arch syndromes (Hallerman-
        Streiff, Treacher Collins)
     H. Neonatal myasthenia

II. Ptosis secondary to myopathy
     A. Myasthenia gravis - Ptosis may be variable and
        asymmetric. May see Cogan's lid twitch sign.
        Improves with edrophonium.
     B. Myopathy restricted to levator palpebrae
        superioris or including external ophthalmoplegia
     C. Oculopharyngeal muscular dystrophy
     D. Myotonic dystrophy
     E. Polymyositis - Conjunctival swelling present.
     F. Aplastic levator muscle
     G. Dysthyroidism
     H. Chronic progressive external ophthalmoplegia
     I. Topical steroid eye drops
     J. Levator dehiscence-disinsertion syndrome. Due to
        aging, inflammation, surgery, trauma, or ocular
        allergy.

III. Ptosis secondary to sympathetic denervation (see
     Horner's Syndrome)

IV. Ptosis secondary to III nerve lesions
     A. Nuclear lesions involving the levator subnucleus
        produce severe bilateral ptosis, medial rectus
        weakness, skew deviation if the IV nerve is
        involved, or upgaze paresis and pupillary
        dilatation if entire III nerve nucleus involved.
     B. Peripheral III nerve lesions produce unilateral
        ptosis with mydriasis, and ophthalmoplegia.
        Isolated ptosis is rare.

V.   Pseudoptosis
     A. Trachoma
     B. Ptosis adiposis
     C. Blepharochalasis
     D. Plexiform neuroma

E. Amyloid infiltration
F. Inflammation secondary to allergy, chalazion, blepharitis, conjunctivitis.
G. Hemangioma
H. Duane's retraction syndrome
I. Microphthalmos phthisis bulbi
J. Enophthalmos
K. Pathologic lid retraction on opposite side
L. Chronic Bell's palsy
M. Hypertropia
N. Decreased mental status
O. Hysterical

Ref: Thompson S, et al. Arch Neurol 39:108, 1982.

Glaser JS. Neuro-ophthalmology. Hagerstown: Harper and Row, 1978, pp 35-8.

PUPIL

Pupils are examined in both light and darkness, with attention to size, shape, and reactivity to a bright light.

Bilateral dilation (mydriasis) may be produced by:
Drugs (see pages 276-277)
Emotional state (startle, fear, pain)
Thyrotoxicosis
Ciliospinal reflex
Bilateral blindness due to severe visual system involvement anterior to the optic chiasm
Parinaud's syndrome
Seizures
During rostral-caudal deterioration due to supratentorial mass lesions

Bilateral constriction (miosis) may be produced by:
Near triad (accommodation, convergence, miosis)
Old age
Drugs (see pages 276-277)
Pontine lesions
Argyll-Robertson pupils

Anisocoria, or unequal pupil size, can be an important localizing sign. A difference of <1 mm exists in approximately 20% of the normal population; >1 mm, in as much as 5%. The asymmetry remains constant in light and dark. Drugs and toxins, including eye drops, may cause constriction or dilation of pupils (see page 277) which is usually symmetric unless agents are applied locally in one eye. Causes of significant anisocoria may be determined clinically and pharmacologically using the flow chart on page 279.

Causes of episodic anisocoria include:
    Parasympathetic paresis
      Incipient uncal herniation
      Seizure
      Migraine
    Parasympathetic hyperactivity
      Cyclic oculomotor paresis
    Sympathetic paresis
      Cluster headache (paratrigeminal neuralgia)
    Sympathetic hyperactivity
      Claude Bernard syndrome following neck trauma
    Sympathetic dysfunction with alternating anisocoria
      Cervical spinal cord lesions
    Benign unilateral pupillary dilatation (involved pupil
      has normal light and near responses)

DRUG EFFECTS ON THE PUPILS

<u>Constriction</u> (Miosis)

SYSTEMIC

Constriction (Miosis)	Dilation (Mydriasis)
Narcotics	Anticholinergics
Morphine and opium alkaloids	Atropine
Meperidine and congeners	Belladonna
Methadone and congeners	Scopolamine
Propoxyphene	Propantheline
Barbiturates	Jimsonweed
Diphenoxylate	Nightshade
Chloral hydrate	Tricyclic antidepressants
Phenoxybenzamine	Trihexyphenidyl
Dibenzyline	Benztropine
Phentolamine	Antihistamines
Tolazoline	Diphenydramine
Guanethidine	Chlorpheniramine
Bretylium	Phenothiazines
Reserpine	Glutethimide
MAO inhibitors	Amphetamines
Alpha methyldopa	Cocaine
Bethanidine	Ephedrine
Thymoxamine	Epinephrine

DRUG EFFECTS ON THE PUPILS (cont.)

<u>Constriction</u> (Miosis)

Indoramin
Meprobamate
Cholinergics
   Edrophonium
   Neostigmine
   Pyridostigmine
   Physostigmine
Cholinesterase inhibitor pesticides
Phencyclidine
Thallium
Lidocaine and related agents
  (extradural thoracic anesthesia)
Marijuana
Phenothiazines

<u>Dilation</u> (Mydriasis)

Norepinephrine
Ethanol
Botulinum toxin
Snake venom
Barracuda poisoning
Tyramine
Hemicholinium
Hypocalcemia
Hypermagnesemia
Thiopental
Lysergic acid
  diethylamide
Fenfluramine (patients
  on reserpine)

LOCAL

Miotics
   Pilocarpine
   Carbachol
   Methacholine
   Physostigmine
   Neostigmine
   Isoflurophate
   Echothiophate
   Demecarium
   Aceclidine

Mydriatics and cycloplegics
   Phenylephrine
   Hydroxyamphetamine
   Epinephrine
   Cocaine
   Eucatropine
   Atropine
   Homatropine
   Scopolamine
   Cyclopentolate
   Tropicamide
   Oxyphenonium

Adapted from Thurston SE, Leigh RJ. The neurological evaluation of the critically ill patient. In: Henning RJ, Jackson DL (eds). Handbook of Critical Care Neurology and Neurosurgery. New York: Praeger, 1985.

Afferent pupillary defects (see page 280), Marcus Gunn pupil, due to a lesion of the optic nerve. Resting pupil sizes are normal. Both direct and consensual pupillary responses are decreased with bright illumination of the involved side, whereas both responses are normal with illumination of the normal side. When alternately stimulating each eye ("swinging flashlight test"), both pupils dilate with stimulation on the abnormal side, both constrict with stimulation on the normal side.

The <u>near reflex</u> should be tested whenever pupils react poorly to light. Have the patient fixate a distant target, then quickly fixate his own finger tip held immediately in front of his nose. Light near dissociation may be seen in:

Severe anterior visual system dysfunction (e.g., severe glaucoma, bilateral optic neuropathy, etc.)
Neurosyphilis (Argyll-Robertson pupil) - associated with miosis, irregular pupils, poor dilation, and, usually, relatively normal vision
Adie's tonic pupil
Rostral dorsal midbrain (Parinaud's syndrome)
Aberrant III nerve regeneration
Diabetes (out of proportion to any retinopathy)
Amyloidosis
Myotonic dystrophy

RADIATION

An acute, dose-related encephalopathy attributed to edema can occur within 24 hours of whole-brain radiation therapy. Symptoms include headache, nausea, vomiting, fever, lethargy, and exacerbation of previous neurological deficits. Herniation occurs rarely. Treatment consists of high-dose steroids.

Sub-acute (early-delayed) demyelination may occur weeks after radiation therapy, especially of head and neck tumors. Brainstem and cerebellar dysfunction predominate. In some there is progression to death, in others, complete or near complete recovery. It is unclear if steroids are of any benefit.

Cerebral radiation necrosis associated with a small vessel vasculopathy and glial proliferation, may occur a few months to years following radiation therapy and is dose-dependent. It can present as an enlarging mass and may be difficult to differentiate from recurrent tumor. Steroids are of unclear benefit. Surgical resection for diagnosis and palliative therapy is commonly undertaken, although the prognosis remains poor.

Radiation therapy and methotrexate in combination in children may cause a decrease in intellectual function, necrotizing leukoencephalopathy, or mineralizing microangiopathy. The necrotizing leukoencephalopathy occurs 4-12 months after radiation therapy. Symptoms include dementia, spasticity, dysarthria, dysphagia, seizures, hemiplegia, and coma. Neurological damage is permanent in most, however, a few recover completely. The mineralizing microangiopathy consists of dystrophic calcification in gray matter, including the putamen, cerebral cortical sulci, and cerebellar folia. It occurs approximately 10 months after

ANISOCORIA

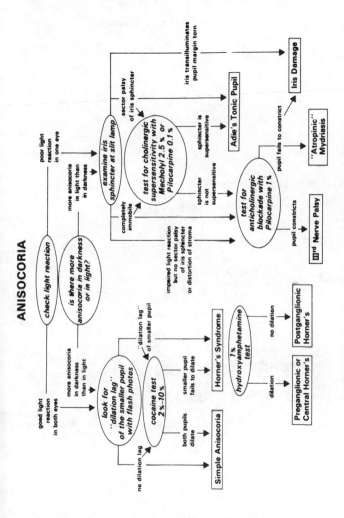

From: Thompson HS, Pilley SJ: Unequal pupils: A flow chart for sorting out the anisocorias. Surv Ophthalmal 21:45-48, 1976. Used by permission.

PUPILLARY LIGHT REFLEX PATHWAYS

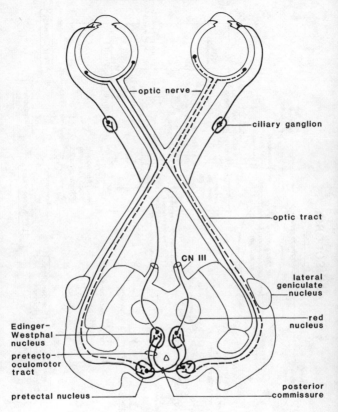

radiation therapy and may be seen on CT scan. Symptoms include headache, focal seizures, perceptual-motor dysfunction and ataxia, or it may be asymptomatic.

Radiation-induced brain tumors, including meningiomas, sarcomas, and gliomas have been reported, although the incidence is low.

A transient myelopathy may occur 2 weeks to several months following radiation therapy, for example, of pharyngeal and laryngeal regions. It frequently presents with Lhermitte's sign, an electric shock-like sensation radiating down the spine following neck flexion which puts mechanical traction on reversibly demyelinated ascending sensory tracts.

Chronic progressive radiation myelopathy occurs 5-30 months after radiation therapy and presents as a transverse myelopathy. Steroids may help. Cranial neuropathies may be radiation-induced. An optic neuropathy can occur months after radiation to the whole brain or pituitary region. It is usually progressive, but can remit. Steroids probably do not help. Other cranial nerves (XII, VII, X, IX, and V, in order of frequency) may be involved, but recurrent tumor should be excluded. Radiation-induced brachial plexopathy may be difficult to distinguish from recurrent tumor (see Brachial Plexus). Severe pain, Horner's syndrome, and lower cervical involvement suggest recurrent tumor. Local CT may help differentiate the two, but, depending on the tumor type, surgical exploration may be necessary. Delayed effects of radiation on blood vessels include carotid occlusion, especially after treatment of neck malignancies, and multiple small vessel occlusions resembling Moyamoya disease.

RADICULOPATHY

Pain, paresthesia or hypesthesia in a dermatomal distribution (see Dermatomes) are most common. Generally, pain occurs more proximally, sensory disturbances more distally. The pain may radiate or "shoot". An isolated root lesion may result in a smaller area of sensory disturbance than expected due to dermatomal overlap. Neck or lower back pain and stiffness are common in cervical and lumbar radiculopathies, respectively. The symptoms are aggravated by the valsalva maneuver during sneezing, coughing, and straining at defecation or with neck or trunk movement. Bedrest usually offers relief. Flattening of the normal lumbar lordosis and straight leg raising sign may be present in cases of lumbar radiculopathy. Crossed straight leg raising usually indicates a larger lesion. Hyporeflexia is restricted to the involved root level. Weakness may occur in the appropriate myotomal distribution (see Myotomes) and may indicate a larger lesion with greater anterior root involvement. Myelopathy (see Spinal Cord) may occur with larger or more centrally located lesions. Central lumbar lesions may result in a cauda equina syndrome. Although herniated intervertebral disc material is the most common cause of radiculopathy, other mass lesions and structural abnormalities should be excluded. Central disc herniation is relatively uncommon.

Common cervical root syndromes:

C5 or C6 radiculopathy (C4-5, C5-6 disc space respectively)
  Pain and sensory loss - shoulder, upper arm, radial
    and anterior aspect of forearm, and first 1-1/2
    digits
  Hyporeflexia - biceps and brachioradialis
  Weakness - clavicular head of pectoralis, supra-
    spinatus, infraspinatus, deltoid, biceps, and
    brachioradialis

C7 radiculopathy (C6-7 disc space)
  Pain and sensory loss - posterior arm and forearm and
    palmar and dorsal second and third digits
  Hyporeflexia - triceps
  Weakness - triceps and wrist extensors

C8 radiculopathy (C7-T1 disc space)
  Pain and sensory loss - inferoposterior aspect of arm,
    ulnar aspect of forearm and dorsal and palmar fourth
    and fifth digits
  Hyporeflexia - possibly triceps
  Weakness - intrinsic hand muscles

Common lumbar root syndromes:

L4 radiculopathy (L3-4 disc space)
  Pain and sensory loss - hip and anterolateral thigh
    (pain), knee, anteromedial leg, medial foot,
    possibly great toe
  Hyporeflexia - quadriceps (patellar)
  Weakness - quadriceps and anterior tibialis

L5 radiculopathy (L4-5 disc space)
  Pain and sensory loss - hip and lateral thigh (mainly
    pain), anterolateral leg, dorsum of foot and medial
    toes (including great toe)
  Hyporeflexia - possibly patellar
  Weakness - peroneus, toe extensors, possibly anterior
    tibialis

KEY NEUROLOGY AND NEUROSURGERY

Editors: Neurology: Russell N. DeJong, M.D., and Robert D. Currier, M.D.
Neurosurgery: Robert M. Crowell, M.D.

AT LAST. . .A quarterly, service-oriented publication is available that will keep you informed of worldwide trends, discoveries, and developments in neurology and neurosurgery with unparalleled timeliness. Each carefully selected article is condensed and critically evaluated by a distinguished group of specialists. **KEY NEUROLOGY AND NEUROSURGERY** delivers abstracts of the most important and clinically oriented articles published in the last 6 to 8 months. These articles are chosen from a literature base of over 650 medical and allied health journals!

—— YES, I would like to become a subscriber to **KEY NEUROLOGY AND NEURO-SURGERY** (KQNR)

—— Practitioner $50.00   —— Resident $35.00   —— Institution $75.00   —— Foreign $50.00

NAME ——————————————————

ADDRESS ——————————————————

CITY —————————— STATE ——————

ZIP —————— PHONE ——————

TO ORDER, mail in this card — or — call **TOLL-FREE 800-621-9262.**

YEAR BOOK MEDICAL PUBLISHERS
35 EAST WACKER DRIVE
CHICAGO, ILLINOIS
60601

Illinois and Tennessee residents will be charged appropriate sales tax. All prices quoted subject to change. A small additional charge will be made for postage and handling.

NO POSTAGE
NECESSARY
IF MAILED
IN THE
UNITED STATES

BUSINESS REPLY MAIL

FIRST CLASS   PERMIT NO. 762   CHICAGO, ILLINOIS

POSTAGE WILL BE PAID BY ADDRESSEE:

Year Book Medical Publishers
35 East Wacker Drive
Chicago, Illinois 60601

S1 radiculopathy (L5-S1 disc space)
    Pain and sensory loss — buttock and posterior thigh
       (mainly pain), posterolateral leg, lateral foot,
       lateral toes, and heel
    Hyporeflexia — ankle (Achilles)
    Weakness — hamstrings, gluteus maximus, plantar
       flexors of foot and toes

S1-5 radiculopathies (see Cauda Equina)

    Diagnostic studies should include plain radiographs
with oblique views. Nerve conduction studies and EMG will
identify evidence of denervation in a root distribution
and exclude more peripheral lesions. Myelogram followed
by CT is being supplanted in many centers by MRI.
    Differential diagnosis includes primary or metastatic
tumors, epidural abscess, rheumatoid spondylosis, brachial
or lumbar plexopathy and peripheral neuropathy.
    Treatment of disc disease should begin conservatively
with bedrest, traction, and nonsteroidal anti-inflammatory
agents. Surgical decompression is indicated when symptoms
are unresponsive to medical therapy, there is progressive
weakness, or when central herniation results in myelopathy
or a cauda equina syndrome. Chymopapain injection is
controversial.

REFLEXES (see also Myotomes)

MUSCLE STRETCH ("DEEP TENDON") REFLEXES

Reflex	Level	Nerve
Jaw (masseter and temporal muscle)	CN, V	Mandibular branch
Biceps	C5, 6	Musculocutaneous
Brachioradialis	C5, 6	Radial
Pectoralis major	C5, 6, 7	Lateral pectoral
Triceps	C6, 7, 8	Radial
Finger flexors	C8	Medial (ulnar)
Adductor	L2, 3, 4	Obturator
Quadriceps (patellar, knee jerks)	L2, 3, 4	Femoral
Internal hamstring	L4, 5, S1	Sciatic
External hamstring	L5, S1	Sciatic
Gastrocnemius-soleus (Achilles, ankle jerks)	L5, S1, 2	Tibial

---

GRADING OF MUSCLE STRETCH REFLEXES

0	Absent, abnormal
1+	Diminished, may or may not be abnormal
2+	Normal
3+	Increased, may or may not be abnormal
4+	Markedly increased, abnormal. May be associated with clonus

Evaluate latency of response, degree of activity, and duration of the contraction. Reflexes should be both observed and palpated. Compare right and left sides. In general, reflexes are not pathological if they are symmetric unless they are absent or 4+.

Hyporeflexia results from dysfunction of any part of the reflex arc. These conditions include neuropathy, radiculopathy, tabes dorsalis, syringomyelia, intramedullary tumors, and spinal motor neuron dysfunction. Hyporeflexia may occur in late stages of primary muscle diseases due to loss of muscle mass. Areflexia with rapidly progressive weakness and only mild sensory loss is the hallmark of Guillain-Barre syndrome. Hyporeflexia is seen transiently in acute upper motor neuron lesions such as cerebral infarction or spinal cord compression (spinal shock). Isolated unilateral hyporeflexia or areflexia is seen in radiculopathy. Symmetric distal hyporeflexia is characteristic of polyneuropathy. Prolongation of both the contraction and relaxation times ("hung-up" reflex) is seen with hypothyroidism. Areflexia may be a component of Adie's syndrome (see Pupil). See also Hypotonic Infant.

Hyperreflexia usually results from an upper motor neuron lesion with loss of corticospinal inhibition. The extrapyramidal system may also play a role. Involvement may occur anywhere from the cortical Betz cell to just proximal to the spinal cord motor neuron. Unilateral hyperreflexia results from a unilateral lesion anywhere along the corticospinal tract, most commonly in the cerebral hemispheres or brainstem. Bilateral hyperreflexia occurs more commonly with myelopathy but also occurs with bilateral cerebral hemisphere or brainstem involvement. Symmetric, 3+ reflexes in the absence of clonus, Babinski, Tromner or Hoffman signs or weakness and with a normal neurological examination is usually benign. Reflexes are variable (usually normal) with extrapyramidal

system dysfunction. Reflexes are normal, slightly
decreased, or pendular with cerebral or cerebellar tract
dysfunction. See also Rigidity, Spasticity.

"Pathological reflexes" (pyramidal tract reflexes)
indicate upper motor neuron dysfunction. The extensor
plantar response (Babinski sign) consists of dorsiflexion
of the great toe and fanning of the remaining toes on
stimulating the plantar surface of the foot. Hoffman and
Tromner signs are elicited by "flicking" the index or
middle finger down or up, respectively, producing flexion
of the thumb; they may be normal if present bilaterally,
especially if reflexes are 3+ and symmetric. Ankle clonus
is the continuing rapid flexion and extension of the foot
elicited by forcibly and quickly dorsiflexing the foot.
Pyramidal tract reflexes are normally present in infants
(see Child Neurology).

CUTANEOUS ("SUPERFICIAL") REFLEXES

Reflex	Level	Nerve
Corneal	Pons	CN V (afferent), VII (efferent)
Pharyngeal	Medulla	CN IX (afferent), X (efferent)
Upper abdominal	T6-9	
Middle abdominal	T9-11	
Lower abdominal	T11-L1	
Cremasteric	L1, 2	Femoral (afferent), genitofemoral (efferent)
Plantar	L5, S1,2	Tibial
Anal	S3,4,5	Pudendal
Bulbocavernosus	S3,4	Pudendal, pelvic autonomics

RENAL DISEASE (see Dialysis, Uremia)

RESPIRATION (see also Coma, Hyperventilation)

Respiratory patterns may reflect many factors. With
careful interpretation, however, they may provide useful
localizing information.

Posthyperventilation apnea is due to impaired forebrain activation of rhythmic breathing when arterial
pCO_2 decreases. The patient is asked to take five deep
breaths, after which the resulting apneic period is timed.

Less than 10 seconds is normal. Greater than 12 seconds is considered abnormal.

Cheyne-Stokes respiration consists of slowly increasing, then decreasing hyperpneic phases, separated by shorter apneic phases. It is believed to result from the interaction of an increased ventilatory drive to pCO_2 and a decreased forebrain stimulus for respiration when pCO_2 is decreased as in posthyperventilation apnea. It suggests bilateral deep cerebral hemispheric or diencephalic dysfunction, but may be exacerbated by a variety of disorders with increased circulation times.

Central neurogenic hyperventilation, attributed to brainstem injury, is very rare in man. Tachypnea, on the other hand, is very common and is usually associated with hypocapnea and hypoxemia. Tachypnea with brainstem disease may be associated with neurogenic pulmonary edema.

Apneustic breathing consists of prolonged "jamming" of respiration in inspiratory and expiratory phases. Although rare, it is seen with dorsolateral pontine lesions at the level of the sensory trigeminal nucleus.

Ataxic breathing consists of generally slow, irregular pattern of respiration of variable amplitude, and can rapidly progress to complete apnea. It is due to bilateral lesions of the reticular formation in the caudal dorsomedial medulla where the respiratory rhythm is generated. Medullary compression, usually from acute lesions, may result in respiratory arrest which typically occurs before cardiovascular collapse. Mechanical ventilation should be readily available. These patients are particularly sensitive to sedative drugs and sleep, both of which may precipitate apnea.

Sleep apnea (Ondine's curse) may result from lesions in the medulla which disrupt the involuntary automatic respiratory outflow pathways (reticulospinal tracts), but leave intact the separate voluntary respiratory pathways from motor cortex. Such a lesion can result in fatal apnea with inattention or sleep. Sleep apnea may also occur in association with a variety of disorders that lack clear evidence of brainstem pathology (see Sleep Disorders). Occasionally, a similar pattern is seen in neuromuscular diseases.

Various respiratory reflexes may be abnormally prominent as a result of central nervous system disease (see Hiccups).

RESTLESS LEGS SYNDROME

Ekbom's Syndrome consists of symptoms of paresthesias or "creeping" sensations in the lower legs, but frequently in the thighs, and, occasionally, in the arms. It is typically bilateral. There is an associated tendency to move the limbs, or walk to avoid the sensation which typically occurs while at rest, is usually intermittent, and lasts from minutes to hours. Familial predisposition (autosomal dominant) as well as a variety of associated conditions have been described, including:

Iron deficiency anemia	Parkinson's disease
Pregnancy	COPD
Distant carcinoma	Amyloidosis
Uremia	Vitamin deficiencies
Diabetes	Caffeine
Exposure to cold	Hyperlipidemia
Acute intermittent porphyria	Barbiturate withdrawal
Prochlorperazine	

Some similarities exist between this syndrome and growing pains in children. Treatment involves correcting, if possible, the underlying condition. A variety of drugs have been tried with variable success, including diazepam, clonazepam, carbamazepine, and amitriptyline.

Ref: Ekbom KA. Neurology 10:308, 1960.

RETINA AND UVEAL TRACT (see also Uveitis)

I. Systemic and neurological disorders associated with retinal pigmentary degeneration.
   A. Typical retinitis pigmentosa changes include early onset nyctalopia, progressive visual loss, bone spicules, narrowing of retinal arterioles, and ERG changes. They may be associated with:
   Myotonic dystrophy (rarely)
   Leber's congenital amaurosis
   Senear-Loken (Leber's + juvenile nephronophthisis)
   Friedreich's ataxia (may also rarely be associated with optic atrophy and deafness)
   Spielmeyer-Vogt's
   Neonatal and childhood adrenoleukodystrophy
   Usher's (vestibulocochlear dysfunction, mutisim)
   Pelizaeus-Merzbacher's (mental retardation, ataxia)
   Hallgren's (mental retardation, ataxia, deafness)

B. Atypical central and peripheral retinal pigmentary changes with variable degrees of visual
impairment. The presumed mechanism in storage
diseases is disruption of pigment epithelial
function by accumulated metabolic material with
secondary retinal receptor degeneration. Primary
rod cone dystrophy may exist in the first 4 of
the following syndromes.
Laurence-Moon-Bardet-Biedl   (hypogenitalism,
   mental retardation, polydactyly)
Biemond's (hypogenitalism, mental retardation,
   iris coloboma)
Alstrom's (hypogenitalism, deafness, diabetes
   mellitus)
Bassen-Kornzweig (abetalipoproteinemia, ataxia,
   acanthocytosis)
Refsum's (polyneuropahy, ataxia)
Sjogren-Larsson (ichthyosis, spastic paresis,
   mental retardation)
Amalric-Dialinos (deafness)
Cockayne's (dwarfism, neuropathy, deafness)
Hallervorden-Spatz (neuropathy, basal ganglia
   degeneration)
Alport's (nephritis, hearing loss)
Hurler's (MPS I), Hunter' (MPS II),
   Sanfilippo's (MPS III), and Scheie's disease
   (MPS V)
C. Postinflammatory
Congenital and acquired syphilis
Congenital rubella (german measles) - "salt and
   pepper fundus"
Congenital rubeola (measles)
D. Avitaminoses and vitamin metabolism disorders
Pellagra
Vitamin B_{12} metabolism disorder associated
   with aminoaciduria
E. Toxic
Chlorpromazine
Thioridazine
Indomethacin

II. Hereditary cerebromacular dystrophies
A. With cherry red spot of the macula
Sphingolipidoses - Tay-Sachs, Niemann-Pick,
   Gaucher's, metachromatic leukodystrophy
   (infantile form), Sandhoff's
Mucolipidoses - GM_1 gangliosidosis, Farber's
Mucolipidosis I
Mucopolysaccharidoses - Hurler's (MPS I), MPS VII
Goldberg's Disease

B. Without cherry red spot
   Ceroid lipofuscinoses - Jansky-Bielschowsky,
   Batten-Mayou, Spielmyer-Vogt,
   Kufs-Hallervorden

III. CNS Vasculitides
   All vasculitides may involve the retinal circulation
   with variable manifestations (arterial occlusive
   retinopathy, hemorrhages, retinal infiltrates, etc.)

IV. Phakomatoses
   A. Vascular malformations of the choroid/retina and
      the CNS
      Von Hippel-Lindau (retinal angiomas and
         cerebellar hemangioblastomas)
      Sturge-Weber (choroidal hemangioma,
         parieto-occipital AVM's)
      Wyburn-Mason (AVM's in the retina and brainstem)
      Retinal cavernous hemangioma (unclassified
         phakomatosis, rarely associated with
         intracranial AVM's)
   B. Retinal and intracranial tumors
      Tuberous sclerosis
      Neurofibromatosis

V. Dystrophies of the uvea
   A. Angioid streaks (ruptures of Bruch's membrane)
      occur in the following diseases which may be
      associated with neurological dysfunction.
      Francois dyscephalic syndrome
      Paget's disease
      Acromegaly
      Sickle cell anemia
   B. Gillespie's (aniridia, ataxia, psychomotor
      retardation)

VI. Retinovitreal syndromes and vitreal involvement
   A. Wagner's vitreoretinopathy (rarely associated
      with encephaloceles)
   B. Dominant familial amyloidosis (diffuse vitreous
      opacification)

RHEUMATOID ARTHRITIS

Neurological complications affecting muscle include
periarticular inflammation, nodular myositis, polymyositis, disuse atrophy, steroid myopathy, denervation, and
vasculitis.

Peripheral nerve involvement is most commonly due to entrapment or compression. Carpal tunnel syndrome is most frequent (20-25%) with peroneal mononeuropathies occurring somewhat less frequently. Involvement of ulnar, posterior interosseus, posterior tibial (in the popliteal fossa due to Baker's cyst or in the tarsal tunnel) and medial and lateral plantar nerves is also seen. A mild distal sensory neuropathy, attributed to segmental demyelination, may be seen in as many as 30% of patients with rheumatoid arthritis, often with milder forms. Ischemic injury due to rheumatoid vasculitis may cause mononeuritis multiplex which may progress to a severe polyneuropathy. This is usually of sudden onset in patients with severe disease. An autonomic neuropathy may also occur.

Central nervous system complications include vertebral subluxation (25-70% of patients with advanced rheumatoid arthritis), and, much more rarely, compressive dural nodules, rheumatoid pachymeningitis, vasculitis, and hyperviscosity syndromes. Anterior atlantoaxial sub-luxation (separation of the anterior arch of the atlas from the dens by >3 mm) is most frequent and occurs in mild or severe disease. Lateral cervical spine films during flexion and extension are usually sufficient to make the diagnosis. The patient, not the technician, should flex and extend the neck. Tomography, myelography and vertebral angiography may be necessary in selected cases. Vertical subluxation of the odontoid process upwards (basilar invagination, see Craniocervical Junction) usually occurs on the background of atlantoaxial subluxation in severe disease and should not be mistaken for improvement. Subaxial subluxation is less common and posterior atlantoaxial subluxation is rare. The course of rheumatoid cervical arthropathy is generally benign and surgical management should be considered cautiously. Indications for surgery include intractable pain or progressive neurological symptoms or signs.

Drugs used to treat rheumatoid arthritis may them-selves produce neurological symptoms. These include chloroquine, gold, salicylates, steroids, and nonsteroidal anti-inflammatory drugs.

RIGIDITY (see also Spasticity)

Rigidity is a form of increased muscle tone that is present throughout the range of motion of a limb (compare with Spasticity). When released, the rigid limb does not spring back to its original position, and rigidity is not associated with increased reflexes. EMG reveals persist-ent motor unit activity during apparent relaxation.

Cogwheel rigidity, seen in extrapyramidal disease, consists of an increased resistance to stretch that is interrupted by rhythmic yielding. **Lead-pipe rigidity** refers to the uniform resistance to movement of a limb, which may retain position; it may be seen in catatonic states. **Gegenhalten or paratonia** refers to increasing tone in response to increasing efforts to move a limb passively throughout its range of motion and is seen in bilateral frontal lobe or medial basal temporal lobe disease, senile dementia of the Alzheimer's type, and certain other disorders with decreased attention.

Although not true rigidity, the following terms are reviewed.

Voluntary rigidity represents agonist-antagonist co-contraction and may be associated with heightened emotional states. **Involuntary rigidity** or **hysterical rigidity** may range from hyperreflexia to opisthotonus. **Reflex rigidity** represents spasm in response to pain, cold or exercise. Rigidity may also be seen in epilepsy, tetanus, hypocalcemic tetany, and the stiff-man syndrome (see also Cramps, Myotonia).

The terms **"decorticate"** and **"decerebrate"** rigidity or posturing are imprecise. **Abnormal flexion** indicates a slow, stereotyped flexion of arm, wrist and fingers with adduction at the shoulder. **Abnormal extension** indicates extension and pronation of the arm with adduction and internal rotation of the leg with plantar flexion of the foot. Abnormal flexion in the arms, with or without extension in the legs, is associated with more rostral, less severe, supratentorial processes. Extension in the arms and legs occurs primarily with more severe forebrain and diencephalic dysfunction, but also with lesions of the midbrain and rostral pons. Extension in the arms with flexion or flaccidity in the legs is associated with lesions of the pontine tegmentum.

ROMBERG SIGN

A test to compare the stability of a patient standing with feet together and eyes open to that with eyes closed. The arms may be at the side or folded against the chest. Normal subjects develop a slight increase in sway with closed eyes. Patients with pathologically increased sway with open eyes, from whatever cause, usually develop an increase in sway with eyes closed but the increase is most marked in patients with proprioceptive and vestibular dysfunction. In the latter, the fall would be towards the side of the slow component of any ongoing primary position nystagmus. Similarly, patients with unilateral cerebellar lesions tend to fall to the side of the lesion.

A pseudo-Romberg, secondary to psychogenic factors, tends to be associated with sway at the hips rather than at the ankles.

The test may be modified by having the patient stand with one foot in front of the other (tandem Romberg) but even normal individuals have difficulty remaining upright during eye closure with this modification.

Ref: Rogers JH. J Laryngol Otol 94:1401, 1980.

SARCOIDOSIS

Sarcoidosis is a generalized noncaseating epithelioid and giant cell granulomatosis involving multiple organs, most frequently mediastinal and peripheral lymph nodes, lungs, liver, skin, phalangeal bones, eyes, and parotid glands. It may be disseminated with adenopathy, anergy, hypercalcemia, uveitis or positive Kveim test, at the time of onset of neurological dysfunction or be clinically limited to the nervous system. It is most common in blacks between ages 20 and 40. High yield biopsy sites include skin lesions, nodes, liver, lip, lung (trans-bronchial) biopsy. Gallium scan or angiotensin converting enzyme may be positive.

Virtually any part of the central or peripheral nervous system may be affected. Cranial nerves most commonly involved are II, VII, VIII, IX and X. The central nervous system is most often involved by a meningitis. Hypothalamic and pituitary dysfunction, encephalopathy, and seizures are not uncommon. Frequent ophthalmological manifestations include uveitis, iritis, chorioretinitis, periphlebitis, and lacrimal gland and optic nerve involvement.

Prednisone is the mainstay of therapy.

SEIZURES (see Antiepileptic Drugs, Epilepsy)

SENSORY EXAM (see Dermatomes, Peripheral Nerve)

SEVENTH NERVE (see Facial Nerve)

SHUNTS

A variety of shunts is available for various clinical circumstances. Ventriculoperitoneal (V-P) shunts are favored in infants and growing children because extra tubing can be left in the peritoneal cavity, allowing for growth and extending the time between shunt revisions. Ventriculojugular (V-J) shunts may be used after major growth is completed; complications are more frequent and serious than with V-P shunts. Lumboperitoneal (L-P) shunts are useful in communicating hydrocephalus. Third ventriculostomy is useful in noncommunicating hydrocephalus. Ventriculo-cisternostomy (ventricle to cervical subarachnoid space) is used primarily for temporary shunting around tumors obstructing the third or fourth ventricle or aqueduct of Sylvius; operative mortality may be as high as 30%.

Valves are used in ventricular shunts and lumbar shunts to control flow rates. Reservoirs allow sampling of ventricular fluid to exclude infections or check pressures.

Complications of shunting are numerous. Mechanical malfunction resulting in increased intracranial pressure may cause headache, lethargy and vomiting. Obstruction proximal to the reservoir is common. It may result from disconnection and separation of the ventricular catheter, blockage of the catheter by choroid plexus or glial tissue, contraction of the ventricle causing the catheter to embed in the ventricular wall or white matter (slit ventricle syndrome), or blockage due to high protein (>1000 mg%). Valves and pumping devices rarely fail if properly checked prior to insertion. Disconnection may occur at the pumping device or distally in 3-piece shunts. Obstruction occurs fairly frequently at the distal end of shunts.

Infection of soft tissue may occur shortly after insertion. There is evidence of sepsis, inflammation at the insertion site, and erythema and warmth along the course of the tubing. Skin necrosis secondary to pressure can also occur. Vascular shunts are more likely to result in septicemia, endocarditis, and septic emboli. Peritoneal shunt infections may cause obstruction of the distal end of the catheter. Infection rate for both is around 7%. Shunt nephritis can occur with either, although usually with vascular shunts, and consists of glomerular immune complex deposits leading to hematuria and proteinuria. Treatment of the infection generally reverses the nephritis. Infected shunts usually need to be removed for antibiotic treatment to be effective, although intrathecal antibiotics have been successfully used without removal.

Seizures develop in 50-75% of shunted patients within 4 years. Lateralized nonparoxysmal and paroxysmal abnormalities on EFG are common in shunted patients. Changes may appear before seizures occur. Some recommend serial EEGs and prophylactic anticonvulsants for patients with a positive EEG or who have porencephalic cysts or cerebral hemorrhage.

Unilateral hematomas or hygromas may cause shift of intracranial structures. Bilateral effusions may be asymptomatic and are commonly seen on CT, possibly reflecting craniocephalic disproportion, and often require no treatment. Craniosynostosis, with or without cerebellar herniation, has been rarely reported following pediatric shunting.

Cardiac complications include vena caval, or right atrial thrombi, bacterial endocarditis, cardiac dysrhythmias, cardiac tamponade, and embolization of tubing to lungs. Pulmonary complications include emboli and consequent pulmonary hypertension.

Peritoneal complications include inguinal hernia (common in children), ascites and cyst formation, perforation of viscus or abdominal wall (with or without peritonitis or ventriculitis), volvulus and intestinal obstruction (rare), and peritoneal metastases (10% in medulloblastoma prior to use of filters).

SIADH (SYNDROME OF INAPPROPRIATE ANTIDIURETIC HORMONE)

The diagnosis of SIADH may be made in a nonvolume depleted patient with normal renal and adrenal function who has serum hyponatremia (see also Sodium) and hypo-osmolarity with an inappropriately high urine osmolarity and inappropriate renal sodium loss (e.g., >25 mEq/l with normal intake). It may be caused by bronchogenic carcinoma, other malignant tumors, and various pulmonary disorders. Neurological causes of SIADH include infarction, subarachnoid hemorrhage, head trauma, intracranial surgery, infection (encephalitis, brain abscess, meningitis), gliomas and metastatic tumors involving the hypothalamus, Guillain-Barre syndrome, acute intermittent porphyria, and hydrocephalus. Drugs which may cause SIADH include carbamazepine, barbiturates, tricyclic antidepressants, phenothiazines, cyclophosphamide, vincristine, chlorpropramide, acetaminophen, and clofibrate.

Treatment begins with removing the cause, if present. Water restriction is usually sufficient for mild cases. More severe involvement may require diuresis and infusion of hypertonic saline. Lithium carbonate or demeclocycline, have been used as adjunctive therapy. Though phenytoin inhibits the release of ADH, it is not of clinical benefit in treatment.

SICKLE CELL ANEMIA

The frequency of neurological manifestations in the hemoglobinopathies is proportional to the propensity to sickle: 6-35% in SS (sickle disease), 6-24% in SC, and 0-6% in AS (trait). Up to 20% of patients with SS first present with neurological complaints. Common

neurological complications of SS disease include cerebrovascular disease, seizures, meningeal signs, coma, and
blindness or blurred vision. Unusual neurological
complications include isolated mental retardation, CNS
infection, radiculopathy, and psychosis. Myelopathy,
peripheral neuropathy, and myopathy are not described.

Cerebrovascular involvement occurs in 14-17%. Under
the age of 20 it is usually ischemic. In adults over 20
subarachnoid and intracerebral hemorrhage tend to occur.
Rarely, fat embolism results from bone marrow infarction.
Anemia is not necessary for cerebrovascular involvement.
Angiography may precipitate sickling, but may be safely
performed after sickle hemoglobin is reduced to less than
20% by repeated or exchange transfusions.

Seizures occur in 8-12% and are usually generalized
tonic-clonic. They frequently occur in the absence of
recognized cerebrovascular involvement or intercurrent
illness, although there may be precipitating factors such
as surgery or anesthesia. In SC disease intercurrent
illness is frequently responsible for seizures.

Coma may be the only neurological manifestation in SS
disease. Intercurrent problems, such as sepsis, may be
responsible. Mortality is approximately 30%. About
50% recover completely. In SC disease, stupor and coma
are less frequent, and are usually associated with crisis.
In almost half, it may be the presenting manifestation of
undiagnosed SC disease with a tendency to occur in older
individuals.

Meningeal signs occur in 6%, either in isolation or
associated with crisis, subarachnoid hemorrhage, or
infectious meningitis.

Visual disturbances are much more frequent in SC than
in SS disease, despite the greater severity of the latter.
About 1/3 of SC patients first present with visual impairment. Visual complications include vitreous, retinal, and
subretinal hemorrhages; central retinal artery and vein
occlusions; retinitis proliferans; and other retinal
vascular changes.

Sickle trait (AS) is unlikely to produce neurological
manifestations, but should be considered, for example,
when they occur following obstetrical and surgical
procedures. Signs of meningeal irritation, subarachnoid
hemorrhage, seizures, and radicular syndromes, should be
attributed to sickle cell anemia only after more common
causes have been excluded.

SIXTH NERVE (see Ophthalmoplegia)

SLEEP DISORDERS

Classification of Sleep Disorders

I. Disorders of initiating and maintaining sleep
   A. Psychological or associated with personality disorders, affective disorders or psychoses
   B. Associated with abuse or withdrawal from drugs or alcohol (depressants or stimulants)
   C. Sleep apnea syndromes
   D. Alveolar hypoventilation, including Ondine's curse
   E. Sleep related myoclonus
   F. Restless legs syndrome
   G. Neurological and medical disorders that interfere with sleep
   H. "Pseudoinsomnia" (subjective symptoms without laboratory evidence of a sleep disturbance)
   I. Normal short sleepers
   J. REM interruptions and other polysomnographic abnormalities

II. Disorders of excessive somnolence
   A. Psychological or associated with personality disorders, affective disorders, or psychoses
   B. Associated with abuse or withdrawal from drugs or alcohol (depressants or stimulants)
   C. Sleep apnea syndrome
   D. Alveolar hypoventilation
   E. Nocturnal myoclonus, restless legs
   F. Narcolepsy
   G. Toxic medical and neurological disorders
   H. Kleine-Levin syndrome
   I. Menstruation-related hypersomnolence
   J. Insufficient sleep
   K. Sleep drunkeness
   L. Normal long sleeper

Sleep apnea syndrome is characterized by daytime somnolence and nighttime or sleep-related apneic periods secondary to either upper airway obstruction (continued diaphragmatic movement), central causes, or both. The typical patient is obese, male, and snores. Recurrent hypoxemia, hypercapnia, cardiac failure, dysrhythmias, and sudden death may result. Diagnosis is made by polysomnographic recording of EEG, air movement, diaphragmatic movement, EKG, and oxygen saturation. Treatment consists of weight loss if possible. Nocturnal home oxygen may improve hypoxemia. Medroxyprogesterone acetate has met with mixed success. Tracheostomy is successful in obstructive apneas, and is reserved for severe, life-threatening disease not responsive to other therapies.

Narcolepsy consists of daytime sleep attacks, hypna-
gogic hallucinations, cataplexy, and sleep paralysis.
Less than 20% have all 4 symptoms. Onset of REM within
ten minutes of sleep onset is evidence for narcolepsy.
Periods of automatic behavior may be confused with complex
partial seizures or transient global amnesia. The
diagnosis is made by the multiple sleep latency test,
consisting of serial EEG monitoring of sleep onset every 2
hours through the day. The incidence is 4 per 10,000. It
is hereditary (probably autosomal dominant) in some cases.

Sleep attacks are treated with methylphenidate,
methamphetamine, or dextroamphetamine, 20-200 mg/day in
2-3 doses. Tolerance may develop, requiring higher doses.
Amphetamines also interfere with normal sleep and may
result in an increased dose requirement. The lowest
effective dose should be used. The abuse potential of
these drugs is high. The side effects are primarily
sympathomimetic or due to other central nervous system
stimulation. Relative contraindications include anxious
or agitated states, glaucoma, hyperthyroidism, motor tics,
Tourette's syndrome, hypertension, and coronary artery
disease. Amphetamines may decrease seizure thresholds and
may interact with a variety of other drugs. Monoamine
oxidase (MAO) inhibitors are very effective in treating
sleep attacks but have many serious side effects.

Cataplexy is treated with the tricyclic antidepressant
imipramine 25 mg tid or up to 100 mg in a single dose.
Imipramine 25 mg tid plus methylphenidate 5-10 mg tid
appears to be a safe combination in patients with sleep
attacks and cataplexy (but blood pressure should be
monitored). Tricyclic antidepressants should never be
used with MAO inhibitors.

SODIUM

Hyponatremia may cause neurological symptoms of
weakness, altered mental status ranging from irritability
and lethargy to coma, myoclonus, and seizures. Neurological symptoms are not usually seen until sodium
concentrations are <125 mEq/l. Symptoms correlate with
the rate of change as well as the absolute concentration.
EEG changes are common but generally nonspecific; there
may be loss of normal α-activity and irregular, high
amplitude slowing (4-7 Hz), greater posteriorly. Acute
symptomatic hyponatremia is a medical emergency and should
be treated with hypertonic saline promptly but cautiously
in order to avoid congestive heart failure or cerebral
hemorrhage. See also SIADH.

Hypernatremia may produce similar neurological manifestations of altered mental status ranging from irritability and lethargy to coma, myoclonus, and seizures. Tone is usually normal although reflexes may be increased. Symptoms generally occur with sodium concentrations >160 mEq/l, but may be related to hyperosmolality >340 mOsm/l. CSF protein may be increased. EEG may be normal or reveal mild background slowing. In some cases there is generalized slowing and in a few there is epileptic activity. Rehydration in chronic hypernatremia should be cautious in order to avoid potentially fatal cerebral edema.

   Hypernatremia (diabetes insipidus) may result from lesions of the supraoptic and paraventricular nuclei or the supraopticohypophyseal tract. Causes include diencephalohypophyseal tumors, trauma, surgery, basilar meningitis, sarcoidosis, and histiocytic disorders. Hypernatremia may result from a variety of other CNS lesions because of inadequate fluid intake due to impaired mental status.

SPASTICITY (see also Rigidity)

   A velocity dependent increase in tonic stretch reflexes (muscle tone) with hyperexcitability and exaggeration of tendon jerks. It is one component of the upper motor neuron syndrome. Other components include flexor spasms, weakness, tonic flexor and extensor dystonia, extensor plantar response (Babinski sign), and loss of dexterity. It results from damage to various descending pathways. Isolated lesions of the pyramidal tract are not sufficient to produce spasticity or the complete syndrome.

   Overall, no medication is particularly useful in relieving the disabling dystonia of cerebral lesions (tightly flexed and adducted upper extremities, extended and adducted lower extremities). Painful flexor spasm can be markedly reduced by baclofen or diazepam. Dantrolene causes mild to moderate muscle weakness in addition to its beneficial effect on spasticity, hyperactive reflexes, clonus, and dystonia. It may be used in bed or wheelchair-bound patients who will tolerate a further decrease in power. All three drugs tend to produce weakness, sedation, and dizziness. Combinations may be more effective with less side effects.

   Baclofen is a GABA agonist (at bicuculline-insensitive presynaptic GABA receptors) and also interferes with the release of excitatory transmitters. Start with 5 mg tid, increase by 5 mg every three days to a maximum of 80-120 mg in 4 doses. Additional adverse effects include mood changes, hallucinations, gastrointestinal symptoms, hypotension, changes in accommodation and ocular motor function, and deterioration in seizure control. Use with care in renal disease. Dose should be reduced slowly to avoid hallucinations or seizures which may occur with abrupt withdrawal.

Diazepam facilitates GABA-mediated post- and presynaptic inhibition. Start with 2 mg bid, increase slowly up to a maximum of 60 mg daily.

Dantrolene sodium interferes with excitation-contraction coupling by decreasing the release of calcium at the sarcoplasmic reticulum. Start with 25 mg qd, increase by 25 mg q3-4 days to a maximum of 100 mg qid. Diarrhea is a frequent side effect. Due to the potential for hepatotoxicity, SGOT, SGPT, alkaline phosphatase and total bilirubin should be obtained prior to beginning therapy. SGOT or SGPT should be monitored during therapy.

Ref: Young RR, Delwaide PJ. NEJM 304:28, 1981.

SPEECH (see Aphasia, Dysarthria)

SPINAL CORD (see also Bladder, Brachial Plexus, Cauda Equina/Conus Medullaris, Craniocervical Junction, Lumbosacral Plexus, Radiculopathy)

Relation of spinal cord segments and roots to the vertebral column is depicted on page 300. Cross-sectional anatomy of the spinal cord (cervical) is depicted on page 301.

Causes of myelopathy

Congenital/developmental: Spinal dysraphism (see Developmental Malformations), craniocervical junction abnormalities, syringomyelia, spinal stenosis.

Traumatic: Vertebral subluxation or fracture, contusion, concussion, hemorrhagic conditions (see below), penetrating injury, birth injury (particularly breech delivery).

Neoplastic: Extra- and intramedullary tumors (see Tumors), carcinomatous meningitis, paraneoplastic.

Infectious: Epidural or subdural abscess, polio-myelitis, viral encephalomyelitides, herpes zoster, rabies, subacute myoclonic spinal neuronitis, syphilis, tuberculoma, typhus, spotted fever, actinomycosis, coccidioidomycosis, aspergillosis, cryptococcosis, trichinosis, malaria, schistosomiasis, various meningitides, postinfectious/postvaccinal.

RELATION OF SPINAL SEGMENTS AND ROOTS
TO THE VERTEBRAL COLUMN

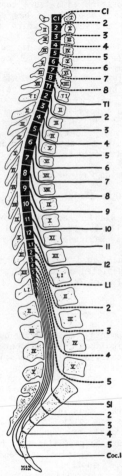

From: Haymaker W, Woodhall B. Peripheral Nerve Injuries:
Principles of Diagnosis. Philadelphia: WB Saunders,
1953, p 32.

CERVICAL SPINAL CORD (Cross-section)

ascending tracts   descending tracts

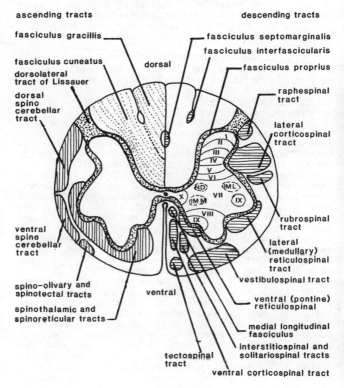

fasciculus gracillis

fasciculus cuneatus

dorsolateral tract of Lissauer

dorsal spino cerebellar tract

ventral spino cerebellar tract

spino-olivary and spinotectal tracts

spinothalamic and spinoreticular tracts

dorsal

ventral

fasciculus septomarginalis

fasciculus interfascicularis

fasciculus proprius

raphespinal tract

lateral corticospinal tract

rubrospinal tract

lateral (medullary) reticulospinal tract

vestibulospinal tract

ventral (pontine) reticulospinal

medial longitudinal fasciculus

interstitiospinal and solitariospinal tracts

tectospinal tract

ventral corticospinal tract

Degenerative: Spondylosis, Japanese disease (calcification of the posterior longitudinal ligament), motor neuron disease, spinocerebellar degenerations.

Vascular: Arterial and venous infarction (see below), hemorrhagic conditions (see below), vasculitides, vascular malformations

Toxic: Clioquinol, ETOH (direct toxicity or secondary to hepatic cirrhosis and portacaval shunting), arsenic, cyanide, lathyrism, intrathecal contrast or chemotherapeutic agents.

Metabolic/Nutritional: Pernicious anemia (B_{12} deficiency), pellagra, chronic liver disease.

Miscellaneous: Radiation myelopathy (subacute form with onset after 6-10 weeks and benign course, chronic form with onset after >1 year progressing to transverse myelopathy), electrical injury, multiple sclerosis, neuromyelitis optica (Devic's disease), arachnoiditis.

Trauma and compression produce various degrees of transverse myelopathy. Spinal cord **hemisection** (Brown-Sequard syndrome) results in ipsilateral segmental sensory loss, reflex loss, and muscle atrophy at the level of the lesion, and spastic paresis, loss of tactile sense and deep sensitivity, transient superficial hyperesthesia, and initial vasomotor abnormalities (overheating, reddening) and sudomotor deficiency below the lesion. Later vasoconstriction, hypothermia, and spinal reflex sweating occur below the lesion. There is contralateral loss of pain and temperature sense 1-3 levels below the lesion. Complete transection acutely (most commonly traumatic) results in spinal shock (lasting weeks to months) with paralysis, anesthesia, and areflexia below the level of the lesion. Loss of higher autonomic control results in bladder and bowel atonia (with maintained sphincter tone) and loss of sexual function, vasomotor tone, sweating and piloerection. Secondary changes such as delayed intramedullary hemorrhage and swelling may result in an ascending level (lower cervical injury with delayed involvement of the phrenic nerve). Return of reflex activity at the spinal level results in exaggerated withdrawal reflexes (flexor spasms), profuse sweating, piloerection, and automatic bladder emptying. **Spinal concussion** denotes a transsection syndrome indistinguishable from the shock phase, but with recovery within hours (or days). **Spinal contusion** also results in spinal shock with variable degrees of recovery.

Anterior cervical cord syndrome is characterized by quadriparesis with mild impairment of exteroception and preserved proprioception. It is most often secondary to disc rupture or vertebral fracture. **Posterior cervical cord syndrome** consists of pain and paresthesias in the neck, arms and trunk, sometimes associated with mild motor impairment of the upper extremities. Central cervical cord syndrome is an incomplete transsection syndrome which usually follows hyperextension injuries of the neck. There is disproportionately more weakness in the upper than lower extremities, bladder dysfunction (retention), and patchy sensory loss below the level of the lesion.

Initial management of spinal cord trauma should include immobilization (long spine board, semirigid plastic collar), correction of hypotension, bladder catheterization, nasogastric intubation, high dose IV corticosteroids, and repeated neurological examination. X-ray studies are directed to the area of interest but generally include cross table lateral and A-P C-spine films (all seven vertebrae), open mouth odontoid film in conscious patients, AP and lateral thoracic and lumbar spine films, and standard chest and abdominal films.

Syringomyelia is characterized by central cavitation of the spinal cord. It is most commonly cervical although extension may occur downwards or upwards to the medulla (syringobulbia). It is frequently associated with developmental malformations of the craniocervical junction, myelomeningocele, cervical ribs, kyphoscoliosis (acquired), and intramedullary tumors (15%). There is segmental loss of pain and temperature sensation (crossing fibers to the contralateral spinothalamic tract), often in a cape-like distribution, with sparing of proprioception ("dissociated loss"). Segmental weakness and atrophy with reflex loss and, often, fasciculations occur in the upper extremities. Expansion of the lesion may lead to Horner's syndrome, lower extremity weakness, ataxia, and urinary incontinence.

Cervical spondylosis causes a painful stiff neck, spastic paraparesis, and paresthesias in the distribution of affected roots. Fasciculations may occur.

Degeneration of the intervertebral discs leads to proliferative changes of bone (osteophytes, spondylitic bars), meninges (fibrosis), and protrusion of the annulus fibrosus. Cervical myelopathy is more likely to develop in patients with congenital narrowing of the spinal cord and results from direct compression, vascular compromise, and repeated trauma by normal flexion and extension of the neck. Lateral C-spine films usually show an A-P diameter of the spinal canal of less than 15 mm (normal 15-22 mm).

Lumbar spondylosis (stenosis) may produce neurogenic claudication. Extension of the back during walking and standing results in weakness, paresthesias, and loss of reflexes in the lower extremities. Pathogenesis is similar to that of cervical spondylosis. More constant symptoms include back and leg pain in 2/3 of the affected patients. Leg weakness and urinary incontinence occur infrequently.

Anterior spinal artery infarction mostly affecting the
mid thoracic region with severe local, radicular and deep
leg pain, paraplegia, dissociated sensory loss (sparing
posterior columns) below the level of infarction,
sphincter disturbance. Sacral sensation may remain
intact. Causes include systemic hypotension, vasculitis,
aortic dissection, embolism, sickle cell disease, or
arterial compression by tumor, disc material, or bone.
Posterior spinal artery infarction is less common and
produces loss of proprioception below the lesion and
variable involvement of lateral corticospinal and spinocerebellar tracts. Venous infarction is less common than
arterial infarction, rarely occurring in the abscence of
an AV malformation. Nonhemorrhagic infarction is of
gradual onset with progression over weeks. Hemorrhagic
infarction (venous emboli or thrombosis) results in sudden
neurological dysfunction and pain. It commonly involves
a larger area than arterial infarction and may progress to
death.

Hematomyelia, hemorrhage into the spinal cord, is seen
most often with blood dyscrasias, anticoagulation, AV
malformations, or trauma. Spinal subarachnoid hemorrhage
presents acutely with severe back pain and variable
neurological deficits. Causes are as for hematomyelia, but
also include intraspinal tumors, especially ependymomas.
Spinal subdural and epidural hemorrhages compress the cord
and present with severe local back pain, paraplegia,
sensory loss, and sphincter impairment. Causes are as
above but also include spinal taps in patients with
clotting abnormalities. Management consists of emergency
myelogram and surgical evacuation after correction of
clotting abnormalities.

Spinal cord tumors are listed by chief location under
"Tumors". They occur predominantly in young and middle
aged adults. Intramedullary tumors are more common in
children. Extramedullary tumors are more common in adults.
Metastases to the spinal cord arise most frequently from
lung, breast, and prostate.

Extramedullary tumors usually involve a few segments
with root compression (especially dorsal) and progressive
compromise of the cord to an incomplete or complete
transsection syndrome. Initial symptoms include focal
pain (good localizing value) and paresthesias followed by
muscular weakness, wasting, and sensory loss in the
distribution of the affected roots. Cord compression
results in variable patterns of spastic paraplegia and
sensory loss below the lesion as well as bladder (less
commonly bowel) dysfunction. Metastases and abscesses
tend to occlude spinal vessels, resulting in vascular
syndromes. Progressive spinal cord compression by

extradural tumor calls for immediate high dose IV corticosteroids, emergency myelogram, and surgical decompression.
Radiation therapy and/or chemotherapy may be utilized,
depending on clinical circumstances.

Intramedullary tumors may extend over multiple levels
causing a clinical picture similar to syringomyelia.
Asymmetric location within the cord results in asymmetric
clinical signs

Ref: Lipton H, Teasdall R. Acute transverse myelopathy
in adults: A follow up study. Arch Neurol 28:252,
1973.

Goodwen-Austen RB, et al. Observations on radiation
myelopathy. Brain 98:557, 1975.

SPINOCEREBELLAR DEGENERATION

CLASSIFICATION
(Adapted from Harding)

			Decade of Onset
I.	Disorders with known metabolic or other cause		
A.	Metabolic (all autosomal recessive)		
	1. Progressive, unremitting ataxia		
		a. Abetalipoproteinemia (Bassen-Kornzweig)	1st-2nd
		b. Hypobetalipoproteinemia	2nd-4th
		c. Hexosaminidase deficiency	1st
		d. Glutamate dehydrogenase deficiency	2nd-6th
		e. Cholestanolosis	3rd-6th
	2. Intermittent ataxia		
		a. Pyruvate dehydrogenase deficiency	1st
		b. Hartnup Disease	1st
		c. Intermittent branched chain ketoaciduria	1st
		d. Urea cycle enzyme deficiencies (autosomal recessive and X-linked)	1st
	3. Disorders characterized by defective DNA repair		
		a. Ataxia telangiectasia (Louis-Bar Syndrome)	1st
		b. Xeroderma pigmentosa	1st-2nd
		c. Cockayne syndrome	1st

II. Disorders of unknown etiology
    A. Early onset cerebellar ataxia
       (before 20 yrs)all are autosomal
       recessive unless indicated
       a. Friedreich's ataxia   1st-2nd
       b. Early onset cerebellar ataxia with   1st-2nd
           retained tendon reflexes
       c. With hypogonadism with or without   1st-3rd
           deafness ± dementia
       d. With congenital deafness   2nd-3rd
       e. With childhood deafness and mental   1st
           retardation
       f. With pigmentary retinal degeneration   1st
           with or without mental retardation,
           dementia, or deafness
       g. With optic atrophy, mental retardation   1st
           with or without deafness, or spasticity
           (Behr's Syndrome)
       h. With cataracts and mental retardation   1st
           (Marinesco-Sjogren syndrome)
       i. With myoclonus (Ramsay Hunt Syndrome)   1st-2nd
           (autosomal recessive and dominant)
       j. X-linked recessive spinocerebellar   1st-2nd
           ataxia
       k. Cerebellar ataxia with essential tremor 1st-3rd
           (autosomal dominant)

    B. Late onset cerebellar ataxia (after 20 years,
       all are autosomal dominant)
       a. With optic atrophy, ophthalmoplegia,   3rd-5th
           dementia, amyotrophy, and extrapyramidal
           features (possibly includes Azorean
           ataxia)
       b. With pigmentary retinal degeneration   2nd-4th
           with or without ophthalmoplegia and
           extrapyramidal features
       c. Pure cerebellar ataxia of late onset   6th-7th
       d. With myoclonus and deafness   2nd-5th

The term olivopontocerebellar atrophy is not used in
this classification. It is generally a pathological
diagnosis which may include involvement of the spinal
cord, basal ganglia, or cerebral cortex. Clinically, they
are characterized by ataxia, tremor, involuntary movements
and sensory abnormalities and are often indistinguishable
from the hereditary ataxias classified above.

    Friedreich's ataxia is the most common of the spino-
cerebellar degenerations of unknown etiology. Symptoms
develop from 18 months to 24 years, consisting of

progressive limb and truncal ataxia, dysarthria, and areflexia in the lower extremities. Pyramidal signs, and loss of position and vibration sense eventually appear. Kyphoscoliosis with restricted lung function, and cardio-myopathy are seen in over two thirds. Pes cavus, optic atrophy, distal amyotrophy, and horizontal nystagmus are less common. Sensory conduction is absent in lower extremities and slowed in upper extremities. Diabetes may be present. Ambulation is usually lost by 25 years and death occurs in the fourth or fifth decade of life.

Pathologically, Friedreich's ataxia is characterized by a narrowed spinal cord with gliosis and cell loss in the posterior columns and corticospinal and spinocere-bellar tracts. Clarke's column, and dorsal root ganglia are depleted. Cranial nerve nuclei VIII, X, and XII are depleted, as may be dentate nuclei and superior cerebellar peduncles. Myocardial fibers are degenerated.

<u>Early onset cerebellar ataxia with retained reflexes</u> is not uncommon and is often confused with Friedreich's. Reflexes are normal or brisk. Optic atrophy, cardio-myopathy, diabetes and skeletal deformities are not seen. Life span is considerably longer.

Ref: Gilman S, et al. Disorders of the Cerebellum. Philadelphia, FA Davis, 1981.

Harding AE. Classification of the hereditary ataxias and paraplegias. Lancet May 21, 1983, p 1151-54.

STATUS EPILEPTICUS (see Epilepsy)

STROKE (see Amaurosis Fugax, Hemorrhage, Ischemia, Lacunar Syndromes)

STUPOR (see Coma, Delirium)

SUBARACHNOID HEMORRHAGE (see Hemorrhage)

SUBDURAL HEMORRHAGE (see Hemorrhage)

SYNCOPE (see also Autonomic Nervous System, Dizziness, Vertigo)

Brief loss of consciousness and postural tone secondary to decreased cerebral perfusion. Recovery is rapid and without sequelae. Presyncope or faintness refers to a preceding state or incomplete faint on the same physiologic basis as a completed attack. The following is a more general differential diagnosis of fainting.

I. Orthostatic syncope is usually preceded by marked
    autonomic dysfunction (diaphoreses, peripheral
    vasoconstriction, pallor), apprehensiveness, and
    bradycardia. Myoclonus and convulsive phenomena
    may occur, especially in younger patients.
    Attaining recumbency may prevent progression or
    result in recovery.

A. Vasodepressor (vasovagal) syncope is associated
    with little or no pathology in younger
    patients. Occurrence is related to pain (more
    common in men), emotional distress (more common
    in women), prolonged fasting, stress, fatigue,
    and standing immobile while overheated.

B. Defective vasopressor response (impaired
    splanchnic and peripheral vasoconstriction)
    1. Drugs (elderly are more vulnerable):
        antihypertensive agents, tricyclic anti-
        depressants, phenothiazines, L-dopa, lithium
    2. Autonomic neuropathy: diabetes mellitus,
        uremia, familial amyloidosis, porphyria,
        Guillain-Barre syndrome, acute autonomic
        neuropathy, familial dysautonomia, Riley-
        Day syndrome
    3. Central dysautonomia: Parkinsonism, Shy-
        Drager syndrome
    4. Following prolonged confinement to bed or
        systemic viral illness
    5. Extensive sympathectomy
    6. Sympathotonic orthostatic hypotension
    7. Hyperbradykininemia

C. Reflex hypotension and other inappropriate
    vagal stimuli
    1. Micturition syncope (mostly men standing
        during micturition)
    2. Defecation syncope
    3. Glossopharyngeal neuralgia
    4. Hypersensitive carotid sinus: stimulation
        results in bradycardia, sinus arrest, AV
        block, or hypotension alone (splanchnic
        vasodilation)
    5. Swallowing cold fluids
    6. Mediastinal masses
    7. Gallbladder disease
    8. Severe vestibular dysfunction

D. Hypovolemia: chronic dialysis, dehydration,
    Addison's disease, hemorrhage, rarely during
    blood donation (may also be vasovagal)

II. Cardiac disease, unrelated to posture. Often preceded by sensation of lightheadedness and chest discomfort. Autonomic dysfunction and incontinence are uncommon. Dysrhythmias are frequently present throughout episode.
   A. Dysrhythmias: mostly paroxysmal tachycardia, bradydysrhythmias (Stokes-Adams)
   B. Decreased cardiac output: pericardial effusion (uremia), myocardial infarction, pulmonary embolism (vagal stimulation), congestive heart failure, aortic and subaortic stenosis (exertional syncope), congenital heart defects
   C. Cardiac tumors (atrial myxoma)

III. Increased intrathoracic pressure. Presumed mechanisms include reduction of cardiac output and increased intracranial pressure with impairment of intracranial circulation.
   A. Cough syncope: prolonged coughing in presence of chronic obstructive pulmonary disease
   B. Sneezing syncope
   C. Weight lifting syncope

IV. Vascular causes
   A. Vertebrobasilar TIA. Diagnosis should only be made when there is other evidence of brainstem ischemia.
   B. Pulmonary hypertension
   C. Pulseless (Takayasu's) disease, subclavian steal
   D. Dissecting aortic aneurysm

V. Hypoglycemia: Slow onset. Pallor and bradycardia persist throughout the attack. Convulsive phenomena and urinary incontinence may occur. Duration is variable. Episode may not be self limited. See also Glucose.

VI. Epilepsy. Mainly akinetic seizures in children. Other seizure phenomena are usually present in adults.

VII. Hyperventilation. Cerebral vasoconstriction may result from severe hypercapnia.

VIII. Hindbrain herniation may be induced by coughing and sneezing in Arnold Chiari malformation, syringomyelia, or foramen magnum mass lesions

IX. Functional

Evaluation should exclude autonomic dysfunction
and neuropathy. EEG should be done if seizures are
suspected. Resting EKG (low yield), prolonged EKG
monitoring (dysrhythmias in as little as 10%), or
invasive cardiac electrophysiologic evaluation (up
to 56% yield of discovering cardiac conduction
abnormalities in syncope of undetermined cause) may
prove helpful. If indicated, stress EKG, echocardiography, cardiac catheterization, carotid sinus
massage, and cerebral and arch angiography may be
performed. Retrospective studies have determined
causes of syncope in 53 to 95% of cases.

Syncope due to cardiovascular disease may be
associated with a one year mortality as high as
30% with a high incidence of sudden death.

Ref: Kapoor WN, et al. A prospective evaluation and
      follow-up of patients with syncope. NEJM 309:4 and
      197, 1983.

SYPHILIS

Neurosyphilis may be asymptomatic or present as acute
lymphocytic meningitis (syphilitic meningitis), ischemic
infarction (meningovascular syphilis), meningoencephalitis
(general paresis), or myeloneuropathy (tabes dorsalis).
Less common forms include optic neuropathy, meningo-
myelitis, spinal meningovascular syphilis, and syphilitic
nerve deafness. Though classified into different types,
neurosyphilis commonly exists in mixed forms with a
spectrum of involvement.

All forms of neurosyphilis begin as a meningitis which
is usually asymptomatic. The diagnosis is made by positive
serum or CSF serologic tests and abnormal CSF with mildly
increased protein (40-20 mg/100 ml), normal glucose, and a
mild, usually lymphocytic, pleocytosis (50-400 cells/
mm3). CSF gamma globulins may be increased. Neurological
signs are absent. Asymptomatic neurosyphilis usually
occurs within two years of primary infection. If left
untreated, 10-25% of patients with syphilis will develop
neurosyphilis. LP, therefore, should be done in all
patients in whom a diagnosis of syphilis is made beyond
the primary stage or in whom the primary cannot be
established. Normal CSF 5 years after infection reduces
the risk of developing CNS syphilis to 1%.

Meningeal neurosyphilis presents with headache,
meningeal irritation and confusion. If the base of the
brain is involved, cranial nerve palsies, especially VII

and VIII, but also II, III, and VI, may occur. Hydrocephalus may result from vertex involvement. Seizures may occur. Syphilitic meningitis usually occurs within 2 years of the primary infection; 10% occur with the rash of secondary syphilis.

Meningovascular syphilis results from an arteritis with inflammation and disruption of the muscular, elastic and adventitial layers of the meningeal and parenchymal arteries. There is also subintimal proliferation (Heubner's arteritis). Ninety percent of patients are between 30 and 50 years old. Presentation is that of ischemic infarction with hemiparesis and other cerebral cortical signs. TIA's may occur. Meningovascular involvement usually occurs 5-10 years after the primary infection, but may occur as early as 6-12 months. Serum and CSF serology are usually positive, but CSF serology may be negative (see below).

Meningoencephalitic (paretic) neurosyphilis is the result of an active treponemal cortical cerebritis. Although there is no characteristic clinical picture, progressive dementia is common. Tremors of the face, tongue, and extremities, as well as delusional thinking, higher cortical deficits, seizures, myoclonus, pyramidal tract signs, and other neurological signs may be seen. Meningoencephalitic neurosyphilis should be excluded in all cases of dementia regardless of the focality of signs. General paresis usually occurs 15-20 years after the primary infection; if untreated, death usually occurs within 3-5 years. If begun early, treatment (see below) is usually effective in arresting progression of the disease. Symptomatic cure occurs in the majority of early treated cases. Seizures may be difficult to control (as compared to seizures in meningovascular neurosyphilis).

Tabetic neurosyphilis results from a mononuclear meningeal infiltrate with inflammation and demyelination of the dorsal columns of the spinal cord and dorsal spinal roots. Inflammation and demyelination of cranial nerves, especially I, III, V and VIII, may also occur. The classic triad of symptoms consists of lightning pain, dysuria, and ataxia. The classic triad of signs consists of Argyll-Robertson pupils, arreflexia (mainly in the lower extremities), and absent proprioception. Later involvement includes visceral crises, optic atrophy, ocular motor palsies, Charcot joints, and foot ulcers. Tabes dorsalis usually occurs 15-20 years or longer after the primary infection. Early treatment usually arrests the progression and may reverse some of the symptoms.

The most common serologic tests for syphilis are the VDRL (Venereal Disease Research Labs) and RPR (Rapid Plasma Reagin), which depend on nonspecific reagin detection, and the FTA-abs (Fluorescent Treponemal Antibody-absorbed), which depends on specific treponemal detection. The nontreponemal tests are less specific and sensitive than the treponemal test. A nonreactive VDRL may be seen in as many as 1/4 of the patients with late neurosyphilis. Biological false positive nontreponemal tests (titers usually less than 1:8) are associated with a variety of collagen vascular disorders, following infectious illnesses and after immunization; rarely, they are associated with leprosy, old age, and drug addiction. The serum FTA-abs is the most sensitive test for neurosyphilis (least seronegativity). The CSF VDRL and RPR are more specific for neurosyphilis (least biological false positives). Essentially every patient with a positive CSF FTA-abs has a positive serum FTA-abs. A normal serum FTA-abs virtually excludes CNS syphilis and makes lumbar puncture unnecessary except in the case of late neurosyphilis. Approximately 5-10% of late neurosyphilis patients may have a negative FTA-abs. Nevertheless, because the FTA-abs remains reactive in as many as 95% of patients, it is useful in the evaluation of late syphilis. The FTA-abs is not useful in evaluating patients after treatment. On the other hand, the quantitative VDRL titer declines approximately fourfold at three months and eightfold at six months after antibiotic therapy (except in the late "serofast" cases).

Treatment of all forms of neurosyphilis should consist of aqueous penicillin G, 4 million units IV, q4h for 14 days. High CSF penicillin levels have also been reported with penicillin G procaine, 2.4 million units IM qd, given with probenecid, 5 gm PO for 14 days. Alternative antibiotics in case of penicillin allergy (in order of preference) include tetracycline hydrochloride 500 mg PO qid for 30 days, erythromycin 500 mg PO qid for 30 days, or chloramphenicol 1 gm IV qid for 14 days.

After treatment, patients should be seen in follow-up every 3 months and serologic tests for syphilis obtained. CSF should be obtained every 6 months for 2 years. The CSF cell count and protein should return to normal. Persistent CSF abnormality or a persistently elevated or rising VDRL or RPR titer requires retreatment. Clinical progression (with the exception of lightning pains, visceral crises, and arthropathy) requires retreatment. A persistent weakly positive VDRL or RPR associated with normal CSF is insignificant.

Ref: Simon RP. Arch Neurol 42:606, 1985.

TASTE

Ageusia and dysgeusia (distortions and abnormal perception of taste) occur in a wide variety of disorders. Unilateral loss of taste over the anterior 2/3 of the tongue results from proximal lesions of cranial nerve VII (see Facial Nerve). Lingual nerve lesions (1/3) are associated also with tongue anesthesia in the same distribution. Lesions of cranial nerve IX cause loss of taste and anesthesia over the posterior third of the tongue. Diffuse impairment of taste may result from xerostomia, head trauma, heavy smoking, postinfluenzal damage of taste buds, hepatitis, viral encephalitis, myxedema, diabetes, hypogonadism, Prader-Willi syndrome, cancer, Vitamin A and B_{12} deficiency, and disordered zinc metabolism. Dysgeusia occurs with many medications including griseofulvin, amitriptyline, penicillamine, vincristine, vinblastine, chlorambucil, and antithyroid drugs. Gustatory hallucinations (rare) may occur as an aura in psychomotor epilepsy, or in alcohol-induced delirium and is usually associated with olfactory hallucinations.

TEMPORAL ARTERITIS (see Vasculitis)

THALAMIC SYNDROMES

The two major thalamic syndromes are: bilateral paramedian infarction and thalamic pain.

The syndrome of bilateral paramedian thalamic infarction consists of transient, followed by an apathetic hypersomnolent state. In addition, there is often a Korsakoff's-type amnesia and a vertical gaze palsy.

The thalamic pain syndrome (Dejerine-Roussy) occurs contralateral to the side of a thalamic lesion (usually infarction). The pain is described as aching, boring, or burning. It is usually omnipresent and punctuated by paroxysmal increases of hypersensitivity and dysesthesias. The pain is best treated by tricyclic antidepressants (amitriptyline 50-100 mg qhs or anticonvulsants such as phenytoin or carbamazepine). Anticonvulsants should be used as in treating epilepsy, achieving appropriate blood levels.

THIRD NERVE (see Ophthalmoplegia)

<u>THYROID</u> (see also Graves' Ophthalmopathy)

<u>Hyperthyroidism</u>
   <u>Myopathy</u>: Severe myopathy seen in "chronic thyrotoxic myopathy" is rare. Weakness is a common complaint. Deep tendon reflexes may appear brisk due to a shortened relaxation time. The EMG may reveal shorter duration, somewhat polyphasic motor unit potentials. CPK is normal or decreased. Light and electron microscopic changes have been described. Muscle power becomes normal as the patient becomes euthyroid. "Acute thyrotoxic encephalomyopathy" has been used to describe an acute presentation of bulbar palsy of uncertain pathophysiology.
   <u>Neuropathy</u> is extremely rare.
   <u>Thyrotoxic periodic paralysis</u> (see Periodic Paralysis)
   <u>Myasthenia gravis</u>: There is a greater association of myasthenia with thyroid disease (hyperthyroidism or hypothyroidism) and thyroid disease may exacerbate myasthenia.
   <u>Corticospinal tract dysfunction</u> is a rare complication of uncertain pathophysiology which resolves for the most part with therapy.
   <u>Seizures,</u> usually generalized, occur rarely in thyrotoxicosis. Thyrotoxicosis may exacerbate preexisting seizure diorders. Approximately 60% of patients with hyperthyroidism have abnormal EEG's, consisting mainly of generalized slowing and increased alpha activity.
   <u>Psychiatric manifestations</u> are varied, but most commonly there is irritability, emotional lability, and hyperactivity with resultant fatigue. Hyperthyroidism may exacerbate preexisting psychosis. Many of the symptoms may be treated with adrenergic blockers.
   <u>Tremor</u> is very common, occurring in the majority of patients with hyperthyroidism. It occurs primarily in the distal upper extremities. It represents an accentuation of physiological tremor by increased sympathetic tone and may be treated with propranolol (see also Tremor).
   <u>Chorea</u> is very rare. It is possibly due to hypersensitivity of dopaminergic receptors and may be abolished with haloperidol. It resolves spontaneously, however, on becoming euthyroid.
   <u>Thyrotoxic crisis (thyroid storm)</u> is an endocrine emergency which may progress to coma and death if not promptly treated. Management includes thiourea agents, sodium iodide, adrenergic blockers, adrenocorticosteroids, sedatives, body cooling, and fluid and electrolyte management. Crisis may be precipitated by infection or inadequate preparation for thyroid surgery. Mortality may be as high as 30%.
   <u>Cerebral embolization due to atrial fibrillation</u>: Anticoagulation may warrant consideration.

Hypothyroidism

Myopathy: Weakness (mainly proximal), cramps, pain, and stiffness are common complaints. Objective weakness is much less common. CPK may be elevated. EMG findings are nonspecific. Light and electron microscopic changes have been noted.

Deep tendon reflexes have slowed relaxation time ("pseudomyotonia"). This may also be seen with hypothermia, leg edema, diabetes, Parkinsonism, neurosyphilis, sarcoidosis, sprue, pernicious anemia, and a variety of drugs.

Myoedema is a local mound of contracted muscle that slowly relaxes following percussion. The contraction is electrically silent on EMG. Myoedema may also be seen in emaciated patients and in normal subjects.

Muscle hypertrophy is a rare and nonspecific finding in adults (Hoffmann's syndrome) and children (Kocher-Debre-Semelaigne). There may be enlarged, firm muscles with slow, weak movements, a feeling of stiffness, and painful muscle cramps. Pseudomyotonia may be differentiated from myotonia by electrical silence on EMG.

Peripheral neuropathy: 80% of patients complain of distal paresthesias. Median neuropathies at the wrist (carpal tunnel syndrome) are most common. Polyneuropathy is much less frequent.

Cranial neuropathies: (see also Graves' Ophthalmopathy). Blurred vision and diplopia are common complaints, although objective signs may be subtle. Ptosis, attributed to decreased sympathetic tone, occurs in 50-75%. Atypical facial pain occurs infrequently. Chronic, recurrent, generalized headaches are much more common. Tinnitus and decreased hearing are common and are probably cochlear in origin. Vertigo has been reported, but is of uncertain pathophysiology. Speech abnormalities most frequenty consist of decreased pitch and hoarseness due to mucopolysaccharide infiltration of the vocal cords, or "dyslalia", and impairment of articulation, due to infiltration of the tongue and soft tissues of the mouth. True dysarthria is rare.

Ataxia: Impaired tandem gait and appendicular incoordination is common and is usually attributed to involvement of the cerebellar system.

Psychosis and dementia: Irritability is fairly common. Paranoia with auditory hallucinations is less frequent. Psychosis may occur in as many as 3-5% of patients. Decreased level of awareness may occur with more severe disease. In the elderly there may be a mental deficiency resembling senile dementia. Thyroid function should be monitored carefully in those patients taking lithium.

<u>Coma</u> occurs rarely (less than 1%), usually in chronic, severe, undiagnosed disease. Other signs of hypothyroidism are associated with altered mental status, hypothermia (as low as 24°C/75°F) without shivering, and respiratory depression. Seizures may occur. Emergency management consists of thyroid replacement; corticosteroids; treatment of hypoglycemia, fluid and electrolyte abnormalities, and hypothermia; and ventilatory support, if needed.

<u>EEG changes</u> include slowing of alpha activity and decreased photic driving responses with high frequency stimulation. These changes may only be apparent when compared to a recording from the same patient while euthyroid. Markedly decreased background amplitude may be seen with hypothermia.

<u>Cerebrospinal fluid</u> protein is elevated in 40-90% of hypothyroid patients, occasionally to >100 mg/ml. The gamma globulin concentration may be increased.

Ref: Swanson JW, et al. Mayo Clin Proc 56:504, 1981.

<u>TIA</u> (see Amaurosis Fugax, Ischemia)

<u>TIC DOULOUREUX</u> (see Neuralgia)

<u>TONE</u> (see Dystonia, Reflexes, Rigidity, Spasticity)

<u>TORTICOLLIS</u> (see Dystonia)

<u>TRANSVERSE MYELITIS</u> (see Spinal Cord)

<u>TREMOR</u>

Regular, rhythmic oscillations produced by alternating contraction of agonist and antagonist muscles. It usually affects the distal extremities (especially fingers and hands), head, tongue, or jaw, and, only rarely, the trunk. It is present only during wakefulness. In any one individual, the frequency of the tremor is usually fairly consistent in all the affected parts, regardless of the size of the muscles involved. It is important to observe the amplitude, frequency, and rhythm of the tremor as well as the effects of physiologic and psychologic factors (see below).

Tremor can be categorized according to behavior at rest and during voluntary activities. Tremors at rest typically occur with Parkinson's disease or related conditions. Action tremors occur during voluntary activity and can be subdivided into 3 types. Postural tremors are most prominent during the maintenance of a sustained antigravity posture, such as out-stretched arms. Intention tremors occur during goal-directed movement of limbs, as in finger-to-nose testing. Contraction tremors are evident during isometric contraction, such as while making a fist.

Physiologic tremor is seen in normal individuals and is of small amplitude and high frequency (6-12 Hz). It may be made evident by placing a sheet of paper on outstretched hands. A physiologic tremor may be exaggerated by psychological factors, endocrine disturbances, or a variety of chemical agents. Psychological factors include stress, anxiety, fright, and fatigue. Endocrine disturbances include thyrotoxicosis, hypoglycemia, and pheochromocytoma. Causative drugs include lithium, tricyclics, phenothiazines, epinephrine, theophylline, amphetamines, thyroid hormone, isoproterenol, hypoglycemic agents, steroids, sodium valproate, L-dopa, and butyrophenones. Toxic agents include mercury, lead, arsenic, bismuth, carbon monoxide, and methyl bromide. Dietary factors include caffeine, monosodium glutamate (MSG). Alcohol withdrawal also exacerbates physiologic tremors. Management depends on the causative agent. Stress-reduction techniques may be necessary. Beta-blockers (e.g., propranolol) have been used with some of the accentuated physiologic tremors, especially performing artists with "stage fright".

Parkinsonian tremor is characterized by a coarse frequency of 3-7 Hz and variable amplitude over time. It may be asymmetric. It occurs at rest and disappears with sleep. It is most prominent in the hands. Patients may have flexion-extension or abduction-adduction of fingers, or pronation-supination of the hands. (Flexion-extension of the fingers in combination with adduction-abduction of the thumb results in the so called "pill-rolling tremor"). Patients may also develop flexion-extension movements of the feet, up and down movements of the jaw, or pursing movements of the lips. Emotional stress or mental concentration may make the tremor worse. Increasing rigidity reduces it. The tremor is diminished with voluntary movement. Patients with Parkinson's disease may also have other tremors, (e.g., postural or contraction). Parkinsonian tremors may improve with medication, especially anticholinergics (see Parkinson's Disease). In addition to idiopathic Parkinson's disease, this type of tremor occurs in Parkinsonism due to other disorders - postencephalitic, drug/toxic (phenothiazines, reserpine, carbon monoxide, manganese, carbon disulfide), tremor, trauma, vascular disease, metabolic (hypoparathyroidism, chronic hepatocerebral degeneration). Other disorders with Parkinsonian features include progressive supranuclear palsy, striatonigral degeneration, olivoponto-cerebellar atrophy, Shy-Drager disease, Wilson's disease, Huntington's disease and, occasionally, normal pressure hydrocephalus.

Essential tremor is mainly postural but often increases with action or intention. It is usually of the flexion-extension type, with a frequency of 7-11 Hz. It is usually localized to the fingers and hands initially, but may progress proximally. It may involve the head and neck horizontally (side to side) or vertically (up and down), or may involve the jaw, tongue, or voice. Occasionally the tremor begins in the head and neck. It is exacerbated by emotional and physical stress, as well as by those factors exacerbating physiologic tremor listed above. It diminishes with rest, mental concentration, and alcohol. The tremor is probably of central origin. It may occur sporadically, with autosomal dominant inheritance, in a senile form, in association with some hereditary neuropathies, or in association with other movement disorders (Parkinson's disease, torsion dystonia, torti-collis). Treatment begins with avoiding precipitating factors. Propranolol is started with low doses of 10-20 mg tid-qid and slowly increased as needed. Up to 320 mg per day may be necessary. Congestive heart failure, asthma and diabetes are contraindications to the use of nonselective β-blockers. Metoprolol has been used successfully and with less potential for bronchospasm. Patients with essential tremor often get significant relief for several hours after a single glass of wine or an ounce of liquor. Clearly, this type of therapy cannot be encouraged indiscriminately.

Cerebellar tremor is an intention tremor that occurs during the performance of an exact, projected movement. It becomes worse as the action continues (e.g., as the patient's finger approaches the examiner's finger in finger-to-nose testing). The oscillation usually originates proximally and occurs at right angles to the plane of movement at a frequency of 3-5 hz. There may be a tremor of the head or trunk (titubation). These patients may also display postural tremors. Causes of intention tremors include lesions of the cerebellar pathways, cerebellar degenerations, Wilson's disease, and drugs or toxins such as phenytoin, barbiturates, lithium, alcohol, mercury, and 5-fluorouracil. Action tremors have been reported with acquired polyneuropathies (Guillain-Barre, chronic recurrent polyneuropathy) as well as with hereditary neuropathies.

Ref: Jankovic J, Fahn S. Ann Int Med 93: 460, 1980.

<u>TRIGEMINAL NEURALGIA</u> (see Neuralgia)

<u>TUMORS</u> (see also Chemotherapy, Paraneoplastic Syndromes, Radiation, Spinal Cord)

Nervous system neoplasms are of many histologic types and occur in many different locations. Symptoms and signs are characteristically progressive. Focal manifestations are highly variable, depending upon the location of the lesion. Focal signs may not be apparent with some tumors such as those occurring in the anterior frontal lobes, nondominant temporal lobe, third ventricle, or, occasionally, the posterior fossa. Many intracranial tumors are associated with increased intracranial pressure causing headache, and occasionally, nausea and vomiting. Acute or subacute changes in neurological status may be due to seizures, brain edema, or, less frequently, hemorrhage into the tumor. Hemorrhage occurs most often with glioblastoma multiforme and metastatic tumors, especially lung, choriocarcinoma, and melanoma).

CHIEF LOCATIONS OF MOST FREQUENT INTRACRANIAL TUMORS

Supratentorial
    Cerebral hemispheres (superficial and deep)
            Gliomas
            Meningiomas
            Metastases
    Sellar region
            Pituitary adenomas
            Craniopharyngiomas
Infratentorial (adults)
    Cerebellopontine angle
            Acoustic schwannomas
    Other sites
            Brainstem gliomas
            Metastases
            Hemangioblastomas
            Meningiomas
Infratentorial (children)
    Midline
            Medulloblastomas
            Ependymomas
    Cerebellar hemispheres
            Astrocytomas

CHIEF LOCATIONS OF MOST FREQUENT
SPINAL AXIS TUMORS

Extradural
    Spinal
            Vertebral metastases
            Primary malignant or benign
            Bone tumors
    Intraspinal
            Epidural metastases
Intradural
    Extramedullary
            Meningiomas
            Schwannomas
            Neurofibromas
    Intramedullary
            Ependymomas
            Astrocytomas
            Glioblastomas

PRIMARY TUMORS OF THE NERVOUS SYSTEM
(From Escourolle and Poirier)

Histological elements normally present within the cranial and/or spinal cavity:

    Cellular deviations of the normal tube
        Glial cells
            Astrocytes
              Astrocytomas
              Glioblastomas
            Oligodendrocytes
              Oligodendrogliomas
            Ependymocytes
              Ependymomas
              Choroid plexus papillomas
              Colloid cysts
        Neurons
              Medulloblastomas
              Ganglioneuromas
              Gangliogliomas
        Pinealocytes
              Pineocytomas
              Pineoblastomas

```
Cellular derivatives of the neural crest
    Schwann cells
                Schwannomas
                Neurofibromas
    Arachnoid cells
                Meningiomas
    Melanocytes
                Melanomas
Other cells
    Connective tissue cells
                Sarcomas
    Reticuloendothelial (? microglial cells)
                Reticulum-cell sarcomas-
                microgliomas
    Vascular cells (?)
                Hemangioblastomas
    Glomus jugulare cells
                Glomus jugulare tumors
    Adenohypophyseal cells
                Pituitary adenomas
Intracranial and/or intraspinal embryonal remnants:
    Ectodermal derivatives
                Craniopharyngiomas
                Cholesteatomas
    Notochord
                Chordomas
    Adipose cells
                Lipomas
    Germ cells
                Germinomas
    Derived from the three germ layers
                Teratomas
```

Ref: Escourolle R, Poirier J. Manual of Basic Neuro-
       pathology. 2nd ed. Transl. Rubinstein LJ.
       Philadelphia: WB Saunders 1978; 21.)

   Metastatic tumors to the nervous system are often multiple but may be solitary. Although certain locations are more common, such as the cerebral gray-white junction, metastases may be seen virtually anywhere. The most frequent types are lung (especially in males), breast in females, kidney, alimentary tract, and malignant melanoma. Meningeal carcinomatosis is also more common with tumors such as breast, lung and melanoma, but is also seen with lymphoma and leukemia. The most common source of vertebral metastases is the prostate, followed by lung, kidney, breast, and bowel.

Diagnosis depends upon clinical history, neurological examination, and radiologic evaluation. CT, without and with contrast, is the most useful study for detecting the majority of intracranial tumors. It also provides information regarding cerebral edema, size of ventricles, and shift of intracranial contents. A normal CT does not exclude all tumor types. Magnetic resonance imaging (MRI) may be superior in detecting certain intracranial, as well as spinal-axis tumors. Skull films remain useful in evaluating sellar lesions and bony metastases. Angiography is useful in defining the vascular anatomy in preparation for surgery. Myelography remains the initial procedure of choice in the neuroradiological evaluation of spinal cord or root compression. CT cisternography or myelography following the installation of metrizamide may provide additional information. After a mass lesion has been excluded, lumbar puncture may be necessary to establish the diagnosis of meningeal carcinomatosis.

The management of nervous system tumors depends upon many factors including type, location, size, clinical behavior, and other clinical factors. The major therapeutic approaches are reduction of intracranial pressure, surgery, radiation therapy, and/or chemotherapy. Clinical worsening due to surrounding edema may be reversed with high-dose steroids, resulting in improvement within 24-48 hours, maximal by day 4-5. For acute lesions, such as spinal cord compression, dexamethasone is given in a loading dose as high as 100 mg IV, then 24 mg q6h which is then tapered over a few days to 4 mg q6h (see also Intracranial Pressure). Surgical management includes biopsy for a histologic diagnosis, shunting for obstructive hydrocephalus, decompression for symptomatic improvement, and total resection of certain tumor types (e.g., various extra-axial tumors) which may be curative. Depending on clinical circumstances, evaluation and management is often done in an emergency setting.

ULNAR NEUROPATHY (see also Peripheral Nerve)

Ulnar neuropathy at the elbow results from compression of the ulnar nerve as it courses between the medial ligament of the elbow in the aponeurosis between the two heads of the flexor carpi ulnaris. It commonly results from extrinsic compression such as from leaning on the elbow (especially in patients with a shallow ulnar groove) or from malpositioning of the arms on operating room tables or the arm rests of wheelchairs. So-called "tardy ulnar palsy" occurs following an old elbow fracture. Other causes include arthritis, ganglion cysts, lipomas, and Charcot joints. Clinically there is pain in the elbow and forearm, numbness and paresthesias of the fifth and ulnar half of the fourth digits and ulnar aspect of the hand, and weakness and wasting of the hypothenar and intrinsic hand muscles. Ulnar innervated muscles of the hand are the adductor pollicis, flexor pollicis brevis, first dorsal interosseus, third and fourth lumbricals, flexor digiti minimi, and abductor digiti minimi. There may be a resultant claw-hand deformity. Marked weakness of the flexor carpi ulnaris suggests a lesion above the elbow. Tenderness or enlargement of the ulnar nerve may be palpable in the epicondylar groove. Differential diagnosis includes C8,T1 radiculopathy, lower trunk brachial plexopathy, and polyneuropathy. Nerve conduction studies should reveal evidence of slowing at the elbow. The EMG may reveal denervation of ulnar innervated muscles. Conservative follow-up is usually sufficient in mild cases without motor involvement. Surgical decompression may be necessary. Anterior transposition of the ulnar nerve is usually not required. Surgery is not indicated in acute compressive ulnar neuropathy.

Ulnar neuropathy at the wrist or hand (Guyon's canal) consists of variable involvement of the deep and superficial branches of the ulnar nerve to the hand while sparing the dorsal cutaneous branch which supplies sensation in the dorsal aspect of the ulnar sensory distribution. There are multiple causes, including ganglion cysts, occupational and sports (e.g., cycling) trauma, fractures, and lacerations. Diagnosis depends on ulnar motor and sensory nerve conduction studies, including motor conduction in the deep palmar branch (latency from the wrist to the first dorsal interosseus).

Ref: Miller RG. Muscle Nerve 7:427, 1984.

UREMIA (see also Dialysis, Neuropathy)

Uremic encephalopathy is related most closely to the rate of progression of uremia rather than to the absolute BUN and creatinine. Early there is sensorial clouding, clumsiness, tremor, and asterixis. Later there is defective cognition, hallucinations, impaired recent memory, and increased tone and reflexes (may be asymmetric). Tetany may occur which does not respond to calcium. Later still there is multifocal myoclonus, stupor or coma, posturing, and seizures. The EEG is characterized by low voltage slowing early; later there may be generalized paroxysmal slowing. Triphasic waves or epileptiform activity are not uncommon. Spinal fluid protein may be normal or increased and there may be mild pleocytosis.

Seizures in renal failure are usually generalized but may be focal. Seizures may occur with uremic encephalopathy, water intoxication with hyponatremia, hypocalcemia, hypomagnesemia, hypertensive encephalopathy, dialysis dysequilibrium syndrome, and penicillin toxicity. Treatment is aimed at the underlying metabolic problem. Seizures due to uremic encephalopathy often respond to dialysis. Failing this, phenytoin is given in the usual doses (total levels decrease, but unbound fraction increases). Phenobarbital levels should be followed and dosage adjusted accordingly (usually decreased). Lidocaine has proven useful in the management of uremic seizures. Hemodialysis patients with seizures secondary to dysequilibrium should have more frequent, shorter duration dialysis and should be maintained on phenytoin.

Uremic neuropathy occurs in 2/3 of those beginning dialysis. It is a distal, symmetric sensorimotor polyneuropathy which may be painful. Abnormal nerve conduction studies may precede clinical symptoms and signs. The neuropathy progresses with great variability over months. It stabilizes or improves slowly with hemodialysis; peritoneal dialysis may be more beneficial. Most improvement seems to occur with renal transplantation. Carbamazepine in anticonvulsant doses may alleviate pain.

Ref: Raskin NH, Fishman RA. NEJM 294:143 and 204, 1976.

UROLOGY (see Bladder)

UVEITIS (see also Retina and Uveal Tract)

See page 325 for table of disorders involving both the uveal tract and the central nervous system. Adapted from Finelli PF, et al. Whipple's disease with predominantly neuro-ophthalmic manifestations. Ann Neurol 1:247-252, 1977.

VACCINATION (see Immunization)

DISEASES THAT MAY INVOLVE THE UVEAL TRACT
AND CENTRAL NERVOUS SYSTEM
(Adapted from Finelli, et al)

Infections
  Bacterial
    Meningococcus   Brucellosis
    Syphilis   Leptospirosis
    Tuberculosis   Listeriosis
    Whipple's disease
  Parasitic
    Trypanosomiasis   Ameliosis
    Toxoplasmosis   Malaria
  Viral
    Cytomegalovirus   Rubella
    Herpes simplex   Rubeola
    Herpes zoster   Subacute sclerosing
    Varicella   panencephalitis
    Mumps
Variola
  Fungal
    Aspergillosis   Histoplasmosis
    Candidiasis   Mucormycosis
    Cryptococcosis
Granulomatous disease
  Sarcoidosis
  Wegener's granulomatosis
Collagen vascular disease
  Systemic lupus erythematosus
  Temporal arteritis
  Polyarteritis
Neoplasms
  Leukemia
  Metastatic carcinoma
  Reticulum cell sarcoma
Other
  Behcet's syndrome
  Multiple sclerosis
  Sympathetic ophthalmia
  Trauma
  Uveal effusion
  Vogt-Koyanagi-Harada (uveomeningoencephalitic)
    syndrome
  Bing's syndrome (chorioretinitis, ophthalmoplegia,
    macroglobulinemia)
  Romberg's syndrome (posterior uveitis,
    ophthalmoplegia, trigeminal neuralgia,
    seizures, unilateral facial atrophy)

VASCULITIS

Refers to a wide spectrum of clinicopathological processes characterized by inflammation of blood vessels. Noninfectious vasculitides that have neurological manifestations are summarized below.

Cranial (temporal) arteritis occurs in the elderly (> 60) and is typically characterized by headache, masseter claudication, polymyalgia rheumatica, malaise, weight loss, fever and various cranial neuropathies. Visual loss is a common complication (may be presenting symptom) which may be prevented by early institution of steroids. The diagnosis is supported by an elevated ESR and positive temporal artery biopsy, although either may be negative. When the diagnosis is suspected clinically, prednisone 60-80 mg is begun immediately and then biopsy of an adequate length of artery is obtained as soon as possible.

Polyarteritis (periarteritis) nodosa most commonly involves the nervous system peripherally, presenting as a mononeuropathy, mononeuropathy multiplex, or symmetric polyneuropathy. CNS involvement usually occurs late. Headache, visual disturbances, and seizures are most common. A variety of neurological symptoms may result from multiple microinfarcts. Large infarctions are much less common.

Systemic lupus erythematosus involves the central nervous system in as many as 75% of cases. Most any neurological symptoms may occur due to multiple micro-infarcts anywhere throughout the nervous system. Disturbances of mental function (including "psychiatric" symptoms), seizures, and cranial neuropathies are common. Stroke-like syndromes also occur. Peripheral neuropathy is not uncommon. Myelopathy is rare, but well recognized. Steroid and immunosuppressive therapy generally improve neurological symptoms although they may worsen muscle weakness, seizures, or psychosis.

Granulomatous angiitis is a rare form of arteritis involving small leptomeningeal and parenchymal vessels presenting clinically with a low-grade aseptic meningitis and/or diffuse or multifocal CNS involvement. Diagnosis may be established in life by brain biopsy. Steroid therapy is recommended.

Wegener's granulomatosis may produce a peripheral neuropathy (polyneuropathy or mononeuropathy multiplex) or multiple cranial neuropathies. Prednisone and cyclophosphamide, chlorambucil, or azathioprine produce dramatic improvement in 90-95% of cases.

VENOUS THROMBOSIS

Cortical vein thrombosis results in headache, focal
seizures and focal signs. Subarachnoid hemorrhage (rupture
of congested veins or extension of hemorrhagic infarction)
or papilledema may also occur. Thrombosis may involve the
following dural sinuses: cavernous (usually secondary to
facial or orbital infection, and characterized by facial
pain, proptosis, and involvement of CN III, IV, VI, and
V), superior petrosal (secondary to otitis media, facial
pain is prominent), inferior petrosal (Gradenigo's
syndrome, with retro-orbital pain and CN IV palsy),
lateral (increased intracranial pressure, ear pain), or
internal jugular (secondary to catheters or pacemakers,
involvement of CN IX, X and XI). Sagittal sinus thrombosis
is the most common and, if the parieto-occipital portion
is involved, may produce elevated pressure, somnolence,
and CN VI palsy. Retinal hemorrhages may be seen. Vein
of Galen thrombosis in neonates following trauma or
infection may result in extensor posturing, fever, tachycardia, tachypnea and death. Survivors have bilateral
choreoathetosis.

Causes of venous thrombosis include:

Trauma: injury, neck surgery, indwelling lines
Infection: middle ear, sinuses, meningitis
Endocrine: pregnancy, contraceptives
Volume depletion: hyperosmolar coma, inflammatory
  bowel disease, diarrhea, postpartum, postoperative
Hematologic: polycythemia vera, disseminated
  intravascular coagulation, sickle cell disease,
  cryofibrinogenemia, paroxysmal nocturnal hemoglobinuria,
  thrombocytosis, antithrombin III deficiency,
  thrombocytopenia, transfusion reaction
Impaired cerebral circulation: arterial occlusion,
  congenital heart disease, congestive heart failure,
  anesthesia in seated position, sagittal sinus webs,
  pseudotumor cerebri
Neoplasm: leukemia, lymphoma, meningeal spread,
  meningioma
Other (Wegener's, polyarteritis nodosa, Behcet's
  syndrome, Logan's syndrome, homocystinuria)

CT scan with contrast may show "negative delta" sign
or nonfilling defect in confluent sinus, parasagittal
hemorrhages, gyral enhancement, slit ventricles, or
tentorial venous enlargement. LP, if not contraindicated
by mass effect, is nonspecific and may reveal increased
pressure, increased protein, polymorphonuclear leukocytes

(if infection is present), and/or red blood cells (if hemorrhage has occurred). Angiography (venography) may show absent filling. Digital subtraction angiography may be sufficient to visualize the dural sinuses. Skull and sinus films may reveal sinusitis. Management includes antibiotic treatment of infection, drainage of abscesses, and supportive care. Anticoagulation is often contra-indicated because of hemorrhagic infarction. Intracranial hypertension should be controlled (see also Intracranial Pressure, Abscess). In uninfected thromboses, the prog-nosis is better, and considerable recovery may occur.

VERTIGO (see also Calorics, Dizziness, Syncope)

Visual, vestibular, proprioceptive, and somatosensory information are necessary to maintain posture and the sense of awareness of body position in relation to the environment. Vertigo, an illusion of self or environmental motion, can be produced by processes that disrupt or cause mismatch among any of these sensory systems. Disease of the semicircular canals or their central connections tends to produce rotational vertigo, while disease of the otoliths or their central connections tends to produce illusions of body or environmental tilt or linear sensations (impulsion, of levitation). Vertigo is often accompanied by nausea, vomiting, or feelings of weakness. Oscillopsia is an illusion of movement of a viewed scene due to slip of visual images across the retina.

Physiological vertigo is induced by external stimu-lation or mismatch of the normal sensory inputs. Vertigo during head extension while standing or while bending over occurs because the otoliths are functioning beyond their optimal physiologic range. If sensory input varies further, e.g. while standing on an unstable ladder, symptoms worsen. Motion sickness is generated by accelerations to which the person is not yet adapted or by a mismatch between conflicting vestibular and visual stimuli, such as in the back seat of a moving vehicle or the closed cabin of a ship. Height vertigo may occur when the distance between the observer and visible stationary objects in the environment become critically large. Visual vertigo may occur when there is a mismatch between the visual sensation of movement and corresponding vestibular and somatosensory inputs such as during the viewing of movie automobile chases.

Pathological vertigo may be classified as acute, recurrent, or posturally-induced, although there may be overlap between groups.

Acute vertigo

Acute peripheral vestibulopathy (other terms include viral labyrinthitis, vestibular neuronitis, and peripheral vestibulopathy) is associated with spontaneous vertigo, nystagmus (fast phase away from the lesion), nausea, and/or vomiting (see page 331). The environment seems to move in the direction of the fast phase (away from the lesion). There is a subjective sense of self motion in the direction of the fast phase. The patient may fall to the side of the lesion during Romberg testing. Past pointing is to the side of the lesion. Symptoms and signs may be brought on by hurried movement ("positioning"), but not necessarily by maintaining a particular position ("positional"). It may last hours to days. Hearing is usually normal. A variable residual deficit of one peripheral vestibular system (labyrinth, nerve, or both) may persist. With a unilateral fixed deficit, central compensatory mechanisms intervene and vertigo and nystagmus decrease and may resolve. Vestibular "exercises" consisting of head movements that induce vertigo, may enhance this compensation. Acute peripheral vestibulopathy may recur (see below). Viral causes are held to be most common. Bacterial suppurative ear infection should be excluded.

Traumatic vestibulopathy is of controversial pathogenesis. It may be secondary to peripheral end-organ damage (symptoms similar to positional vertigo of peripheral type) or brainstem dysfunction. It may be related to fracture of the petrous bone, and, when symptoms are delayed, may result from hemorrhage into the labyrinth. Onset may occur days to weeks following trauma. Recovery (central compensation) usually occurs in weeks to months.

Perilymph fistula is usually secondary to spontaneous rupture of the inner ear membranes with resultant vertigo that may be aggravated by changes in position. It is associated with a fluctuating hearing loss. The fistula may occur during strenuous activity or Valsalva. The patient may hear a "pop" in the ear at the moment of rupture. The attacks are discrete and short lived. The therapy is bedrest. If this fails, surgery may be required. The patient should be evaluated by an otologist.

Central vestibular vertigo results from lesions of the vestibular nuclei or vestibulocerebellar pathways. Vertigo and nystagmus are usually accompanied by other CNS symptoms or signs such as diplopia, dysarthria, weakness, sensory loss, and pathological reflexes. Characteristics of vertigo and nystagmus which help distinguish between central and peripheral causes are outlined on page 331.

Central causes include brainstem ischemia or infarction, multiple sclerosis, cerebellar hemorrhage or infarction, trauma, basilar migraine, and tumors of the brainstem, cerebellum, or eighth cranial nerve. Acoustic neuromas are usually associated with hearing loss, tinnitus, and, occasionally involvement of other cranial nerves including VII and V.

Alcohol diffuses into the cupula, and, initially, produces nystagmus and vertigo when the subject lies down. Approximately 3-5 hours after the cessation of drinking there is a period during which there is no positional vertigo. Approximately 5-10 hours after cessation of drinking, when there is a falling blood level, nystagmus and vertigo recur. Positional vertigo may persist for hours after the blood alcohol level is zero as alcohol continues to leave the endolymph.

Other drugs which involve the peripheral end-organ or nerve include aminoglycosides, furosemide, ethacrynic acid, anticonvulsants (phenytoin, phenobarbital, carbamazepine, primidone), some anti-inflammatory agents, salicylates, and quinine. Drugs may produce only dysequilibrium when the damage is bilateral, but can produce vertigo when the damage is asymmetric. Some agents also produce hearing loss.

Recurrent vertigo

Meniere's disease, due to endolymph hydrops, is characterized by severe episodic vertigo, vomiting, fluctuating or progressive hearing loss, distortions of sound, tinnitus, and pressure or fullness in the ears. Recovery is usually within hours to days. The interval between attacks often ranges from weeks to months. Therapy is controversial, but low salt diet and diuretics are considered most helpful. Surgical therapy (endolymphatic drainage or vestibular nerve section) may give lasting relief, but should be considered only as a last resort.

Other causes of recurrent vertigo include otosclerosis (conductive hearing loss and tinnitus), syphilis (congenital and acquired), Cogan's syndrome (deafness, interstitial keratitis, and signs of systemic vasculitis), Arnold-Chiari syndrome (may be associated with Valsalva), idiopathic vertigo of childhood (vertigo, pallor, and sweating), hypothyroidism, and recurrent forms of central vertigo. Vestibular seizures (vertiginous epilepsy) may be secondary to focal discharges in temporal lobe or parietal association cortex. A familial syndrome of ataxia, vertigo, and nystagmus has been described.

Posturally induced vertigo

Benign paroxysmal positional vertigo is a symptom that usually indicates benign peripheral (end-organ) disease. Vertigo and nystagmus, often with systemic symptoms such as nausea and vomiting, occur when certain positions of the head are assumed, such as lying down on the back or side. Symptoms are usually transient (<60 seconds). Latency is usually several seconds but may be as long as 30-45 seconds. Signs and symptoms fatigue after onset and do not recur until there is a change in position. Nystagmus is most commonly torsional toward (upper pole) the undermost ear during Nylen-Barany testing (see below). With repetitive maneuvers, signs and symptoms lessen (habituate). Therapy consists of repetitive positioning exercises to stimulate central compensation. Elderly patients compensate more slowly. Vestibular suppressant medications generally do not help.

Other causes of posturally induced vertigo include central vertigo (may have postural features), alcohol, and physiologic vertigo.

Other forms of vertigo

Visual vertigo may occur with incorrect or recent changes in refractive correction.

Psychogenic vertigo has features of rotational or linear movement rather than isolated lightheadedness. It often begins gradually, is associated with anxiety, and terminates abruptly. Forced hyperventilation may provoke vertigo. A patient complaining of severe rotational vertigo without nausea or nystagmus suggests a psychogenic cause. Patients with chronic, constant dizziness are usually non-organic.

Clinical evaluation of the dizzy or vertiginous patient

First, classify the patient's symptoms (see Dizziness). The history should establish the date and details of the first attack, what the patient was doing at the time, the frequency and duration of subsequent attacks, the time and pattern of occurrence, relation to stress, whether onset was abrupt or gradual, precipitating or contributing factors (medications, certain positions or movements), association with Valsalva maneuvers, association with hyperventilation, and relation to diet (large amounts of sodium may trigger attacks of Meniere's). A history of associated symptoms should be sought. These include tinnitus (especially if unilateral or occurs or changes with attacks of vertigo), fluctuations in hearing,

a feeling of pressure in the ears, nausea, vomiting,
shortness of breath, paresthesias, chronic anxiety, or a
history of ear dysfunction, including change in hearing,
pain, discharge, history of trauma, therapy with ototoxic
medication, occupational exposure to loud noise, or family
history of ear disease.

Physical exam is done with special attention to the
heart rate and rhythm, pulses, bruits, and lying and
standing blood pressure. Careful otologic exam is
essential. Neurological exam should include evaluation of
nystagmus (may need to use Frenzel lenses), past-pointing,
Romberg sign, and brainstem and cerebellar function. The
exam is also aimed at precipitating and documenting the
nature of the dizziness. Helpful maneuvers include
Valsalva, head turns while sitting and standing with eyes
opened and closed, sudden turns while walking, hyperventilation for at least three minutes (may also be done with
postural testing), and Nylen-Barany testing. The latter
is performed by abruptly moving the patient from a sitting
to a lying position, with the head hanging 45° over the
end of the examining table and rotated 45° to one side.
This is repeated with the head rotated to the opposite
side. The development of vertigo and the time of onset,
duration, and direction of the fast phase of nystagmus is
noted. Frenzel lenses may be necessary to observe
vestibular nystagmus. The patient is also asked to
perform any other maneuver that he feels may trigger his
dizziness. Ophthalmoscopy provides a sensitive way to
evaluate vestibular function. Have the patient fixate a
stationary object with one eye while viewing the optic
disc of the other. Nystagmus is seen as drift of the disc
with corrective quick phases. Transiently cover the
fixating eye and note if the rate of drift increases.
Typically, nystagmus due to a peripheral vestibular lesion
increases in intensity when fixation is removed. Finally,
evaluate the vestibulo-ocular reflex (VOR) by having the
patient maintain steady fixation; then rotate his head
back and forth through a 10° range at about 1-2 cycles
per second. If the VOR is normal, eye movements will be
equal and opposite to head movements, and the optic discs
will not appear to move. If the VOR is inadequate, the
ocular fundus will appear to move in the opposite
direction to head movement.

Laboratory evaluation consists of quantitative ocular
motor and vestibular testing. Audiometric testing and
brainstem auditory evoked potentials assess auditory
pathways. A search for a cause may include CBC, FTA,
VDRL, temporal bone films and tomograms, CT of the head
with views of the internal auditory canal and base of the

skull. The necessity of any of these tests depends on the clinical presentation and differential diagnosis of each patient.

Generally management during acute vertigo includes bedrest, avoiding sudden head movements, clear fluids or light diet if tolerated, and reassurance. Vestibular suppresssant medications (see page 335) and antiemetics may be useful in acute peripheral vestibulopathy, in acute brainstem lesions near the vestibular nuclei, and for prevention of motion sickness. These agents are of no proven benefit in chronic vestibulopathies. Specific therapy depends on the underlying pathology. After the acute phase (approximately 1-3 days), a graded program of exercises may hasten the adaptive recalibration of the vestibular system to provide better ocular motor and postural control.

VESTIBULAR NYSTAGMUS AND VERTIGO
(Adapted from Daroff et al.)

	Peripheral	Central
Direction of nystagmus	Unidirectional, fast phase opposite lesion, uniplanar	Bi- or uni-directional. May change planes with gaze
Pure horizontal without rotary component	Uncommon (usually horizontal or vertical with rotary component)	Common
Vertical or purely rotary	Never present	May be present
Visual fixation	Inhibits nystagmus and vertigo	No inhibition
Vertigo	Marked	Mild to moderate
Environmental movement	To fast phase	Variable
Past pointing	To slow phase	Variable
Romberg fall	To slow phase	Variable
Head turning	Changes Romberg fall	No effect
Duration of symptoms	Finite (minutes, days, weeks). May be recurrent.	May be chronic
Tinnitus and/or deafness	Often present	Usually absent
Latency to nystagmus and vertigo after position change	Present	Absent
Habituation, fatigue of response	Present	Absent

MEDICATIONS USEFUL IN TREATING VERTIGO

Dimenhydrinate (Dramamine)	50-100 mg q4-6h	PO, IM, IV, PR
Diphenhydramine (Benadryl)	25- 50 mg tid-qid	PO, IM, IV
Meclizine (Antivert)	12.5-25 mg bid-qid	PO
Promethazine (Phenergan)	25 mg bid-qid	PO, PR, IM, IV
Hydroxyzine (Vistaril)	25-100 mg tid-qid	PO, IM
Cyclizine (Marezine)	50 mg q4-6h	PO, IM

Ref: Brandt T, Daroff RB. Ann Neurol 7:195, 1980.

Drachman DA, Hart CW. Neurology 22:323, 1972.

Leigh RJ, Zee DS. The Neurology of Eye Movements. Philadelphia: FA Davis, 1983, Chapters 2, 9.

Daroff RB, et al. Nystagmus and related ocular oscillations. In Glaser JS. Neuro-ophthalmology. Hagerstown: Harper and Row, 1978, Chapter 11.

VESTIBULO-OCULAR REFLEX (see also Calorics, Vertigo)

Reflex eye movements in response to vestibular stimulation. The term is used commonly to refer specifically to the oculocephalic reflex in which a head rotation in any direction is associated with a compensatory conjugate movement of the eyes in the opposite direction. The sum of the movements results in steady gaze (eye position in space). Following the head movement, the eyes are normally held steady in the orbit.
The reflex is elicited after neck injury has been excluded by quickly rotating the head horizontally or vertically and holding it in its new position for several

seconds. With head flexion, the lids elevate (doll's head response) in association with upward movement of the eyes. The reflex may be sensitively tested in alert patients using ophthalmoscopy (see Vertigo). Head rotation in unconscious patients without other brainstem signs will result in compensatory controversive eye movements, but the eyes do not remain in their new position and drift back towards primary position. This suggests dysfunction in the brainstem reticular formation and cerebellar connections involved in maintaining gaze. Other abnormalities of vestibular eye movements are very useful in localization (see Calorics).

VISUAL FIELDS

Visual field defects may be caused by obstruction of optical pathways to the retina or by disorders of the retina itself. Such defects may be of any shape and occur in one or both eyes. The cause is usually visible on ophthalmoscopy.

Defects also result from disturbed conduction along neural pathways. The characteristic features of these defects allow more precise localization. Arcuate defects occur with segmental lesions of the optic nerve. Centro-cecal defects suggest a lesion in the axis of the nerve. Hemianopic defects (respecting the vertical meridian) may be bitemporal, indicating chiasmal involvement, or homonymous, indicating postchiasmal involvement.

Ref: Ellenberger C. Perimetry: Principles, Techniques, and Interpretation. New York: Raven, 1980.

VITAMIN DEFICIENCY AND TOXICITY (see Nutritional Deficiency Syndromes)

WILSON'S DISEASE

Eponymic designation of hepatolenticular degeneration. It is an autosomal recessive disorder secondary to copper deposition in multiple organs especially the liver, cornea and brain. Patients ultimately develop hepatic dysfunction and 40% have neurological abnormalities. The latter consists of tremor, dysarthria, rigidity, chorea, and a variety of psychiatric disturbances. The diagnosis is made by observing Kayser-Fleischer rings in the cornea, a low serum ceruloplasmin, increased copper in liver biopsy, and elevated 24-hour urinary copper.

The treatment consists of D-penicillamine, 250 mg qid with the addition of pyridoxine 25 mg qd. A low copper diet is also required. Patients who do not respond to penicillamine or who develop side effects represent difficult treatment problems which are best handled by physicians who specialize in this disorder.

Ref: Scheinberg IH, Sternlie BI. Wilson's Disease. Philadelphia: WB Saunders, 1984.

WRITER'S CRAMP (see Dystonia)

ZOSTER

Herpes zoster (shingles) may represent reactivation of latent varicella zoster (chickenpox). Its incidence increases with age and immunocompromised states, particularly with lymphomas, immunosuppressive therapy and radiation therapy. A vesicular skin eruption is preceded by radicular pain within 3-4 days. Clear vesicles become cloudy in several days and dry and crusted after 5-10 days. Any spinal or cranial sensory ganglia may be involved, but T5-T10 is most common, followed by craniocervical levels. Usually a single dermatome is involved, although occasionally 2 or more contiguous levels may be affected. Generalized involvement is rare and is usually associated with malignancy. Pain and dysesthesias usually last 1-4 weeks, but in some, may persist for months or even years. Decreased sensation in the involved dermatome is common. Segmental weakness and atrophy occurs in less than 5%. CSF may reveal an elevated protein and mild lymphocytic pleocytosis. Diagnosis can be established by immunofluorescence of biopsied skin lesions.

Herpes zoster ophthalmicus is the most common cranial herpetic syndrome (>90%), usually occurring in the first division of the trigeminal nerve (>65%) unilaterally. There is a significant risk of corneal involvement with anesthesia and scarring. There may be associated external and/or internal ophthalmoplegias, iridocyclitis, or, rarely, optic neuropathy. The prognosis for improvement of ocular motor disturbances is usually excellent, whereas the prognosis for visual improvement after the optic neuropathy is usually poor. A less common manifestation of cranial zoster is the Ramsay-Hunt syndrome consisting of peripheral VII nerve palsy associated with vesicles in the external auditory meatus, with or without auditory and/or vestibular symptoms. Encephalitis, myelitis, and cerebral angiitis are rare complications of cranial zoster. Treatment consists of analgesics and local skin care. Corticosteroids decrease the incidence of postherpetic neuralgia but do not alter the acute course. Steroids are contraindicated in patients with ophthalmic zoster, malignancy, immunosuppression, or

who were on steroids prior to the zoster infection.
Antiviral agents such as adenine arabinoside (vidarabine)
or acyclovir, decrease pain and shorten the acute course
but do not decrease the incidence of postherpetic
neuralgia. Ophthalmic zoster may be treated with oral
acyclovir. Postherpetic pain and dysesthesia eventually
subsides, even in severe, protracted cases. Symptomatic
treatment with carbamazepine, phenytoin, or tricyclic
antidepressants may be of help.

Ref: Bean B, et al. Lancet 2:118, 1982.

        Whitley RJ, et al. NEJM 294:1193, 1976.

EPONYM INDEX

Haff disease (182)
Hallerman-Streiff syndrome (274)
Hallervorden-Spatz disease (68,100,200,288)
Hallgren's syndrome (287)
Hartnup's disease (305)
Henoch-Schonlein purpura (69)
Hering's law (125)
Hoffmann syndrome (184,315)
Hoffmann's sign (284)
Horner's syndrome (24,30,133,145,274)
Hounsfield number (76)
Hunt-Hess scale (140)
Hunter's disease (288)
Huntington's chorea, disease
     (26,68,87,100,117,176,200,248,318)
Hurler's disease (288)
Jackson's syndrome (38)
Jakob-Creutzfeldt (see Creutzfeldt-Jakob)
Jansky-Bielschowski disease (117,289)
Joseph's disease (Motor Neuron Disease) (176)
Kallmann's syndrome (234)
Kaposi sarcoma (3)
Kayser-Fleischer ring (336)
Kearns-Sayer-Daroff syndrome (180,235)
Kleine-Levin syndrome (296)
Klippel-Feil anomaly (82)
Klumpke (Klumpke-Dejerine) palsy (30)
Kocher-Debre-Semelaigne syndrome (315)
Koerber-Salus-Elschnig syndrome (36)
Korsakoff's psychosis (4,225)
Krabbe's disease (85,152)
Kuf's disease (117,289)
Kugelberg-Welander-Wohlfart disease (151,175)
Kuru (113)
Lafora body disease (117,200)
Lambert-Eaton syndrome (193,197)
Landau reflex (66)
Landau-Kleffner syndrome (118)
Landouzy-Dejerine dystrophy (179,187)
Landry-Guillain-Barre syndrome (see Guillain-Barre)
Laurence-Moon-Biedl syndrome (288)
Leber's disease (88,240,287)
Leigh's disease, syndrome (226)
Lennox-Gastaut syndrome (117,199)
Lesch-Nyhan syndrome (68)
Lhermitte's sign (178,281)
Lisch nodule (210)
Louis-Bar syndrome (305)
Lundborg (Intracranial Pressure) (117)

Maddox rod (124)
Marchiafava-Bignami disease (5,87,226)
Marcus-Gunn pupil (277)
Marfan's syndrome (152,180)
Marinesco-Sjogren syndrome (306)
McArdle's disease (181,185,203)
McGregor's line (81)
Meige syndrome (99)
Melkersson-Rosenthal syndrome (128)
Meniere's disease (137,330)
Millard-Gubler syndrome (37,127)
Mobius syndrome (128,179)
Mollaret's meningitis (173)
Mollaret's triangle (200)
Moro reflex (66)
Morvan's disease (217)
Moya-moya (162,281)
Niemann-Pick disease (288)
Nothnagel syndrome (36)
Nylen-Barany maneuver (332)
Osler-Rendu-Weber disease (161)
Paget's disease (39,80,81,135,241,288)
Parinaud's syndrome (36,129,275,278)
Parkinson's disease (25,26,100,176,248,308,317)
Pelizaeus-Merzbacher disease (68,84,287)
Peyronie's disease (154)
Phelan's sign (44)
Pick's disease, lobar atrophy (87)
Pompe's disease (181,203)
Prader-Willi syndrome (153,313)
Raeder's paratrigeminal neuralgia, syndrome (145)
Ramsay-Hunt syndrome (117,127,200,306,337)
Raymond's syndrome (37)
Raymond-Cestan syndrome (37)
Refsum's disease (215,217,288)
Riley-Day syndrome (24,154,218,308)
Rinne's test (137)
Romberg sign (24,292)
Romberg's syndrome (Horner's syndrome) (325)
Rosenthal, basal vein of (8,9)
Roussy-Levy syndrome (216)
Sandhoff's disease (117,288)
Sanfilippo's disease (287)
Santuavori-Haltia-Hagberg disease (117)
Scheie's disease (288)
Schilder's disease (87)
Schilling test (228)
Schwabach's test (137)
Schwartz-Jampel syndrome (100,109,181)
Senear-Loken (287)

Sheehan's syndrome (269)
Shy-Drager syndrome (25,26,145,176,248,308,318)
Sjogren's syndrome (162,183,204)
Sjogren-Larsson syndrome (288)
Spielmeyer-Vogt-Sjogren disease (117,288)
Sprengel's deformity (80)
Stevens-Johnson syndrome (19)
Stokes-Adams attacks (238,309)
Strachan's syndrome (225)
Sturge-Weber syndrome (40,211,289)
Sydenham's chorea (69)
Takayasu's disease (162,309)
Tangier disease (215,221)
Tapia's syndrome (39)
Tarui's disease (203)
Tay-Sachs' disease (2,117,288)
Thomsen's disease (181,207)
Tinnel's sign (44)
Todd's palsy, paralysis (158)
Tolosa-Hunt syndrome (236)
Tourette's syndrome (297)
Treacher Collins syndrome (274)
Tromner's sign (284)
Trousseau's sign (41,165)
Uhtoff's phenomenon (179)
Unverricht-Lundborg syndrome (200)
Usher's syndrome (287)
Van Gierke disease (181)
Vernet's syndrome (38)
Vogt-Koyanagi-Harada syndrome (325)
Von Gierke disease (181)
Von Hippel-Lindau disease (211,289)
Von Recklinghausen's disease (210)
Waldenstrom's macroglobulinemia (137,162)
Wallenberg's syndrome (38,145)
Weber's syndrome (36)
Weber's test (137)
Wegener's granulomatosis (162,214,325,326,327)
Werdnig-Hoffmann disease (152,175)
Wernicke's disease, encephalopathy (4,26,74,225)
Wernicke-Korsakoff syndrome (4,168,224,234)
West syndrome (117)
Whipple's disease (324)
Wilson's disease (69,86,100,200,248,318,336)
Wohlfart-Kugelberg-Welander disease (151,175)
Wyburn-Mason syndrome (289)